Academic Clinical Nurse Educator Review Book

The Official NLN Guide to the CNE®cl Exam

Academic Clinical Nurse Educator Review Book

The Official NLN Guide to the CNE®cl Exam

Edited by

Teresa Shellenbarger, PhD, RN, CNE, CNEcl, ANEF

National League
for **Nursing**

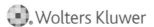

Philadelphia • Baltimore • New York • London
Buenos Aires • Hong Kong • Sydney • Tokyo

Vice President and Publisher: Julie K. Stegman
Director of Nursing Content Publishing: Renee Gagliardi
Director of Product Development: Jennifer K. Forestieri
Senior Development Editor: Meredith L. Brittain
Marketing Manager: Katie Schlesinger
Editorial Assistant: Molly Kennedy
Design Coordinator: Steve Druding
Senior Production Project Manager: David Saltzberg
Manufacturing Coordinator: Karin Duffield
Prepress Vendor: Aptara, Inc.

Library of Congress Cataloging-in-Publication Data

ISBN-13: 978-1-97515-401-1
Library of Congress Control Number: 2019916474
Cataloging in Publication data available on request from publisher.

shop.lww.com   www.NLN.org

About the Editor

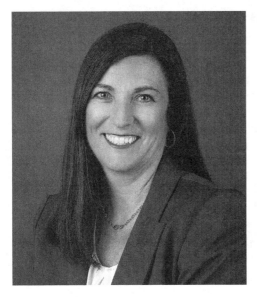

Teresa Shellenbarger, PhD, RN, CNE, CNEcl, ANEF is Distinguished University Professor and the Doctoral Program Coordinator in the Department of Nursing and Allied Health Professions at Indiana University of Pennsylvania, Indiana, PA. She received her bachelor's degree in nursing from The Pennsylvania State University, master of science in nursing from Southern Connecticut State University, and her PhD in nursing from Widener University.

As an experienced nurse educator of more than 25 years, Dr. Shellenbarger has taught a variety of theoretical and clinical courses at the bachelor's, master's, and doctoral levels. She has published and presented extensively on topics related to innovative teaching strategies, faculty role development, technology use in nursing education, and clinical nursing education. She is coauthor of the popular book *Clinical Teaching Strategies in Nursing*. Dr. Shellenbarger also edited the National League for Nursing publication *Clinical Nurse Educator Competencies: Creating an Evidence-Based Practice for Academic Clinical Nurse Educators*. She is a member of the editorial boards for *Nursing Education Perspectives* and *Nurse Educator*, as well as serving as a reviewer for various other nursing publications.

Dr. Shellenbarger has been active in the National League for Nursing (NLN), having served as a member of the Board of Governors for 6 years and as the NLN Secretary for 3 years. She also participates as a member on various NLN task groups and committees. Additionally, Dr. Shellenbarger is an NLN-certified nurse educator and was inducted as an inaugural fellow into the NLN Academy of Nursing Education.

Contributors

Audrey M. Beauvais, DNP, MSN, MBA, RN
Associate Dean and Associate Professor
Egan School of Nursing and Health Studies
Fairfield University
Fairfield, CT

Jennifer Chicca, MS, RN
PhD Candidate and Graduate Assistant
Department of Nursing and Allied Health Professions
Indiana University of Pennsylvania
Indiana, PA

Kristy Chunta, PhD, RN, ACNS, BC
Professor
Department of Nursing and Allied Health Professions
Indiana University of Pennsylvania
Indiana, PA

Kaitlin Cobourne, MSN Ed, RN
Program Coordinator
School of Nursing
Pittsburgh Technical College
Oakdale, PA

Nicole Custer, PhD, RN, CCRN-K
Assistant Professor and Chairperson
Department of Nursing
Mount Aloysius College
Cresson, PA

Jenna Davis, MSN, RNC-NIC
PhD Candidate and Graduate Assistant
Department of Nursing and Allied Health Professions
Indiana University of Pennsylvania
Indiana, PA

Taylor Edwards, PhD, RN
Assistant Professor
Department of Nursing and Allied Health Professions
Indiana University of Pennsylvania
Indiana, PA

Megan Gross, PhD, MPH, RN
Assistant Professor
Department of Nursing
Messiah College
Mechanicsburg, PA

Sara K. Kaylor, EdD, RN, CNE
Assistant Professor
Capstone College of Nursing
The University of Alabama
Tuscaloosa, AL

Monica M. Kidder, DNP, RN-BC, CNE
Curriculum Coordinator
Covenant School of Nursing
Covenant Health System
Lubbock, TX

Joan M. Krug, MSN, RN, CCRN, CNEcl
Nursing Instructor
College of Nursing
The Pennsylvania State University
Altoona, PA

Melissa L. Mastorovich, DNP, RN, BC
Senior Clinician
STAT Nursing Consultants, Inc.
Pittsburgh, PA

Donna S. McDermott, PhD, RN, CHSE
Associate Professor, Department Head
Robert Morris University Department of Nursing
Robert Morris University
Moon Township, PA

Jacquelyn McMillian-Bohler, PhD, CNM, CNE
Assistant Professor
Duke University School of Nursing
Duke University
Durham, NC

Angela G. Opsahl, DNP, RN, CPHQ
Assistant Professor
Indiana University School of Nursing
Indiana University
Bloomington, IN

Cristina M. Perez, PhD, RN
Associate Professor
Nursing Programs
Ramapo College of New Jersey
Mahwah, NJ

Susan G. Poorman, PhD, RN, CNS-BC, ANEF
Professor Emeritus
Department of Nursing and Allied Health Professions
Indiana University of Pennsylvania
Indiana, PA
President
STAT Nursing Consultants, Inc.
Pittsburgh, PA

Katherine A. Raker, MSN, RN, CNM
PhD Candidate
Department of Nursing and Allied Health Professions
Indiana University of Pennsylvania
Indiana, PA
Assistant Professor
Department of Nursing
Bloomsburg University
Bloomsburg, PA

Maren M. Reinholdt, MSN, RN
PhD Candidate
Department of Nursing and Allied Health Professions
Indiana University of Pennsylvania
Indiana, PA
Clinical Faculty
Master's Entry into Nursing Program
Johns Hopkins University School of Nursing
Baltimore, MD

Meigan Robb, PhD, RN
Assistant Professor
Department of Nursing
Chatham University
Pittsburgh, PA

Kristy A. Sands, PhD, RN
Assistant Professor
Department of Nursing
Bloomsburg University
Bloomsburg, PA

Aaron M. Sebach, DNP, MBA, RN, AGACNP-BC, FNP-BC, NP-C, CEN, CPEN, FHM
Associate Professor and Chair, Doctor of Nursing Practice Program
College of Health Professions
Wilmington University
New Castle, DE

Teresa Shellenbarger, PhD, RN, CNE, CNEcl, ANEF
Distinguished University Professor and Doctoral Program Coordinator
Department of Nursing and Allied Health Professions
Indiana University of Pennsylvania
Indiana, PA

Amy Stoker, PhD, RN
Director, School of Nursing
West Penn Hospital School of Nursing
Allegheny Health Network, West Penn Hospital
Pittsburgh, PA

Lauren Succheralli, MS, RN
Instructor and PhD Candidate
Department of Nursing and Allied Health Professions
Indiana University of Pennsylvania
Indiana, PA

Phillip M. Timcheck, MSN, MBA, RN
Instructor
Division of Nursing/School of Health Sciences
Winston-Salem State University
Winston-Salem, NC

Meagan White, PhD, RNC-MNN
Senior Operations Manager
Practice Transition Accreditation Program (PTAP)
American Nurses Credentialing Center (ANCC)
Washington, DC

Malinda Whitlow, DNP, RN, FNP-BC
Assistant Professor, Program Director
Department of Nursing
George Washington University
Ashburn, VA

Heather Zonts, PhD, RN
Assistant Professor
Department of Nursing
Mount Aloysius College
Cresson, PA

Foreword

This book is an essential resource for nurse educators preparing for the National League for Nursing (NLN) Certified Academic Clinical Nurse Educator Examination (CNE®cl). This official NLN guide is the premier preparation book for this certification examination that aligns with the NLN core competencies for academic clinical nurse educators and the test blueprint. As such, this review book is essential in preparing academic clinical nurse educators for the certification exam. Potential test candidates will benefit from the more than 500 multiple-choice questions and accompanying rationales. These questions, which follow best practices for test construction, will be indispensable for reviewing test content and identifying areas needing further study.

Academic clinical education is a specialty practice that requires its own unique set of teaching and learning strategies and evaluation approaches. The primary role of the academic clinical nurse educator is to facilitate student learning in the clinical component of academic programs, including simulation. Earning the CNE®cl certification demonstrates the nurse educator's commitment to excellence and professional expertise in the role of an academic clinical nurse educator.

Brenda Morris, EdD, RN, CNE
Clinical Professor of Nursing
Edson College of Nursing and Health Innovation
Arizona State University
Phoenix, AZ

Preface

The National League for Nursing (NLN) has led initiatives to advance nursing education and recognize the specialized advanced practice role of nurse educators. The academic nurse educator certification and examination is one example of this work. Since the initial academic nurse educator certification examination was offered in 2005, nearly 7,000 academic nurse educators have been certified (Malone, 2019). However, it became clear to NLN leadership and members that there were unique aspects of clinical nursing education that were not fully addressed in the academic nurse educator core competencies and test blueprint. Nurse educators also serve in academic roles that focus primarily on clinical teaching and do not encompass the full academic practice of the nurse educator. The unique aspects of clinical nursing education were not adequately captured in the scope of practice for academic nurse educators. Although some overlap exists with the academic nurse educator responsibilities, the academic clinical nurse educator has a distinct skill set and practice area.

Academic clinical nurse educators facilitate the learning of nursing students through the clinical component of an academic nursing program (National League for Nursing, 2019). They help learners gain the knowledge, skills, and attitudes needed to ensure delivery of safe and effective care, and they assist students in translating theory to practice. Academic clinical nurse educators help ensure that graduates are prepared for the practice profession. The work they do as academic clinical nurse educators is critical for preparing a qualified workforce that can address client problems and can use clinical reasoning and problem-solving skills effectively. To fully articulate these roles and responsibilities, the NLN convened a task group that helped to identify the specific core competencies and task statements that delineated the work of the academic clinical nurse educator (Christensen & Simmons, 2019). Their work, along with a practice analysis, resulted in the core competencies that serve as the test plan for the academic clinical nurse educator exam and certification offered by the NLN.

Like academic nurse educators, many in the academic clinical nurse educator role will want to pursue certification to demonstrate their knowledge and expertise. They may be searching for resources that will assist them as they prepare for the academic clinical nurse educator certification examination. This book continues to follow in the path of the NLN's commitment to advancing academic clinical nurse educators. It serves as another example of preparation support that will help promote certification success and excellence in nursing education.

This book provides an invaluable resource by offering preparatory materials and more than 500 practice questions that can be used for exam preparation. These materials can be part of an applicant's test preparation review and study plan. Using this book does not guarantee certification success, but it should assist candidates with preparation.

Chapter 1 provides an overview and background information about the academic clinical nurse educator (CNE®cl) exam and certification process. Because many individuals may experience test anxiety when taking certification or other high-stakes exams, Chapter 2 offers a useful guide for test-taking preparation and suggests testing strategies to address test anxiety and promote success. This chapter also makes suggestions for better studying and test-taking approaches.

Chapters 3 through 8 are organized by the core competencies for the academic clinical nurse educator. Each chapter offers numerous practice test questions representing all task statements found on the test blueprint. The questions reflect best practices used for item writing and provide an accurate reflection of the types of questions likely to be on the CNE®cl exam. Each question, derived from scholarly references about clinical teaching, provides a justification for the correct answer as well as an explanation about the incorrect options. The questions are labeled according to the CNE®cl test blueprint, and all questions are coded for the cognitive level assessed. Like the CNE®cl, three cognitive levels or codes are identified, and each question is labeled as recall, application, or analysis.

The majority of the CNE®cl exam questions are written at the application level or higher; the same is true of the questions in this review book. Users of the book are encouraged to review each question, either while studying alone or in a study group, and use the questions and rationales to identify areas that may need additional review.

It is hoped that readers of this official NLN guide will find these materials useful and this book may help test takers to achieve the CNE®cl credential and obtain recognition for the excellent and important work that they do as academic clinical nurse educators.

Teresa Shellenbarger, PhD, RN, CNE, CNEcl, ANEF
September 2019

References

Christensen, L. S., & Simmons, L. E. (2019). Development of the core competencies of clinical nurse educators. In T. Shellenbarger (Ed.), *Clinical nurse educator competencies: Creating an evidence-based practice for academic clinical nurse educators* (pp. 1-5). Washington, DC: National League for Nursing.

Malone, B. (2019, March 20). NLN CEO update on Certification day and NLN Day on the hill. *NLN member update.* Retrieved from http://www.nln.org/newsroom/newsletters-and-journal/nln-update/newsletter/nln-member-update/2019/03/20/march-20-2019-certification-day-and-nln-day-on-the-hill

National League for Nursing. (2019). Certification for Nurse Educators. Retrieved from www.nln.org/Certification-for-Nurse-Educators

Acknowledgments

There are numerous people who assisted in the completion of this book who deserve acknowledgment and my sincere appreciation. First, I offer my thanks to the National League for Nursing (NLN) leadership team for identifying the need for this review book. Beverly Malone, Linda Christensen, Larry Simmons, Elaine Tagliareni, Janice Brewington, and Barbara Patterson have been instrumental in advancing this work and offering support. Special thanks to Larry Simmons for sharing the best practice guidelines for test writing that served as the foundation for test item construction and for answering questions about the certification exam. Amy McGuire, staff member at the NLN, served as a vital connection to Wolters Kluwer and was very helpful as I encountered questions during the publication process.

I also offer my thanks to the many nurse educators who served as contributors. I am so grateful they shared their knowledge about clinical nursing education expertise and willingly constructed hundreds of test questions for this book. I am fortunate to have some amazing educator colleagues and friends.

Lastly, I would like to offer my most sincere appreciation and a very special thanks to Indiana University of Pennsylvania PhD nursing candidate Jennifer Chicca for her meticulous proofreading, careful editing, and thoughtful critique. She offered many valued suggestions that enhanced and clarified these review questions. I am so very grateful for her assistance and hard work.

Teresa Shellenbarger, PhD, RN, CNE, CNEcl, ANEF

Contents

1

Introduction to the CNE®cl Examination

Teresa Shellenbarger, PhD, RN, CNE, CNEcl, ANEF

The United States Department of Labor Bureau of Labor Statistics (2018) reports that approximately 55,580 nurse educators are employed in postsecondary settings, working primarily in colleges, universities, and professional schools. These nurse educators engage in a variety of activities that help prepare learners for future nursing roles, including teaching in the classroom, guiding learners in simulation activities, practicing care skills with students in learning laboratories, and coaching learners in client care delivery in clinical settings. Nurse educators guide learners in professional practice experiences in a variety of settings, such as hospitals, long-term care facilities, schools, clinics, client homes, and in the community. Learners have opportunities to provide care in these settings to clients across the life span.

CHALLENGES

Clinical nurse educators face numerous challenges that impact the work they do in these diverse learning settings. One challenge involves the changing health care environment. Hospitals, a common site for clinical learning experiences, offer a rich learning environment as clients needing health care present with complex health conditions that require advanced delivery of care. These clients, many of whom are aging, frequently have multiple health care concerns arising from their acute and chronic health problems. Care providers must address these critical health issues in a rapidly changing environment.

Health care agencies have also become more complex as they confront the ongoing challenge of providing quality care amid financial restraints associated with increasing costs and decreasing reimbursements. Additionally, many institutions may not have enough experienced nurses needed to meet the demands of the health care system and provide expert care (Institute of Medicine [IOM] of the National Academies, 2011). This further impacts available staff qualified to mentor nursing learners. Clinical nurse educators teaching in these settings also face the struggles of adapting to the rapidly changing environment, confronting the ongoing knowledge explosion, and learning to use new technology in client care areas.

Clinical nurse educators also encounter issues and challenges in the academic setting as they work with learners, many of whom have limited past clinical experience and struggle to deliver care in a fast-paced and stressful environment. They must guide learners to interpret client needs and problems, make carefully thought-out decisions while providing intimate care, and complete invasive procedures that

1

often cause client discomfort. Clinical nurse educators help these learners develop the high-level thinking and problem-solving skills needed to deliver appropriate client-centered sensitive care. Educators must help foster clinical reasoning and decision-making skills and ensure that learners can translate abstract concepts learned in the classroom into real-life practice situations (Benner, Sutphen, Leonard, & Day, 2010).

Clinical teaching is further complicated as nursing programs confront the increased costs of educational delivery amid shrinking budgets. Learners present with unique educational needs and represent various cultural groups with diverse demographics. Many college students report having inadequate social and interpersonal skills to communicate effectively, and growing numbers experience anxiety and stress (American College Health Association, 2018). Additionally, clinical nurse educators work with learners who have competing interests for their time, such as work demands or family responsibilities.

These challenges make it difficult for clinical nurse educators as they attempt to balance clinical site needs, expectations and needs of the learner, and demands of higher education. The traditional approach and most common model used in clinical nursing education involves one educator working directly with a small group of learners (8–12) while spending short amounts of time on a clinical unit (Giddens & Caputi, 2020). The clinical nurse educator guides and evaluates learners while working in conjunction with the staff nurse. Although this traditional model is widely used, many nursing programs are exploring alternative approaches, such as immersion experiences, preceptorships, and dedicated education units. Simulation is another growing educational trend that has gained widespread acceptance and is frequently used as part of clinical nursing education (Oermann, Shellenbarger, & Gaberson, 2018). Lastly, as health care continues to shift from acute care to community-based settings, clinical nurse educators will be further challenged to adapt and incorporate new clinical learning experiences.

The title used by these clinical nurse educators may vary across clinical and academic settings and institutions. Educators are called various names—including *faculty*, *instructor*, *educator*, or *teacher*—or they may be referred to by their employment status and have titles such as *adjunct* or *part-time faculty*. Regardless of their title, these educators coach learners and guide the learning process as they facilitate student learning throughout clinical components of an academic nursing program (National League for Nursing, 2019). In this book, these individuals will be referred to as *clinical nurse educators* and those they teach will be referred to as *learners*. The people they serve in clinical settings will be referred to as *clients*.

CLINICAL NURSE EDUCATOR ROLE

Given the multiple changes and challenges in nursing education, it is even more crucial to have adequately prepared clinical nurse educators who can confront these issues while ensuring that learners gain opportunities for growth. Clinical nurse educators are vital in helping to ensure the success of learners. They are critical for the preparation of the emerging workforce that will deliver quality nursing care.

Nurse educators influence learning by helping learners develop clinical reasoning and practice skills. Educators also serve as role models, imparting the professional values that socialize learners into the nursing profession. Moreover, clinical nurse educators play a pivotal gatekeeping role in providing educational leadership that will ensure that learners possess the knowledge, skills, and attitudes needed to deliver safe, quality care and meet the needs of the populations they serve. Ultimately, they help strengthen the health care workforce and address the ongoing nursing shortage.

CERTIFICATION

Since this role demands expertise and advanced knowledge to navigate the complex issues in health care and academia successfully, it is logical to expect that those serving in this role would want recognition for the work they do. One way to demonstrate their expertise is to pursue certification, the official recognition of knowledge and skills in a specialty area. Certification as a clinical nurse educator offers validation, through testing, that an individual has met established standards associated with the role (Institute for Credentialing Excellence, 2019).

The National League for Nursing (NLN) offers two certifications for nurse educators. The first certification validates expertise with the Certified Nurse Educator® Exam. This test aligns with the *Scope of Practice for Academic Nurse Educators 2012 Revision* (National League for Nursing, 2012) and represents the full scope of the academic nurse educator role, including the following core competencies: facilitating learning; facilitating learner development and socialization; using assessment and evaluation strategies; participating in curriculum design and evaluation of program outcomes; pursuing continuous quality improvement; engaging in scholarship, service, and leadership; functioning as a change agent and leader; engaging in the scholarship of teaching; and functioning effectively within the institutional environment and academic community. However, not all nurse educators participate in the full scope of this role. Instead, many educators in the academic setting function as clinical nurse educators. In this role, there is some overlap with the academic nurse educator, but there are also some different tasks and unique responsibilities for the clinical nurse educator role. Clinical nurse educators function in distinct nursing roles that focus on the following core competencies: function within the education and health care environments; facilitate learning in the health care environment; demonstrate effective interpersonal communication and collaborative interprofessional relationships; apply clinical expertise in the health care environment; facilitate learner development and socialization; and implement effective clinical assessment and evaluation strategies (National League for Nursing, 2018).

Even though the original NLN Nurse Educator Certification has been an essential part of nursing education for over 10 years, it has been only recently that the clinical nurse educator core competencies were identified. Beginning in 2015, a task group of nursing leaders used an iterative process to identify and refine the emergent six core competencies and task statements associated with the clinical nurse educator role. A verification process that sought input from NLN members helped the task group further refine the competencies and related task statements (Christensen & Simmons, 2019a). These competencies and task statements serve as the basis for the Certified Academic Clinical Nurse Educator (CNE®cl) test plan and are found in Appendix A. Presently, the NLN CNE®cl is the first and only certification for academic clinical nurse educators. Pilot testing was completed, and this new certification exam was offered for the first time to eligible candidates in fall 2018 (Christensen & Simmons, 2019b). Fifty-eight clinical nurse educators successfully passed the exam during piloting and were the first to use the CNE®cl designation (Malone, 2018). Given the large number of nurse educators engaged in this teaching role, it is expected that many more will pursue certification and take this certification examination.

Individuals interested in pursuing CNE®cl certification are encouraged to consult the NLN website (www.nln.org) and the *Certified Academic Clinical Nurse Educator (CNE®cl) Examination Candidate Handbook* (National League for Nursing, 2018). The candidate handbook, available on the NLN website, serves as a useful guide that provides an overview of the exam, outlines eligibility criteria, provides the current test blueprint (see Appendix A), and offers resources helpful for examination preparation. It also describes the test form, application deadlines, exam scheduling, testing locations, and other relevant policies. It is important for potential test takers to consult the NLN website and obtain the candidate handbook, as the exam and associated policies and procedures are regularly updated. The website will provide the most up-to-date guide needed for potential candidates.

Currently, to be eligible for the exam, candidates must document nursing licensure, educational qualifications, and have the appropriate practice experience. Applicants with a graduate degree with a focus in nursing education do not need to demonstrate academic teaching practice. However, candidates with a baccalaureate degree (or higher) in nursing without a focus in nursing education must demonstrate two years of teaching experience within the academic setting during the last five years (National League for Nursing, 2018).

Individuals interested in taking the clinical nurse educator certification exam will want to be prepared, and this book can help candidates. After this introductory chapter, Chapter 2 discusses strategies that test takers can use to prepare for the examination and approaches for overcoming test anxiety. Next, practice exam questions for each of the six clinical nurse educator competencies are offered. Each practice question provides a source and explanation that supports the correct answer. Additionally, incorrect answers are explained so that readers can understand why these options are wrong. All questions were peer-reviewed and represent best practices in clinical nursing education and testing. The questions in this book represent all items on the test plan. Each question is labeled according to the task statements found on the test plan. Some questions could align with more than one task statement; however, contributors made recommendations for question labeling, and these recommendations were generally followed.

Readers are encouraged to practice test taking with this book. A review of the questions and rationales can help identify topics for further study. Candidates are then encouraged to devise a study plan that meets their learning needs. Some may find it helpful to read and review relevant sources. Others may prefer to discuss content areas in study groups. Regardless of the method chosen, this book can assist candidates to review and identify relevant topics for further study. For additional practice, candidates may also want to complete the NLN Self-Assessment Examination (SAE). The computer-based SAE provides additional questions for practice with test taking but with the added benefit of computer-based testing. This delivery format allows candidates to become accustomed to the electronic delivery that will be used during testing. The SAE will also provide a score report that can be used to direct additional study. Using these resources can help candidates identify areas they need to review before taking the exam. Candidates are encouraged to develop a study approach and schedule that will ensure adequate review. It is hoped that, with adequate practice and review, test takers will be successful in achieving certification and will become recognized for their advanced knowledge as clinical nurse educators.

References

American College Health Association. (2018). National college health assessment reference group executive summary. Retrieved from https://www.acha.org/documents/ncha/NCHA-II_Fall_2018_Reference_Group_Executive_Summary.pdf

Benner, P., Sutphen, M., Leonard, V., & Day, L. (2010). *Educating nurses: A call for radical transformation.* San Francisco, CA: Jossey-Bass.

Christensen, L. S., & Simmons, L. E. (2019a). Development of the core competencies of clinical nurse educators. In T. Shellenbarger (Ed.), *Clinical nurse educator competencies: Creating an evidence-based practice for academic clinical nurse educators* (pp. 1–5). Washington, DC: National League for Nursing.

Christensen, L. S., & Simmons, L. E. (2019b). The academic clinical nurse educator. *Nursing Education Perspectives, 40*(3), 196. doi:10.1097/01.NEP.0000000000000509

Giddens, J. F., & Caputi, L. B. (2020). Conceptual teaching strategies in clinical education. In J. F. Giddens, L. B. Caputi, & B. Rodgers (Eds.), *Mastering concept-based teaching* (pp. 101–117). St. Louis, MO: Elsevier.

Institute for Credentialing Excellence. (2019). What is credentialing? Retrieved from http://www.credentialingexcellence.org/p/cm/ld/fid=32

Institute of Medicine of the National Academies. (2011). *The future of nursing: Leading change, advancing health.* Washington, DC: National Academies Press.

Malone, B. (2018, December 12). NLN CEO update on NLN—a year in review and a glimpse of the achievements on the horizon. NLN Member Update. Retrieved from http://www.nln.org/newsroom/newsletters-and-journal/nln-update/newsletter/nln-member-update/2018/12/12/december-12-2018-nln-ceo-update-on-nln-a-year-in-review-and-a-glimpse-of-the-achievements-on-the-horizon

National League for Nursing. (2012). *Scope of practice for academic nurse educators 2012 revision.* Washington, DC: Author.

National League for Nursing. (2018). *Certified academic clinical nurse educator (CNE®cl) examination candidate handbook.* Washington, DC: Author.

National League for Nursing. (2019). Certification for nurse educators. Retrieved from http://www.nln.org/Certification-for-Nurse-Educators

Oermann, M. H., Shellenbarger, T., & Gaberson, K. B. (2018). *Clinical teaching strategies in nursing* (5th ed.). New York, NY: Springer.

United States Department of Labor Bureau of Labor Statistics. (2018). Occupational employment and wages, May 2017. Retrieved from https://www.bls.gov/oes/2017/may/oes251072.htm

2

Preparing for the Exam

Susan G. Poorman, PhD, RN, CNS-BC, ANEF
Melissa L. Mastorovich, DNP, RN, BC

Preparing for any exam can seem like an overwhelming task. The meaning of the exam to the person taking it can also further add to that feeling. If the exam has a significant personal value, it can be even more daunting. For example, a student's SAT results may be used in part to determine which college the student can attend (Clinedinst & Koranteng, 2017). As another example, passing the National Council Licensure Examination (NCLEX-RN®) is required to practice as a registered nurse; thus, passing this exam represents a major career milestone. Graduate Record Examination (GRE) scores are often used as one of the criteria for admission into graduate programs (Patzer et al., 2017). These high-stakes examinations impact life and career options, intensifying the meaning of the exam and increasing stress and feelings of being overwhelmed.

The National League for Nursing (NLN) certification exam for academic clinical nurse educators (CNE®cl) can also carry significant meaning to someone who currently teaches or wants to teach clinical nursing. However, there are many things that a CNE®cl candidate can do to properly prepare for the certification exam which will hopefully lead to success. This chapter will provide specific information and helpful strategies that may help the candidate prepare for this exam.

HOW TO GET STARTED

The first thing a candidate preparing to take the CNE®cl exam should do is find out as much about the test as possible. In addition to using this book, one of the best ways to start is to obtain the *Certified Academic Clinical Nurse Educator (CNE®cl) Examination Candidate Handbook* (National League for Nursing, 2018), which is available on the NLN website at www.nln.org. The handbook includes important information about the exam and offers a good starting point for test preparation. The candidate handbook includes a detailed blueprint that serves as a guide to major content areas on the exam. Begin your preparation by reviewing the test plan. Consider how well you know these topics. Have you learned about the content areas? Are the topics familiar or unfamiliar? As you consider the test blueprint, try to identify your strengths and weaknesses. The handbook also includes a list of helpful resources, both books and journals, that you can use to study for this test (National League for Nursing, 2018). Familiarize yourself with the topics, major content areas, and core competencies that are found on the test. Read about the candidate application process, eligibility criteria, exam administration, and other test-related policies to prepare for the examination process.

PREPARATION AND TEST-TAKING STRATEGIES

A variety of approaches can be used to prepare for the examination. These strategies can be implemented when studying alone or in a group. Some candidates may prefer to prepare for the exam in isolation while others may prefer to study with others in study groups. Decide which approach may work best for you and use the following test-taking strategies to help facilitate your review.

Practice, Practice, Practice

One of the most important steps in test preparation is practicing as many sample test questions as possible. When you practice questions, you are actively participating in your learning instead of just passively reading information. Practicing questions will also help improve your ability to problem solve and can enhance your performance on the actual exam. Finally, it can desensitize you to answering questions, thus decreasing your anxiety for the actual test.

Start with the sample questions that are included in the candidate handbook. Then, complete the practice questions in this book. You may also want to consider completing the Self-Assessment Examination (SAE) that is available from the NLN. The SAE is similar to the CNE®cl exam and gives test takers practice with computer-based testing. Use practice questions and assessments to further identify areas of weakness that can then serve as a guide for focused study. If rationales are provided with practice questions, as in this book, use them to help understand why an answer is correct and why others are wrong. Use the list of helpful resources available in the candidate handbook to identify books, articles, and journals to find information about the specific content you need to study.

Timing

You may also want to time yourself when you practice questions. A candidate will have three hours to complete the exam. A digital clock with the amount of testing time left can be found on the computer screen. The total exam contains 150 questions. If you are a fast test taker and your scores are good, you may not need to be concerned about timing. However, for some test takers, answering too quickly can lead to errors, such as misreading. Slower test takers run the risk of running out of time. If a candidate runs out of time on the NLN CNE®cl exam, the test is terminated. A good way to pace yourself is to check your time every 15th question. We suggest averaging a minute per question. This would still allow time to take breaks. A candidate can take breaks throughout the exam; however, the clock does not stop once you have begun the test.

A Metacognitive Strategy: Think Out Loud

There are other strategies that can be used as part of your test preparation, including the use of metacognitive strategies. Metacognition is described as the experiences and knowledge we have about our own cognitive processes (Flavell, 1979). In other words, metacognition is thinking about thinking and involves having control over the thinking processes that we use in learning (Livingston, 2003; Poorman & Mastorovich, 2016). Using this metacognitive strategy is a good way to hear our thoughts out loud (Poorman, Mastorovich, Molcan, & Gropelli, 2017).

A useful metacognitive strategy is called *think out loud*. This technique is easily implemented. When selecting the answer to practice questions in this book, think out loud. By this, we mean to say out loud why you are choosing an option. For example, "I am going to pick Option B because…." When expressing the rationale for an answer out loud, you can often recognize errors in your thinking. In other words, when you say your rationale out loud, frequently you can hear your thought processes in a more objective way. After thinking out loud, look at the rationale for the correct answer. If you answered the question incorrectly, look at how your rationale differed from the rationale for the correct answer. Consider where your thinking went wrong. Identifying the questions you are answering incorrectly will help you determine what areas to review and study.

This strategy can also be used with a study partner or study group. Research suggests that when learners collaborate using think-aloud protocols, they increase their ability to critically think and problem solve (Kaddoura, 2013; Siddiq & Scherer, 2017). When you listen to each other think out loud, you can help identify errors in thinking but also work together to arrive at the correct answer.

What Is This Question Asking?

Another helpful strategy is to rephrase the question stem—or sentence that asks the question—into your own words. This will help ensure that you understand what the questions are asking you. Often, people miss questions for reasons other than lack of knowledge. Sometimes it is because what you thought was being asked is different than what the item writer intended. Ask yourself, "What do they want me to know? What is the question asking me?" As you read the question stem, also pay attention to keywords that can impact responses. For example, words such as *best*, *first*, or *most* ask you to prioritize responses. All items may be correct, but these keywords require you to consider order and impact. Most of the examination questions are testing higher cognitive thinking, including the application or analysis level of thinking; only a small number will test recall of specific knowledge. As you read test questions or when reviewing content, consider how the information can be applied in clinical nursing education.

Eliminate Options and Trust Your "Glimmer"

After you are sure what the question is asking, look at the four possible answers. First, try to identify any options that you automatically know are wrong. If you can eliminate even one option at this point, you will increase your chances of selecting the right answer. Then, review the question again. If you still do not know which option is correct, then trust your "glimmer." Your glimmer is that first flicker of thought about which option is correct. It is often the correct answer because you have not had time to contaminate it with your other thoughts. Rather than spending valuable time changing your mind and worrying about which option is correct, trust your glimmer.

Don't Rely Only on Personal Experience

An important strategy to keep in mind is that the way you have personally handled clinical situations is not necessarily the widely practiced or correct theoretical-based approach. Remember, rationales for the questions on this exam are taken from nursing articles and books. When you get a question that you are unsure of, ask yourself this: "What do the scholarly references say?" When you find yourself thinking,

"I know the answer to this question—a situation just like this happened to me a couple of weeks ago with my learners and here's how I handled it," you may not be answering correctly. Keep reminding yourself to consider the literature and available evidence; then, consider what the references say about this type of situation.

Test takers can use these strategies for preparation and test taking to help them plan and practice for the exam. Box 2.1 provides an example of how these strategies may be applied when answering a test question.

BOX 2.1 Putting Test-Taking Strategies Together

Now that you understand some general test-taking strategies, let's see an example of how these strategies all work together. In this example, we demonstrate how a candidate might use the suggested test-taking strategies when answering a sample question.

Question
A novice clinical nurse educator is conducting a clinical conference. The learners are interrupting each other and there is no educational purpose to their conversation. What is the best action by the clinical nurse educator?

A. Ask the learners to settle down and have them suggest an agreeable topic for discussion.
B. Interrupt the learners and ask an open-ended question about the clinical experience.
C. Start to discuss a specific clinical topic and ask the learners to take notes.
D. Wait for the learners to stop talking and ask if they have any questions from today's experience.

Using Test Taking Strategies
To think through this sample question, the candidate could start by paraphrasing the stem. The candidate may ask "**What is this question asking me?** The question is asking what the clinical nurse educator should do to redirect the focus of this clinical conference. Consider **which is the best action**. Once the question has been carefully paraphrased, I can consider **which option(s) I can eliminate**. I know the answer isn't Option A. *Telling people to settle down rarely works. Also, having everyone agree on a topic or issue is not the purpose of a clinical conference. I think Option D might be correct. I've done that before during clinical conference. I just stare at them until they are quiet. But wait, just because I've done that before doesn't mean I have evidence that this is the correct answer. It's just my personal experience. I realize that I need to stop answering questions from personal experience.* When I am not sure of the answer, **I will trust my glimmer**. So now with my choices narrowed down to Options B and C, I reread the question and I am still not sure of the answer. What was my first thought when I read the question? *I think Option B was my glimmer response, so I am going to pick B as the correct answer.*"

As you can see from the rationale that follows, by using the test-taking strategies to think and reason through the options, often candidates can choose the correct answer even if they aren't entirely certain.

Rationale
The correct answer is B. The purpose of the clinical conference is to have a discussion that focuses on some aspect of clinical practice. Asking open-ended questions, Option B, encourages the learners to talk and understand multiple perspectives regarding a clinical issue. Option A is incorrect because the role of the educator is to help learners examine and critique different perspectives of care, not to get total agreement from the group (Oermann, Shellenbarger, & Gaberson, 2018). Option C is incorrect because clinical discussions are not intended to be a lecture, nor are they effective as such. Option D is incorrect because waiting for the learners to stop talking and interrupting each other may not be effective; it is also wasting valuable learning time.

TEST ANXIETY

Another problem that some candidates may have is test anxiety. Test anxiety is a type of performance anxiety that impairs a learner's ability to prepare for and take an exam (Poorman et al., 2017). Test anxiety has been defined by many researchers. Gibson (2014), for example, identified test anxiety as a multidimensional state that involves physical, behavioral, and cognitive components. However, many researchers define test anxiety in simpler terms that include the components of worry and emotionality (Duty, Christian, Loftus, & Zappi, 2016; Putwain & Symes, 2018; Shen, Yang, Zhang, & Zhang, 2018).

Symptoms of test anxiety can vary widely. Some test-anxious people report physical symptoms such as a feeling of butterflies in their stomachs, nausea, diarrhea, palpitations, headaches, sweaty palms, or even blurred vision. Others have feelings of uneasiness and dread. Many people experience negative thoughts, such as: "I didn't study enough for this test, I'll never pass, I'm just not smart enough. Everyone else is finished and I'm still working on my test." Some individuals report only one or two symptoms that cause mild discomfort and a few missed questions on an exam. Others discuss a variety of symptoms that severely impair their test performance. Fortunately, there are several techniques available to combat this type of anxiety.

Cognitive Restructuring

Recent test-anxiety research has identified that the cognitive component or worrisome thoughts can impair test performance (Duty et al., 2016; Khalaila, 2015; Thomas, Cassady, & Heller, 2017). It is for this reason that many researchers recommend some form of cognitive treatment when addressing test anxiety (Brodersen, 2017; Gibson, 2014; Killu & Crundwell, 2016; Reiss et al., 2017; von der Embse, Barterian, & Segool, 2013).

Cognitive restructuring, based on Beck's model (Beck, 1976), is easy to learn and implement (Burns, 2009). One of the principles, according to Beck (2011), is that cognitive restructuring is educative and the person becomes one's own therapist. It requires that individuals become aware of their cognitions or thoughts before and during an exam. People with test anxiety often experience many negative and distracting thoughts while preparing for and taking an examination (Kamel, 2018; Putwain & Pescod, 2018; Putwain & Symes, 2018; Raufelder & Ringeisen, 2016). Examples of these negative thoughts could include the following: "I don't know the answer to this question, I can't remember all the information that I need for this test. There's just too much to learn." These worrisome thoughts often increase the individual's feelings of stress and anxiety, making it more difficult for the candidate to focus and be successful on an exam.

Unfortunately, many people are not aware of the thoughts that occur while they study or take an exam. Thus, the first step of cognitive restructuring is to learn to identify your thoughts. What most test-anxious individuals first recognize as a problem are the feelings of anxiety and stress that are produced by the thoughts they are having. These thoughts not only create difficulties when taking a test but also when preparing for it. Test-anxious individuals often have feelings of anxiety and dread when they are studying for an exam. These feelings are uncomfortable and can decrease focus, which can lead to avoidance behaviors or not studying at all. According to Custer's (2018) descriptive study of 202 prelicensure nursing students representing diploma, associate degree, and baccalaureate programs, there

Table 2.1

Restructuring Thoughts

Worrisome Thought	Restructured Neutral or Positive Thought
"These questions are dumb."	"I don't usually fail tests. I can do this."
"I'll never pass this test."	"Take it slow, one question at a time."
"Where do they get these questions?"	"I need to think about the theory of nursing education."
"I have been a clinical nurse educator for five years. I should know the answers to these questions."	"Just because I am not sure about the answer doesn't mean I'm not a good educator."
"Why don't I know this?"	"I need to think about what the nursing literature reports."

is a small but statistically significant relationship between test anxiety and procrastination. In a larger exploratory study of 534 undergraduate students, Thomas et al. (2017) found that test-anxious learners used avoidance behaviors as a coping mechanism. These behaviors prevent the learners' ability to process, store, or retrieve academic information while studying for or taking a test.

To identify your thoughts, you need to consciously become aware of them. The best place to start is during test preparation. Keep a notepad with you when you study and write down your thoughts and feelings. Once you identify your negative or unrelated thoughts, you can review them and ask yourself whether these thoughts are true. If you believe they are true, ask yourself whether you have any evidence to support them. Most of the time, thoughts are distorted and can even be catastrophic. For example: "If I fail this test, I will never get a job teaching nursing." After you learn to recognize negative thoughts, you can ask yourself the questions above and learn to restructure the thoughts. Table 2.1 illustrates restructuring negative thoughts to neutral or positive ones. When you learn to evaluate your negative thoughts and restructure them to positive or neutral thoughts, they have much less power and will not impact your ability to prepare for and take an examination.

Progressive Muscle Relaxation

Another approach to overcoming test anxiety involves progressive muscle relaxation. This technique requires individuals to actively contract a muscle group, and then release the muscles in a progressive manner to decrease anxiety (Zargarzadeh & Shirazi, 2014). High anxiety can affect test performance, specifically impairing concentration, organization, memory, and attention (Killu & Crundwell, 2016). Since physical tension and relaxation cannot occur simultaneously, this technique is especially helpful for people who experience physical symptoms related to test anxiety. Progressive relaxation is a behavioral technique; therefore, it must be practiced daily for several weeks. It will not be very helpful if you start using it several days before the test. Many scripts and tapes are available for implementing progressive muscle relaxation for individuals with test anxiety (Bourne & Garano, 2016; Davis, Eshelman, & McKay, 2019; Poorman et al., 2017).

Visual Imagery

Visual imagery, another approach to decreasing test anxiety, can also help improve your ability to take a test. It is a technique of seeing yourself being successful (Ellis, 2018). Visualize positive changes in yourself. When you practice visualizing these changes, performance can be improved (Bourne & Garano, 2016; Debarnot, Clerget, & Olivier, 2011; Schussel & Miller, 2013). Specifically, visualization has been found to decrease test anxiety (Brodersen, 2017; Quinn & Peters, 2017; Reiss et al., 2017).

There are many ways to practice visual imagery. You can write down what you would like to improve or change in your life, then practice that change in your imagination (Ellis, 2018). Start visual imagery by sitting in a comfortable chair or lying down, shutting your eyes and relaxing. There are also many different types of visualizations that you can record and listen to daily. Alternatively, you might prefer to use a phone or computer application that offers visual imagery and is easy to access and use. Many of these visualization scripts start with helping you relax. There are short scripts and longer ones depending on your personal preference (Bourne & Garano, 2016; Davis et al., 2019; Poorman et al., 2017).

Thought Stopping

Thought stopping is a behavioral technique that is useful for individuals who experience anxiety, including test anxiety. It can be especially helpful for people who have repetitive or intrusive thoughts that are unrealistic and unproductive. Thought stopping is considered a specific type of thought suppression. In thought suppression, the individual tries not to think about a specific topic (Slepian, Oikawa, & Smyth, 2014). In thought stopping, the individual is encouraged to stop the negative or bothersome thoughts and replace them with neutral or more positive ones. This technique involves a group of procedures designed to increase a person's ability to block a response sequence at the cognitive level (Bakker, 2009).

While there are many ways to use thought stopping, there is one way that is easy to learn. In the beginning, you will want to practice thought stopping when you are calm and relaxed. Sit in a comfortable chair where you have privacy (McKay, Davis, & Fanning, 2011). An easy way to practice thought stopping is by using a rubber band as a stimulus. Wear a rubber band on your wrist at all times. When you determine that your thoughts are negative or unproductive, you want to lightly snap the rubber band, just as a small stimulus. Then say the word *stop*. As soon as you say the word *stop*, try to immediately stop the negative thoughts. Empty your mind of these negative thoughts just for a few seconds. Now, replace the thoughts with neutral or positive ones. For example: "I don't know if I got that last question right. That makes three in a row, I am not sure of the answers." (Snap the rubber band.) "STOP. You can do this." Focus on the question in front of you. What is it asking?

You may find that the thoughts may stop for a few seconds and then reoccur. If that happens, snap the rubber band and say *stop* again. As you become better at using this technique, you can say the word *stop* quietly to yourself (Poorman et al., 2017). It is recommended that you work on one negative thought at a time and practice thought stopping throughout the day for at least three days to a week (Bourne, 2015; Wehrenberg, 2012).

APPROACHING THE TEST

Although we suggest practicing questions and reading books and journal articles as often as you can to prepare for the exam, you may want to just relax the evening before the test. Try to do something that will help you stay calm. Some people find that watching a movie, going to dinner with a friend, or taking a yoga class, for example, are relaxing. These activities help you focus on something other than the exam and may help you get a good night's sleep before the test. Another suggestion for the day before the test is to travel to the testing center, especially if you are not familiar with where it is located. Practicing getting to the testing site can save stress and anxiety since you will be familiar with the site and how to get there.

Be mindful of whom you talk to the day before or the morning of the test. Often, without meaning to, friends can make you more nervous, especially if they are also taking the test. Find supportive and encouraging friends who boost your confidence before testing.

Additionally, if you are easily distracted by noises when you take an exam, wearing earplugs may be beneficial. Practice wearing them while you are studying and practicing questions so that you get used to how they feel. Make sure you eat something before the exam. You do not want to be distracted by hunger during the exam. Taking a test when you are hungry can decrease your focus and ability to concentrate. If you do get nervous during the exam, do not forget to use the strategies that you have learned in this chapter. If you have practiced them on a regular basis, they will be helpful to you when you are taking the test.

CONCLUSION

With the suggestions offered for preparation—adequate review, use of helpful test-taking strategies, and techniques to reduce test anxiety—you have the needed tools to enhance success on the NLN academic clinical nurse educator examination. Your certification will demonstrate to others the advanced knowledge and expertise you have in this specialized field.

References

Bakker, G. M. (2009). In defence of thought stopping. *Clinical Psychologist, 13*(2), 59–68. doi:10.1080/13284200902810452

Beck, A. T. (1976). *Cognitive therapy and emotional disorders.* New York, NY: International Universities.

Beck, J. S. (2011). *Cognitive behavior therapy: Basics and beyond* (2nd ed.). New York, NY: Guilford.

Bourne, E. J. (2015). *The anxiety and phobia workbook* (6th ed.). Oakland, CA: New Harbinger.

Bourne, E. J., & Garano, L. (2016). *Coping with anxiety: 10 simple ways to relieve anxiety, fear and worry* (2nd ed.). Oakland, CA: New Harbinger.

Brodersen, L. D. (2017). Interventions for test anxiety in undergraduate nursing students: An integrative review. *Nursing Education Perspectives, 38*(3), 131–137. doi:10.1097/01.NEP.0000000000000142

Burns, D. D. (2009). *Feeling good: The new mood therapy* (reprint ed.). New York, NY: HarperCollins Publishers.

Clinedinst, M., & Koranteng, A. (2017). *2017 State of college admission.* Arlington, VA: National Association of College Admission Counseling.

Custer, N. (2018). Test anxiety and academic procrastination among prelicensure nursing students. *Nursing Education Perspectives, 39*(3), 162–163. doi:10.1097/01.NEP.0000000000000291

Davis, M., Eshelman, E. R., & McKay, M. (2019). *The relaxation and stress reduction workbook* (7th ed.). Oakland, CA: New Harbinger.

Debarnot, U., Clerget, E., & Olivier, E. (2011). Role of the primary motor cortex in the early boost in performance following mental imagery training. *PLoS ONE, 6*(10), e26717. doi:10.1371/journal. pone.0026717

Duty, S. M., Christian, L., Loftus, J., & Zappi, V. (2016). Is cognitive test-taking anxiety associated with academic performance among nursing students? *Nurse Educator, 41*(2), 70–74. doi:10.1097/ NNE.0000000000000208

Ellis, D. (2018). *Becoming a master student* (16th ed.). Boston, MA: Cengage Learning.

Flavell, J. H. (1979). Metacognition and cognitive monitoring: A new area of cognitive-developmental inquiry. *American Psychologist, 34*(10), 906–911. doi:10.1037/0003066X.34.10.906

Gibson, H. A. (2014). A conceptual view of test anxiety. *Nursing Forum, 49*(4), 267–277. doi:10.1111/nuf.12069

Kaddoura, M. (2013). Think pair share: A teaching learning strategy to enhance students' critical thinking. *Educational Research Quarterly, 36*(4), 3–24.

Kamel, O. M. (2018). The relationship between adaptive/maladaptive cognitive emotion regulation strategies and cognitive test anxiety among university students. *International Journal of Psycho-Educational Sciences, 7*(1), 100–105.

Khalaila, R. (2015). The relationship between academic self-concept, intrinsic motivation, test anxiety, and academic achievement among nursing students: Mediating and moderating effects. *Nurse Education Today, 35*(3), 432–438. doi:10.1016/j.nedt.2014.11.001

Killu, K., & Crundwell, R. M. A. (2016). Students with anxiety in the classroom: Educational accommodations and interventions. *Beyond Behavior, 25*(2), 30–40. doi:10.1177/107429561602500205

Livingston, J. S. (2003). Metacognition: An overview. Retrieved from https://files.eric.ed.gov/fulltext/ED474273.pdf

McKay, M., Davis, M., & Fanning, P. (2011). *Thoughts & feelings: Taking control of your moods & your life* (4th ed.). Oakland, CA: New Harbinger.

National League for Nursing. (2018). *Certified academic clinical nurse educator (CNE®cl) candidate handbook.* Washington, DC: Author.

Oermann, M. H., Shellenbarger, T., & Gaberson, K. B. (2018). *Clinical teaching strategies in nursing* (5th ed.). New York, NY: Springer.

Patzer, B., Lazzara, E. H., Keebler, J. R., Madi, M. H., Dwyer, P., Huckstadt, A. A., & Smith-Campbell, B. (2017). Predictors of nursing graduate school success. *Nursing Education Perspectives, 38*(5), 272–274. doi:10.1097/01.NEP.0000000000000172

Poorman, S. G., Mastorovich, M. L., Molcan, K. L., & Gropelli, T. (2017). *A good thinking approach to the NCLEX® and other nursing exams* (3rd ed.). Pittsburgh, PA: STAT Nursing Consultants.

Poorman, S. G., & Mastorovich, M. L. (2016). Using metacognitive wrappers to help students enhance their prioritization and test-taking skills. *Nurse Educator, 41*(6), 282–285. doi:10.1097/NNE.0000000000000257

Putwain, D. W., & Pescod, M. (2018). Is reducing uncertain control the key to successful test anxiety intervention for secondary school students? Findings from a randomized control trial. *School Psychology Quarterly, 33*(2), 283–292. doi:10.1037/spq0000228

Putwain, D. W., & Symes, W. (2018). Does increased effort compensate for performance debilitating test anxiety? *School Psychology Quarterly, 33*(3), 482–491. doi:10.1037/spq0000236

Quinn, B. L., & Peters, A. (2017). Strategies to reduce nursing test anxiety: A literature review. *Journal of Nursing Education, 56*(3), 145–151. doi:10.3928/01484834-20170222-05

Raufelder, D., & Ringeisen, T. (2016). Self-perceived competence and test anxiety: The role of academic self-concept and self-efficacy. *Journal of Individual Differences, 37*(3), 159–167. doi:10.1027/1614-0001/a000202

Reiss, N., Warnecke, I., Tolgou, T., Krampen, D., Luka-Krausgrill, U., & Rohrmann, S. (2017). Effects of cognitive behavioral therapy with relaxation vs. imagery rescripting on test anxiety: A randomized controlled trial. *Journal of Affective Disorders, 208*, 483–489. doi:10.1016/j.jad.2016.10.039

Schussel, L., & Miller, L. (2013). Best self visualization method with high-risk youth. *Journal of Clinical Psychology, 69*(8), 836–845. doi:10.1002/jclp.22019

Shen, L., Yang, L., Zhang, J., & Zhang, M. (2018). Benefits of expressive writing in reducing test anxiety: A randomized controlled trial in Chinese samples. *PLoS ONE, 13*(2), e0191779. doi:10.1371/journal.pone.0191779

Siddiq, F., & Scherer, R. (2017). Revealing the processes of students' problem solving task: An in-depth analysis of think-aloud protocols. *Computers in Human Behavior, 76*, 509–525. doi:10.1016/j.chb.2017.080070747-5632/.08.007

Slepian, M. L., Oikawa, M., & Smyth, J. M. (2014). Suppressing thoughts of evaluation while being evaluated. *Journal of Applied Social Psychology, 44*(1), 31–39. doi:10.1111/jasp.12197

Thomas, C. L., Cassady, J. C., & Heller, M. L. (2017). The influence of emotional intelligence, cognitive test anxiety, and coping strategies on undergraduate academic performance. *Learning and Individual Differences, 55*, 40–48. doi:10.1016/j.lindif.2017.03.001

von der Embse, N., Barterian, J., & Segool, N. (2013). Test anxiety interventions for children and adolescents: A systematic review of treatment studies from 2000–2010. *Psychology in the Schools, 50*(1), 57–71. doi:10.1002/pits.21660

Wehrenberg, M. (2012). *The 10 best-ever anxiety management techniques workbook.* New York, NY: W.W. Norton.

Zargarzadeh, M., & Shirazi, M. (2014). The effect of progressive muscle relaxation method on test anxiety in nursing students. *Iranian Journal of Nursing and Midwifery Research, 19*(6), 607–612.

3

Function Within the Education and Health Care Environments

1. Which preclinical activity would best ensure that learners are prepared for client care?
   A. Completing flash cards for the medications that their assigned client takes
   B. Discussing the pathophysiology of the client's diagnosis and two interventions
   C. Completing a reflection journal entry focused on feelings about caring for their assigned client
   D. Writing a five-page paper detailing their client's diagnosis and pathophysiology with references

   Correct Answer: B

   Rationale: Learners should be expected to complete some cognitive preparation before clinical practice, but extensive, detailed written preparation assignments are unrealistic and often shift focus away from learning during clinical activities (Oermann, Shellenbarger, & Gaberson, 2018, p. 77). Option B gives learners an opportunity to apply classroom learning (pathophysiology) in the preparation for clinical experiences (interventions). Options A and D require excessive preclinical writing that would be unnecessary and may be distracting. Learners should complete more realistic preparation that would better facilitate their learning without the extensive writing. Option C focuses on reflection and may be more appropriate for an assignment after caring for their client.

   Test Blueprint: 1 A 1
   Cognitive Code: Application

2. Which action best facilitates the learner's ability to apply theory to practice?
   A. Asking the learners to share what was taught in the previous class
   B. Requesting the weekly course content outline from the lead course educator
   C. Selecting client assignments based on potential clinical skills needed
   D. Asking the nursing staff to suggest "interesting" clients

   Correct Answer: B

   Rationale: If the clinical nurse educator is aware of the course content taught in the classroom, then clinical assignments can be made that can align with the course content. This practice will allow for the clinical nurse educator to facilitate discussions and clinical activities to apply classroom knowledge to practice (Oermann et al., 2018). Obtaining the information from the lead course educator would be optimum, as in Option B. Option A is relying on learner recall and may not accurately indicate the classroom content. Option C is based on the possibility of performing clinical skills rather than specific knowledge taught in the classroom. Option D does not consider current classroom content.

Test Blueprint: 1 A 1
Cognitive Code: Application

3. Which question facilitates application of theory to clinical practice best?
   A. "What risk factors does your client have that are related to the client's diagnosis of pneumonia?"
   B. "Is nasopharyngeal suctioning a clean or sterile procedure?"
   C. "What is the mechanism of action of the prescribed nebulizer treatment?"
   D. "What did the client's chest x-ray indicate?"

Correct Answer: A

Rationale: Application of classroom knowledge is essential in clinical practice (Oermann et al., 2018, p. 28). By asking the learner to analyze the client's past medical and social history and determine what risk factors increased the risk for pneumonia development, the learner needed to recall the theory information and compare the client's information, thus making Option A the correct response. Options B, C, and D are all lower-level questions that do not require application of theory to practice.

Test Blueprint: 1 A 1
Cognitive Code: Application

4. Which action bridges the theory-practice gap best?
   A. Completing the learners' summative clinical evaluations
   B. Being a member of the program's curriculum committee
   C. Working part-time at one of the program's clinical sites
   D. Providing exam questions for the theory examination

Correct Answer: B

Rationale: Clinical nurse educators make a valuable contribution to the learning process. Involving the clinical nurse educator in the curriculum process, as in Option B, is a valuable method to improve the theory-practice gap in nursing education (Akram, Mohamad, & Akram, 2018, p. 881). Option A reflects one of the responsibilities of the clinical nurse educator but does not necessarily help bridge the theory-practice gap. Option C may increase the clinical nurse educator's understanding and comfort related to the clinical site but does not affect the theory portion of nursing education. Providing exam questions, as in Option D, does not help learners apply theory to practice.

Test Blueprint: 1 A 1
Cognitive Code: Application

5. Which learning activity emphasizes nursing roles related to health promotion and disease prevention best?
  A. Completing preclinical assignments, including a care plan and concept map
  B. Administering influenza vaccinations to educators
  C. Shadowing a school nurse during a pediatric clinical rotation
  D. Collaborating with a social worker to plan home care visits

Correct Answer: B

Rationale: Clinical learning experiences are selected and planned to provide learners with opportunities to work across settings. They also help learners manage care for varied populations, with emphasis on applying theory content from the classroom to the clinical experiences. Clinical experiences should include an emphasis on the nursing roles related to health promotion and disease prevention (Gubrud, 2016, p. 286). Option B provides an example of preventive care that will allow learners to engage in health promotion and disease prevention activities. Preclinical assignments, Option A, and shadowing a school nurse, Option C, are not necessarily related to health promotion or disease prevention. Planning home care visits, as in Option D, may decrease readmission rates, but is not necessarily the best representation of preventing disease or promoting health.

Test Blueprint: 1 A 1
Cognitive Code: Analysis

6. Which question would best promote reflection during a simulation debriefing session?
  A. "What was the client's heart rate?"
  B. "Where did you chart the intake and output?"
  C. "What were you thinking about during the simulation?"
  D. "Did you transfer the client from chair to bed safely?"

Correct Answer: C

Rationale: The use of probing, open-ended questions will help to engage learners in reflective conversations (Oermann et al., 2018, pp. 147–148). Asking about the client's heart rate, Option A, yields a simple numerical response. Where the learner charted the intake and output, Option B, requires a closed-ended response. Asking whether the learner transferred the client safely, Option D, likely yields a yes or no response. Only Option C is open-ended and promotes reflective thinking.

Test Blueprint: 1 A 2
Cognitive Code: Analysis

7. Which statement or question would foster reflection and learner professional growth best?
  A. "What diagnostic tests were completed?"
  B. "Tell me what went well during the Foley catheter insertion."
  C. "What are the steps for mixing insulin?"
  D. "Tell me about the client's medications."

Correct Answer: B

Rationale: One key strategy of teaching for salience is helping learners reflect on practice to identify what is important in a given situation (Oermann et al., 2018, p. 167). By asking the learner to share what went well during a Foley catheter insertion, the clinical educator is prompting the learner to reflect on actions. This reflective activity will help promote learner growth. Options A, C, and D are seeking factual information and are not the best way to facilitate clinical reasoning and learner reflection.

Test Blueprint: 1 A 2
Cognitive Code: Application

8. A clinical group assigned to a pediatric emergency department witnesses the demise of a preschooler following an automobile accident. Several of the learners are visibly upset after observing the efforts that were made to save the child. Which is the best initial action by the clinical nurse educator?
   A. Notifying the program administration of the incident and canceling the rest of the clinical day
   B. Providing the contact information of the agency grievance counselor to the learners
   C. Sending the learners to the cafeteria for a break before completing the clinical day
   D. Transferring client care to the unit nurses and initiating an impromptu clinical conference

Correct Answer: D

Rationale: Clinical nurse educators need to recognize the importance of debriefing and guided reflection to support learners following the death of a client in the clinical setting (Heise & Gilpin, 2016). A clinical conference, as suggested in Option D, allows for the support and debriefing needed by the learners. Option A does not address the learners' needs to discuss the situation. Option B may be completed by the clinical nurse educator, but it is not the best action for immediate learner support. Option C does not acknowledge the learners' feelings or the need to debrief.

Test Blueprint: 1 A 2
Cognitive Code: Application

9. Which statement or question would best support learner self-assessment?
   A. "Tell me about the health problems your client was experiencing."
   B. "Tell me about your experience during this clinical day."
   C. "I listened to your report to your primary nurse. Next time, could you include the most recent set of vital signs?"
   D. "Were you able to complete all of the required assessments and paperwork on your assigned client?"

Correct Answer: B

Rationale: The clinical nurse educator is a resource for learners. By asking open-ended questions and supporting learner responses, the educator encourages learners to arrive at their own decisions and to engage in self-assessment about clinical practice (Oermann et al., 2018, p. 199). Asking about the client's health problems, as in Option A, is an open-ended statement but does not promote learner self-assessment. Asking about vital signs,

Option C, and completion of paperwork, Option D, are closed-ended questions that do not promote learner self-assessment. Only Option B, an open-ended statement, encourages the learner to self-assess following the clinical experience.

Test Blueprint: 1 A 2
Cognitive Code: Application

10. A learner submits a written health assessment that lacks sufficient detail. Which statement represents the most appropriate response?
    A. "You need to refer to class notes and reference your textbook more when completing future assignments."
    B. "This assignment is superficial and lacks detail about your health assessment data collection."
    C. "This health assessment is lacking detail in the cardiovascular and respiratory sections. I would suggest using your textbook for help."
    D. "Your health assessment could use more information, especially in the cardiovascular and respiratory sections."

    Correct Answer: C

    Rationale: Constructive and timely feedback, which promotes achievement and growth, is an essential element of evaluation (Gubrud, 2016, p. 288). Options A, B, and D are not specific and do not provide constructive feedback that will sufficiently guide the learner. Option C involves specific and constructive feedback that provides the learner with a clear understanding of the problems and how to improve.

    Test Blueprint: 1 A 2
    Cognitive Code: Application

11. Which situation provides the highest potential for learning?
    A. After medication administration, the clinical nurse educator tells the learner, "everything went well."
    B. Following a sterile dressing change, the clinical nurse educator tells the learner, "you followed sterile technique but just remember to bring all supplies with you before you begin."
    C. At the end of the clinical day, the clinical nurse educator reminds the learner to complete the preclinical assignment in a timely manner in the future.
    D. During a physical assessment, the clinical nurse educator instructs the learner to inspect for edema.

    Correct Answer: B

    Rationale: Clinical educators have a variety of opportunities to offer feedback in response to performance behaviors relating to psychomotor as well as cognitive and affective actions. Regardless of the action, key considerations should be practiced, including specificity, timing, consistency, continuity, and approach (Gubrud, 2016, p. 289). Option A is incorrect because making general summary statements, such as "everything went well," is not specific feedback that can direct learner improvement. Providing feedback regarding preclinical assignments at the end of the day, as in Option C, is not appropriate timing of feedback. It is also not appropriate to provide learners with performance feedback during a physical assessment, as in Option D. Option B provides the best example of specific, timely, and useful feedback.

Test Blueprint: 1 A 2
Cognitive Code: Application

12. A primary nurse and nursing aide approach the clinical nurse educator, complaining that the learner assigned to their client is working too slowly and has not yet assessed the fasting blood sugar. Which action is most appropriate?
    A. Go to the room, help guide the learner to reprioritize skills, and obtain the fasting blood sugar.
    B. Apologize to the primary nurse and aide and replace the learner with another who works faster.
    C. Send another learner in to take the fasting blood sugar and report it to the primary nurse.
    D. Assess the fasting blood sugar while the learner is out of the room and discuss time management in post-conference.

Correct Answer: A

Rationale: If the clinical nurse educator expects that a learner will not be able to complete client care activities in a timely manner, this is a rich opportunity to help the learner prioritize, organize, complete a complex set of tasks for the client, and work collaboratively with other health care team members (Oermann et al., 2018, p. 67). In Option A, the clinical nurse educator is not preventing the learner from learning a valuable lesson. The other options are limiting to the learner and do not allow the learner the opportunity to engage in client care.

Test Blueprint: 1 A 2
Cognitive Code: Application

13. Which statement or question would help a learner self-reflect and grow professionally best?
    A. "Tell me what you did during your shift with your preceptor."
    B. "Tell me why or why you would not change any of your actions during your shift."
    C. "What are other possible reasons for the client's symptoms?"
    D. "What types of skills did you perform during your shift?"

Correct Answer: B

Rationale: Option B asks learners to not only recall their actions during their clinical shift, but also asks them to critically think and question their own actions and defend their responses. This will help the learner self-appraise and grow professionally. Reflection is key in engaging and developing learners (Popkess & Frey, 2016). Options A and D are not the best ways to elicit self-reflection responses and may likely result in the learner providing a simple list of activities and tasks. Option C is a good question for encouraging critical thinking and clinical reasoning skills (Oermann, 1997; Paul & Elder, 2008), but does not necessarily encourage self-reflection.

Test Blueprint: 1 A 2
Cognitive Code: Application

14. Which technology-based activity is best suited for creating direct clinical practice experiences?
   A. Prerecorded case presentations
   B. Virtual clinical simulations
   C. Quizzing software
   D. Social media sites

Correct Answer: B

Rationale: If the educational intention is direct experience, related technologies include use of electronic health records, virtual reality environments, multi-player online role-playing games, virtual case simulations, or high-fidelity simulations (Oermann et al., 2018, p. 160). Prerecorded case presentations, as in Option A, deliver clinical information to learners but do not create direct clinical practice experiences. Option C, quizzing software, is useful for drill and cognitive practice but not for creating direct practice experiences. Option D, social media sites, can be used for locating clinical information or for discussion and reflection but are not best for direct clinical practice experiences.

Test Blueprint: 1 A 3
Cognitive Code: Analysis

15. What initial action encourages appropriate use of mobile devices as a reference tool in the clinical setting?
   A. Inquiring about available Internet access at the agency
   B. Creating a list of available electronic applications
   C. Determining if all learners have a mobile device
   D. Referring to the agency's policy regarding mobile device use

Correct Answer: D

Rationale: The use of mobile devices in the clinical setting can greatly assist learners and, when used appropriately, can increase ability to access resources to provide more effective and efficient client care (Oermann et al., 2018, p. 162). It is important for clinical educators to first know the clinical agency's policies regarding mobile devices, as in Option D (Oermann et al., 2018, p. 162). Knowing the agency's policy first then allows for further planning and information seeking. Options A, B, and C would be appropriate actions to take after reviewing the agency's policy.

Test Blueprint: 1 A 3
Cognitive Code: Application

16. A learner has just completed a one-day rotation in a hospice unit. During postclinical conference, the learner states, "I spent half the day with the respiratory therapist. It was so boring; I don't understand why that was necessary." Which is the most appropriate response?
   A. "I'm not sure why you were with a respiratory therapist. I'll speak with the unit manager."
   B. "How did working with the respiratory therapist make you feel?"
   C. "Well, what did you do the other half of the day? That might help me understand your experience a bit better."
   D. "Breathing difficulties are common at the end of life. Tell me more about your time with the respiratory therapist."

Correct Answer: D

Rationale: The clinical nurse educator needs to value the contribution of others (health care team members, families, etc.) in helping learners achieve learning outcomes (Shellenbarger, 2019). In Option D, the clinical nurse educator acknowledges the likely reason that a learner was placed with a respiratory therapist in the hospice unit, that is, that breathing difficulties are common at the end of life. This activity values the contribution of another health care team member in helping the learner achieve learning outcomes. The clinical nurse educator then asks the learner to recount the time with the respiratory therapist, helping the learner make the relevancy connection and further supporting learning. Option A does not value the contribution of the respiratory therapist and sounds accusatory. Option B is not helpful because the learner's feelings have already been stated. Option C sounds accusatory and does not address the concern.

Test Blueprint: 1 A 4
Cognitive Code: Analysis

17. Learners in a community health clinical group are assigned with school nurses in local schools. While at the school, they are assigned to interview teachers to gain their perspectives on the health issues facing students. When a learner asks about the assignment purpose, which clinical nurse educator response is most appropriate?
    A. "I want you to see what the teacher knows about student health so you can provide them with further education."
    B. "Since teachers are with students all day, I think they will have valuable insights on health issues."
    C. "It is important to talk to more than just the school nurse to benefit from this learning experience."
    D. "You need to work on your interview skills and talking with teachers will help develop these skills."

Correct Answer: B

Rationale: The clinical nurse educator needs to value the contribution of others (health care team members, families, etc.) and how they can help learners achieve outcomes (Shellenbarger, 2019). In Option B, the clinical nurse educator is valuing teachers and their insights on health issues facing students. This, combined with learner reflections, can help contribute to learning and achievement of outcomes in the community health course. Option A would not reflect the purpose of this assignment; the learner would not be assessing and educating the teacher as part of this assignment. Options C and D may be true, but they do not best describe the purpose of this assignment and do not value the contributions of the teacher in the school health environment.

Test Blueprint: 1 A 4
Cognitive Code: Analysis

18. The clinical nurse educator is assisting the learner in preparing to administer client medications. One of the client's pills is missing from the medication drawer. The learner states that other clients have several of the same pills. Which response best models safe and ethical care?
   A. "In order to comply with medication timing, we will borrow and immediately replace the pill from the other client's drawer."
   B. "Since this medication is a daily standing order, it is acceptable for us to wait and see if it gets delivered this afternoon."
   C. "We need to investigate this now. Let's notify the pharmacy of the discrepancy and obtain the pill for our client."
   D. "Place a call to the physician and explain that the medication is missing. Perhaps we will not have to give it today."

Correct Answer: C

Rationale: Clinical nurse educators can model ethical behavior as well as how nurses should respond to quality and safety issues in the clinical setting, a lesson often easier to learn in context rather than in a classroom (Adelman-Mullally et al., 2013, p. 30). In Option C, the clinical nurse educator is modeling the behavior that promotes safe and ethical care. Options A, B, and D are promoting work-around behaviors, which is not appropriate as work-arounds can present quality and safety concerns.

Test Blueprint: 1 A 5
Cognitive Code: Application

19. Which activity is most appropriate to help ensure that learners provide culturally competent care?
   A. Reviewing the literacy level of teaching materials used with clients
   B. Teaching an international client how to administer an insulin injection
   C. Avoiding the use of slang and colloquialisms when teaching clients
   D. Considering preferences and experiences during client teaching sessions

Correct Answer: D

Rationale: Cultural competence is now considered essential for providing quality care to the increasingly diverse client populations (Bauce, Kridli, & Fitzpatrick, 2014). Options A, B, and C are strategies that may be helpful for learners but do not ensure their development of cultural competence.

Test Blueprint: 1 A 6
Cognitive Code: Application

20. Which is the best strategy to increase success of diverse learners?
   A. Encourage minority nurses to function as role models and mentors for learners.
   B. Require learners to complete an online learning module about diversity in the workplace.
   C. Assign clients from diverse backgrounds for learners to care for during clinical experiences.
   D. Intentionally incorporate culturally appropriate nonpharmacological pain interventions.

Correct Answer: A

Rationale: Practicing minority nurses can be encouraged to function as role models and mentors, as suggested in Option A. Many nursing learners plan to practice in hospital or community settings after graduation; matching them with a practicing nurse is a way to instill confidence that they can be successful (Popkess & Frey, 2016, p. 21). Educating learners about diversity issues, as in Option B, and seeking clients with diverse backgrounds for clinical assignments, as in Option C, are important, but do not focus on increasing the success of diverse learners. Option D incorporates culturally appropriate nursing care but does not necessarily help increase learner success.

Test Blueprint: 1 A 6
Cognitive Code: Application

21. Which clinical learning activity promotes the highest level of cognitive learning related to client-centered, culturally appropriate nursing care?
    A. Observing a simulation that emphasizes cultural awareness
    B. Completing a health history on a client from a different cultural group
    C. Attending a class presentation that focuses on a specific culture
    D. Listening to a panel of guests from different cultures speak during clinical conference

Correct Answer: B

Rationale: Nursing programs have an obligation to help learners develop knowledge, skills, and attitudes needed to care for an increasingly diverse population. Completing a health history is an active learning activity that provides learners with the opportunity to develop communication skills and cultural knowledge (Alexander, 2016, p. 266). Options A, C, and D are also learning activities that may provide information about cultural awareness and knowledge; however, they do not ensure active engagement with a person from another culture and do not guarantee learning.

Test Blueprint: 1 A 6
Cognitive Code: Analysis

22. Which learning activity best encompasses the goal of being learner centered?
    A. Responding to a structured writing prompt
    B. Completing a case study
    C. Developing a learning contract
    D. Participating in a role-play scenario

Correct Answer: C

Rationale: Option C would allow learners to develop their own goals and objectives for a clinical course, which places the learner at the center of the course and allows the nurse educator to tailor experiences. Learning contracts typically include activities to meet goals and objectives as well as evaluation methods and due dates (Oermann & Gaberson, 2017). Learning contracts can be a precourse activity or a remediation activity (Oermann & Gaberson, 2017). Although Options A, B, and D are all appropriate learning activities for engaging learners (Phillips, 2016), they are not as encompassing as a learning contract in the goal of being learner centered.

Test Blueprint: 1 A 6
Cognitive Code: Analysis

23. A clinical nurse educator is asked to evaluate a clinical unit after completing a semester working on the unit with a group of learners. The clinical nurse educator notes that learners did not have many opportunities to engage in client teaching activities, which is an important objective for this course. Which suggestion would best help the nursing program address this issue for future clinical experiences?

A. Eliminate the client teaching objective because not all sites prioritize teaching.

B. Assign the client teaching objective to learners only in the final semester.

C. Consider a unit where client teaching is critical, such as same-day surgery.

D. Avoid assigning learners to that unit again because it wasted learner time.

Correct Answer: C

Rationale: Clinical nurse educators should conduct a careful assessment of potential clinical sites before selecting those that will be used. Criteria in potential clinical agency selection should include the opportunity for learners to achieve learning outcomes (Oermann et al., 2018, p. 68). Option C is the only suggestion that is focused on future site planning. Options A, B, and D are incorrect because they either criticize the learning objective or the clinical site. They do not offer a solution that ensures that learners gain experience or engage in activities supportive of the course objective focused on client teaching.

Test Blueprint: 1 B 1
Cognitive Code: Application

24. When deciding whether a clinical agency will be an appropriate clinical site, which action would be least helpful?

A. Asking to shadow staff for a day to learn unit routines

B. Attending the institution's standardized orientation for new staff

C. Determining unit routines, such as medication, activity, and mealtimes

D. Meeting with the nurse manager to determine average client acuity and length of stay

Correct Answer: B

Rationale: While some of the information presented at standardized orientation is useful—such as the institutional mission and philosophy, organizational structure, and key personnel—much of the information will be irrelevant to the instructional role (O'Connor, 2015, p. 56). Thus, Option B is the least helpful action and the correct response. Option A will allow the clinical nurse educator to become acclimated to the environment, routine, and nuances of the agency. Option C allows the clinical nurse educator to determine the availability of the clients when learners are scheduled for their experience; if the clients are in activities or away from the agency during the scheduled clinical time, the agency may not provide the best experience for the learner. Option D supports the need to collect data related to the client population; it helps to determine the availability of appropriate client assignments based on the learners' educational level and the clinical course.

Test Blueprint: 1 B 1
Cognitive Code: Analysis

25. When evaluating potential clinical sites, which is the lowest priority?
   A. Level of the learner
   B. Location of the agency
   C. Compatibility of philosophies
   D. Availability of role models for learners

Correct Answer: B

Rationale: All of the criteria are included in the assessment of a clinical site; however, the geographical location of the clinical site is usually not the most important selection criterion (Gaberson & Oermann, 2007, p. 29). Options A, C, and D should take priority over location when selecting a clinical site.

Test Blueprint: 1 B 1
Cognitive Code: Application

26. When selecting a clinical agency, which is the most important factor for the clinical nurse educator to consider?
   A. The learners' needs
   B. The average daily census at the agency
   C. The proximity to the school
   D. The clinical nurse educator's relationship with the agency

Correct Answer: A

Rationale: Based on the criteria provided, the congruence between the clinical agency and the learner needs, goals, and outcomes are the most important consideration for clinical placement (Gaberson & Oermann, 2007, p. 29). Options B, C, and D are other factors that should be taken into consideration but do not supersede the importance of agency selection based on the learners' goals and needs.

Test Blueprint: 1 B 1
Cognitive Code: Application

27. Which clinical experience would best prepare learners for transition to practice?
   A. Shadowing an intensive care nurse for a 12-hour shift
   B. Interviewing several clients to allow practice with communication skills
   C. Designing and implementing a care plan during the clinical experience
   D. Providing complete care for three medical-surgical clients

Correct Answer: D

Rationale: Learning goals may help facilitate learners' ability to synthesize information, integrate didactic and clinical knowledge, develop clinical reasoning and judgment skills, and plan care for groups of clients. Assignments that involve planning care for clients with complex needs and for multiple clients, as in Option D, are appropriate and would assist learners preparing for the transition to practice (Gubrud, 2016, p. 287). Shadowing a nurse, Option A, interviewing multiple clients, Option B, and implementing a care plan, Option C, are not the best clinical experiences to prepare learners for transition to practice.

Test Blueprint: 1 B 2
Cognitive Code: Analysis

28. Which action by the clinical nurse educator enables learners to meet clinical objectives best?
    A. Allowing learners to hear the nurses' shift change report
    B. Providing the agency director with a copy of the course syllabus
    C. Introducing the learners to the nurses and other staff working on the unit
    D. Asking the charge nurse about the clients on the unit prior to the learners' arrival

Correct Answer: D

Rationale: Client selection should be based on factors such as the level of the learner and activities learners will perform. Consulting with staff prior to the learners' arrival, Option D, will help ensure that client assignments will best enable learners to meet objectives. The staff nurses can help the clinical nurse educator determine which clients will provide a suitable clinical experience (O'Connor, 2015, p. 113). Option A may be important for learner preparation; however, it does not ensure that learners meet the clinical objectives. Option B provides general information to the agency director but does not provide additional information regarding how this information may or may not be shared with direct bedside staff. Option C is a valuable part of communication but does not ensure that learners will meet clinical objectives.

Test Blueprint: 1 B 2
Cognitive Code: Application

29. The clinical nurse educator wants to use a written assignment to help learners prepare for the clinical day. Which assignment would help learners demonstrate the connection between theoretical concepts and clinical care best?
    A. Portfolio
    B. Concept map
    C. Reflective journal
    D. Evidence-based paper

Correct Answer: B

Rationale: Concept maps are a valuable tool to help learners plan for the clinical experience and visually display the relationships between concepts that include, but are not limited to, assessment data, medications, interventions, and pathophysiology, thus making Option B correct (Gaberson, Oermann, & Shellenbarger, 2015, p. 300; Oermann & Gaberson, 2009, p. 302). Options A, C, and D are appropriate written assignments; however, the use of these strategies is not the best assignment for preclinical preparation and not best for demonstrating links between concepts and client care.

Test Blueprint: 1 B 2
Cognitive Code: Application

30. The clinical nurse educator wants to assess learner needs related to safe medication preparation prior to entering the clinical setting. Which activity will provide the most valuable information for the clinical nurse educator?
   A. Review past clinical evaluations that were completed prior to the start of the clinical experience.
   B. Create an electronic discussion for learners to share stories from past clinical experiences.
   C. Have learners complete a self-assessment prior to the first clinical day.
   D. Require learners to achieve a passing score on a dosage calculation exam prior to the first clinical day.

Correct Answer: D

Rationale: Medication administration presents the largest risk for errors for nurses. Requiring learners to complete a dosage calculation exam prior to entering the clinical setting is a method used to help evaluate one aspect of safety related to medication preparation (O'Connor, 2015, p. 118). Option A could be considered a privacy violation if the review of the learner's records is completed without cause. Options B and C will promote open discussions and self-evaluation but are not the best strategy to assess learner needs related to client safety.

Test Blueprint: 1 B 2
Cognitive Code: Application

31. A clinical nurse educator is assigned to teach a fundamentals course on a step-down trauma unit. Which initial action is most appropriate?
   A. Proceeding with the clinical experience and using the assigned clinical unit
   B. Informing the nurse manager that the clinical unit is too complex
   C. Creating a handout for learners with common equipment used on the nursing unit
   D. Contacting the lead educator for the course, discussing the concern with the assigned unit

Correct Answer: D

Rationale: Both the level of the learner and opportunity to achieve learning outcomes must be considered when selecting appropriate clinical learning settings (Oermann et al., 2018, p. 57). The clinical setting of a step-down trauma unit would be a setting for advanced learners rather than beginning learners. The ability for learners to achieve the learning outcomes may be hindered in this setting. The clinical educator should discuss the assigned clinical unit with the lead educator to address concerns and problem solve solutions, as in Option D. It would be important to discuss first with the lead educator to determine how the learning needs can be met before speaking with the nurse manager, as suggested in Option B. Options A and C would be inappropriate since the clinical unit is probably not a good match for the learning needs.

Test Blueprint: 1 B 2
Cognitive Code: Application

32. A clinical nurse educator is assigned to teach in a new clinical setting. Which action is most appropriate?
  A. Arrive 30 minutes early on the first clinical day to become familiar with the clinical unit.
  B. Contact the agency to schedule an observation experience with a staff nurse prior to the first clinical day.
  C. Develop a list of questions to ask staff during the clinical day.
  D. Review the agency's website for accreditation information.

Correct Answer: B

Rationale: The educator may become familiar with a new clinical setting by working with or observing the staff for a few days prior to returning to the site with learners, as in Option B (Oermann et al., 2018, p. 71). Options A, C, and D do not allow the clinical educator to become adequately familiar with the clinical setting prior to having learners present.

Test Blueprint: 1 B 2
Cognitive Code: Analysis

33. Which represents the most important criterion when making clinical assignments?
  A. Connection to learning outcomes
  B. Learner interest
  C. Educator expertise
  D. Learner ability

Correct Answer: A

Rationale: Each clinical activity should be an integral part of the course or educational program—it is essential that the clinical educator, learners, and staff members understand the goals of each clinical activity. Learning activities should be selected and structured so that they relate logically and sequentially to the desired outcomes (Oermann et al., 2018, p. 122). Learner interest, Option B, educator expertise, Option C, and learner ability, Option D, should be considered when selecting clinical assignments, but they are not the most important criteria.

Test Blueprint: 1 B 2
Cognitive Code: Application

34. Which is the most important consideration when selecting client assignments for learners?
  A. The types of clients on the clinical unit
  B. The availability of nurse preceptors
  C. The potential for practicing psychomotor skills
  D. The learning outcomes for the clinical experience

Correct Answer: D

Rationale: The learning outcomes should direct the learning activities and guide the placement of the learners in the clinical setting, as indicated in Option D (O'Connor, 2015). The types of clients on the unit, as in Option A, is an important consideration, but not more important than the learning outcomes of the course. There are other skills aside from psychomotor skills,

Option C, that need to be mastered by the learner. Therefore, considering the availability of psychomotor skill performance is not the most important aspect when selecting client assignments. The availability of preceptors or staff who can work with learners, as in Option B, should be considered but is not the most important factor when selecting client assignments for learners.

Test Blueprint: 1 B 2
Cognitive Code: Application

35. Which action best helps the clinical nurse educator select client assignments that are appropriate for the learners' education and skill level?
    A. Asking learners which client assignments they are most comfortable having
    B. Reviewing the organizing framework of the curriculum and clinical course objectives
    C. Avoiding assigning complicated clients to learners who are not in upper-level nursing courses
    D. Using the on-campus simulation laboratory experiences to evaluate learner abilities

Correct Answer: B

Rationale: Clinical courses are based on an organizing framework, which provides structure for the program and directs course sequencing and clinical learning experiences. Course configuration must logically build and offer learning opportunities that will enable learners to achieve outcomes (Oermann et al., 2018, p. 5). Option B indicates that the clinical nurse educator is aware that there is a structured plan for learner knowledge and guiding objectives for clinical assignments. Asking learners whom they want to care for, as in Option A, or eliminating clients based on acuity, as in Option C, are not appropriate actions. There are many factors that educators must weigh when selecting learning assignments and acuity of clients is not the only factor to consider. Additionally, individual learner abilities are also not the only factor to consider in client assignments, as in Option D; thus, this is not the best action for selecting appropriate client assignments.

Test Blueprint: 1 B 2
Cognitive Code: Application

36. A clinical nurse educator is reviewing the unit census to create a client assignment for the day. The clients are low to moderate acuity. Most of the learners have already met the objectives of the course. Which action would best challenge learners for the day?
    A. Assigning two learners to each client
    B. Assigning two clients to each learner
    C. Assigning one learner to give medications to all of the clients
    D. Assigning all learners to observational experiences off the unit

Correct Answer: B

Rationale: The client acuity level in a clinical setting affects the selection of learning opportunities for learners. Some learners may be assigned to apply their knowledge in the care of two or more relatively stable clients to develop their prioritization and time management skills (Oermann et al., 2018, p. 134). Option B best meets the needs of most learners in the group.

Option A will not challenge learners who have already met the course objectives. Option C challenges only one learner, and Option D is not appropriate because learners are observing and not participating in care delivery.

Test Blueprint: 1 B 2
Cognitive Code: Application

37. A senior-level learner has difficulty inserting a Foley catheter and is not demonstrating sterile technique despite these skills being taught in a previous course. Which is the best initial action?
    A. Assigning a short paper on how to maintain sterile technique during catheterization
    B. Failing the learner in the course for not mastering this skill
    C. Referring the learner to the nursing lab educator for coaching and practice
    D. Having the learner reflect on strengths and weaknesses in the clinical area in the learner's weekly journal

Correct Answer: C

Rationale: Options A, B, and D would not be appropriate actions because the learner needs to practice this psychomotor skill consistently over time; through skill repetition, the technique will become instinctive. The clinical nurse educator needs to allow time for remediation and coach the learner until the learner becomes proficient, as suggested by Option C (Oermann et al., 2018).

Test Blueprint: 1 B 2
Cognitive Code: Application

38. Which initial action is most appropriate when the clinical nurse educator is assigned to teach a new topic in the clinical skills laboratory?
    A. Perform extensive research on the subject.
    B. Assess personal knowledge and expertise in the subject.
    C. Review similar courses for content.
    D. Consider the use of innovative teaching methods.

Correct Answer: B

Rationale: The clinical nurse educator would first need to discern one's level of knowledge and expertise, Option B, prior to conducting research about the new subject, Option A (Popkess & Frey, 2016). Once the clinical nurse educator has done the knowledge assessment, then it may be appropriate to review similar courses, Option C, and consider teaching methods, Option D.

Test Blueprint: 1 B 2
Cognitive Code: Application

39. A clinical nurse educator is assigning clients to first-semester learners and effective client communication is the objective for the day. Which client assignment is ideal?
    A. 86-year-old female with pneumonia and stage four Alzheimer disease
    B. 60-year-old male who is four days post–hip replacement surgery
    C. 25-year-old male who is on day two of an alcohol withdrawal protocol
    D. 32-year-old female with cervical cancer and scheduled for a hysterectomy

Correct Answer: B

Rationale: The most important criterion for selection of clinical assignments is usually the desired learning outcome (Oermann et al., 2018, p. 133). Yet the learner's abilities and client's needs must be considered as well. Option B is the best client for a learner at this level in terms of learning how to communicate. Option A is a client with dementia; this assignment would pose communication challenges for beginning learners. Options C and D are clients who are in crisis and would not be appropriate for beginning learners.

Test Blueprint: 1 B 2
Cognitive Code: Application

40. In preparation for a postclinical conference, a clinical nurse educator must select one learner to present that learner's client case to the clinical group. Which selection best focuses on learning priorities and aligns with learning outcomes and the nursing curriculum?
    A. The learner who cared for a client with a rare disease who slept all day
    B. The learner who sent a client to dialysis for the entire shift
    C. The learner whose client felt dizzy and fell in front of the learner
    D. The learner whose client was constipated and needed an enema

Correct Answer: C

Rationale: Nurse educators must determine what content is critical and necessary and what information is nice to know but may not be necessary to include (Oermann et al., 2018, p. 9). Prioritizing learning that focuses on client safety is critical in clinical education. Option C presents an opportunity for learners to discuss a common threat to safety: falls. The other options, while interesting and relevant to nursing, are not the learning priority.

Test Blueprint: 1 B 2
Cognitive Code: Application

41. Which action would best help learners achieve the course objective to *effectively complete a system-focused assessment for a client with cardiac disease*?
    A. Preparing a preconference case study on cardiac assessment findings
    B. Assigning learners to care for clients who are recovering from surgery
    C. Selecting clients with cardiac disease and assisting the learners with assessments
    D. Inviting a pharmacist to a preclinical conference to discuss the pharmacokinetics of diuretics used with clients with congestive heart failure

Correct Answer: C

Rationale: Clinical nurse educators should help learners integrate classroom knowledge and expertise in clinical learning. They should provide a real-life perspective for viewing content and skills. When a nurse educator is an established expert, the educator can skillfully provide support and assist learners in meeting the course objectives (Adelman-Mullally et al., 2013, p. 31). Option C offers the best opportunity for the educator to help learners analyze findings in a complicated client and achieve the objective. Option A is repeating didactic experience, Option B does not guarantee that clients have heart disease and so may not align with the course objective, and Option D does not help learners achieve the objective.

Test Blueprint: 1 B 2
Cognitive Code: Application

42. Which is the best way to develop a simulation plan for the semester?
  A. Consider the number of learners and available simulation mannequins
  B. Ask the learners what topic interests them for simulation
  C. Conduct a needs assessment to identify the educational gap
  D. Ask the simulation lab coordinator for some recommended scenarios

Correct Answer: C

Rationale: The needs assessment, Option C, provides a foundation for the simulation experience and requires the clinical nurse educator to examine the knowledge, skills, and attitudes of learners (International Nursing Association for Clinical Simulation and Learning Standards Committee, 2016). Option A is an operational or implementational issue but is not the primary consideration for planning. Option D addresses content without regard to needs of the learners. While Option B incorporates the ideas of the learners, it may not incorporate all aspects required for planning a simulation experience and may not be congruent with the course objectives.

Test Blueprint: 1 B 2
Cognitive Code: Analysis

43. Near the end of the semester, the clinical nurse educator notes that the learners in the clinical group have met the clinical objectives for the course. Which action is most appropriate?
  A. Cancel the final clinical day so that learners can catch up on other course assignments.
  B. Ask the learners what their goals are and what they would like to experience.
  C. Send learners to the operating room or emergency department to observe.
  D. Contact the course coordinator to see what the coordinator would recommend.

Correct Answer: B

Rationale: The enrichment curriculum is used to enhance learning, individualize activities, and motivate learners. Learners who meet essential clinical activities can quickly select additional learning activities to satisfy needs for more depth (Oermann et al., 2018, p. 10). Option B takes the learners' desires into account once the objectives have been met and would provide for additional enriching learning activities. Options A and C are not appropriate as they do not provide planned learning activities. Option D is not necessary because the objectives have been met.

Test Blueprint: 1 B 3
Cognitive Code: Application

44. Which action would best assess learner goals prior to a clinical experience?
  A. Administering a preclinical experience multiple-choice quiz
  B. Requesting a checklist of completed clinical skills
  C. Asking learners to complete a self-assessment
  D. Creating an assignment that seeks learners' areas of interest

Correct Answer: C

Rationale: Self-assessment by learners is a means to evaluate learners' goals at the beginning of the learning process (Bonnel, 2016, p. 443). Option A assesses knowledge rather than goals. Option B provides a list of skills but does not address goals of the learner. Option D will provide the clinical nurse educator with interest areas but not goals of the learner for the clinical experience. Option C provides a means to assess learner's goals.

Test Blueprint: 1 B 3
Cognitive Code: Application

45. Which activity would best help learners become familiar with the nursing unit?
A. Searching for equipment used on the clinical unit
B. Introducing staff by name and title
C. Showing examples of charting with the electronic health record
D. Reviewing clinical assignments and performance expectations

Correct Answer: A

Rationale: A scavenger hunt, like the example of the equipment search suggested in Option A, helps learners locate typical items needed for client care (Oermann et al., 2018, p. 70). The learners could work in pairs to locate a list of pertinent items and become acclimated and familiar with the assigned clinical unit. Options B, C, and D are helpful for learners on the first day of the clinical experience but do not help them to become familiar with the nursing unit.

Test Blueprint: 1 B 4
Cognitive Code: Application

46. When reviewing the roles of learners, educators, and staff members during the first clinical day, which action is best?
A. Reviewing a list of permitted questions to ask staff members
B. Developing and presenting an electronic presentation outlining staff roles
C. Informing learners that staff should not be bothered during the clinical day
D. Preparing a handout summarizing clinical expectations and requirements

Correct Answer: D

Rationale: The clinical nurse educator should review the roles of learners, educators, and staff members with the learners. Handouts summarizing these expectations and requirements, as in Option D, are useful because learners can review them later when their anxiety is lower (Oermann et al., 2018, p. 71). Since learners tend to perceive the first day of the clinical experience as stressful, they may not recall the shared information; therefore, Option A is not the best approach to use for reviewing roles (Oermann et al., 2018, p. 69). Additionally, there may be other questions that learners will need to ask staff; thus, it is unrealistic to have a finite list of allowable questions that learners can ask. Option B does not allow for the learners to review the information later; therefore, given the stressful nature of the first clinical day, the learners may not recall this information if only shared orally.

Option C does not allow for the staff to be part of the clinical experience. All three groups should have interaction.

Test Blueprint: 1 B 4
Cognitive Code: Application

47. A clinical nurse educator wants to allow learners to use mobile devices to access drug information while in the clinical setting. How can the clinical nurse educator best validate the information that learners obtain from personal technology devices?
   A. Provide the learners with a list of credible applications (apps) and websites.
   B. Allow learners access to their devices only under educator supervision.
   C. Have the learners present the information to the primary nurse for approval.
   D. Assign medication administration skills to two learners each week.

   Correct Answer: A

   Rationale: Nurses in clinical practice use technological resources on mobile devices for quick access to information. Learners need to practice using this technology throughout their educational program. Clinical nurse educators can help direct learners to credible apps and websites (Oermann et al., 2018, p. 174). Option A is the only way to ensure that the information found by learners is appropriate while giving learners the space and trust to investigate and learn. Options B and C are not realistic for the clinical nurse educator and staff. Option D does not ensure the use of valid medication information.

   Test Blueprint: 1 B 4
   Cognitive Code: Application

48. A clinical nurse educator is leading a technology-based simulation scenario focused on drug administration. To help learners understand the effects of furosemide (Lasix), which action is best?
   A. Discuss the side effects of furosemide during the presimulation conference.
   B. During the simulation, lower the client's blood pressure after drug administration.
   C. Evaluate the learners' ability to assess vital signs prior to starting the simulation.
   D. Debrief the learners afterwards and ask them what they think should have happened after drug administration.

   Correct Answer: B

   Rationale: A key characteristic of a clinical nurse educator is integrating expertise and providing a real-life perspective for viewing content and skills (Adelman-Mullally et al., 2013, p. 31). Option B provides an opportunity for learners to experience the drug effects during the simulation, while the other options do not offer that "real-life" experience.

   Test Blueprint: 1 B 5
   Cognitive Code: Application

49. A learner is upset about missing an opportunity to participate in a client's wound care because the charge nurse stopped the learner in the hall and said, "I need you to go and help the nursing assistant finish the last two bed baths." Which is the clinical nurse educator's best response?
A. Tell the learner that it was the right decision to follow the charge nurse's request.
B. Ask the learner why the incident was not reported at the time of the occurrence.
C. Discuss the level of the learner and the expected outcomes with the charge nurse.
D. Tell the learner that there will be other opportunities to observe wound care.

Correct Answer: C

Rationale: Communication is one of the most important factors in building and maintaining relationships with a clinical agency and staff. Information about goals, competencies, expected outcomes, the level of learners, practice expectations, and related information, as in Option C, must be shared to enable the clinical agency staff to be able to assist with identifying appropriate learner experiences (Gubrud, 2016, p. 314). Options A and D do not ensure learning. Option B places the learner in a defensive position and may be perceived as placing blame and possibly increasing the learner's anger.

Test Blueprint: 1 B 5
Cognitive Code: Analysis

50. A clinical nurse educator is working with a learner who is a kinesthetic learner. Which learning activity best meets the learner's needs?
A. Allowing the learner to observe the clinical nurse educator preparing insulin
B. Observing the learner preparing insulin in the medication room
C. Having the learner watch a video demonstrating the insulin preparation
D. Providing the learner with a card that includes the step-by-step process for preparing insulin

Correct Answer: B

Rationale: Learners who prefer kinesthetic learning learn best by performing the action. Manipulation of the equipment and the development of motor skills helps the learner to increase understanding and proficiency (Luparell, 2015, p. 42). Options A, C, and D are activities that can be used to support learning for those individuals who prefer visual or auditory learning.

Test Blueprint: 1 B 5
Cognitive Code: Recall

51. When determining clinical assignments, the clinical nurse educator should give priority to selecting which types of clients?
A. Clients requiring the learner to complete many procedures during the clinical day
B. Clients with clinical diagnoses that are like the clients described in the corresponding theory courses
C. Clients identified as a "good client" for the learners by the clinical nursing staff
D. Clients with complex clinical diagnoses that will challenge learners' critical thinking skills

Correct Answer: B

Rationale: The clinical portion of a course should provide opportunities for learners to apply concepts that are learned in the didactic portion of a course (O'Conner, 2015). Although the clinical nurse educator should also consider clients who will provide opportunities for skill building, such as Option A, the priority is to ensure that learners have experiences that will allow them to meet course learning outcomes, as in Option B. Although nursing staff can offer valuable input when making assignments, as in Option C, they are often unfamiliar with the classroom content and would not necessarily identify clients with health problems discussed in the theory courses. Clients with complex diagnoses, as suggested in Option D, can provide valuable learning experiences but care should be taken to ensure that the client diagnoses correspond to classroom content covered. The assignment should not be based solely on client complexity.

Test Blueprint: 1 B 5
Cognitive Code: Application

52. Which statement would best guide learners in clinical practice?
    A. "Since your client is unsteady, I can assist you in ambulating your client."
    B. "I will check your charting to make sure you covered everything."
    C. "Tell me about the next steps you would take in caring for your client."
    D. "I saw you donned personal protective equipment before entering the room; that was excellent."

Correct Answer: C

Rationale: Guiding is a facilitative and supportive process that leads the learner toward achievement of the outcomes. It is a process of supporting and coaching learning. Guiding is not supervision; supervision is a process of overseeing. Effective clinical teaching requires that the clinical nurse educator guide learners in their learning, not oversee their work (Oermann et al., 2018, p. 81). Options A and B suggest tasks or care that the learner needs to complete rather than guiding the learner in determining the best course of action. Option D praises the learner's action but does not guide the learner. Only Option C allows the clinical nurse educator to guide learning.

Test Blueprint: 1 B 5
Cognitive Code: Application

53. A clinical nurse educator is planning education experiences for undergraduate learners. Which learning activity would incorporate collaboration with other health care disciplines?
    A. Interprofessional simulation
    B. Shadow experiences in the emergency department
    C. Attendance at a nurse practice council meeting
    D. Discussion forum with the chief nursing officer

Correct Answer: A

Rationale: Learning to collaborate with the many health care groups involved in client care can be a daunting task. Learners should be provided with opportunities to work as members of interprofessional teams and in practice environments where practice models are used for joint planning, implementation, and evaluation of outcomes of care. Interprofessional simulations may assist learning about the management of a variety of clients and to collaborate with other professions, as in Option A (Gubrud, 2016, p. 287). Shadowing in a department, Option B, attending a nurse council meeting, Option C, and engaging in a discussion forum with a nurse administrator, Option D, do not represent collaboration with other health care disciplines.

Test Blueprint: 1 B 6
Cognitive Code: Recall

54. Which learning activity helps learners develop interpersonal skills best?
   A. Unfolding case study regarding a difficult client
   B. Concept map regarding factors influencing communication with clients
   C. Matching assignment regarding roles of various health care professionals
   D. Simulation using standardized patients

Correct Answer: D

Rationale: Interpersonal skills involve knowledge of human behavior and social systems (Oermann et al., 2018); Option D provides learners with an active learning activity that will require learners to understand behaviors, systems, and communications, and will help them develop their interpersonal skills. Though Options A and B may be considered active learning activities (Phillips, 2016), they do not provide the learner with the best opportunities to develop their interpersonal skills. Option C is not the best representation of an active learning activity nor does it directly help develop interpersonal skills.

Test Blueprint: 1 B 6
Cognitive Code: Application

55. Which learning activity would emphasize the development of interprofessional collaboration and teamwork skills most?
   A. Asking a physician assistant to share the roles and responsibilities of that position with learners
   B. Inviting nursing assistants to participate in postclinical conference
   C. Pairing respiratory therapy and nursing learners for a clinical shift
   D. Requiring learners to shadow the charge nurse for a clinical shift

Correct Answer: C

Rationale: Option C requires learners of nursing and respiratory therapy disciplines to become a team and work together during a clinical shift, requiring them to develop their interprofessional collaboration and teamwork skills, an essential interprofessional competency according to the Interprofessional Education Collaborative (IPEC) Expert Panel (2011). Option A can help meet the interprofessional competency of understanding others' roles and responsibilities (IPEC Expert Panel, 2011), though it will not necessarily help the learners hone their collaborative and teamwork skills. Options B and D may be appropriate learning activities that could help develop collaboration and teamwork skills, though they are not interprofessional in nature since they are within the nursing discipline.

Test Blueprint: 1 B 6
Cognitive Code: Analysis

56. A clinical nurse educator assigns one learner from the clinical group to the operating room to observe the interprofessional health care team. Which question is most appropriate to assess learning related to interprofessional competencies?
A. "What are the roles of the health care professionals in the operating room?"
B. "What did you do for the client while you were in the operating room?"
C. "How did the client tolerate the operative procedure?"
D. "Did you assess the client's vital signs after anesthesia was administered?"

Correct Answer: A

Rationale: The purpose of the clinical team observation is to embed learners in already assembled teams so that they can observe how a team in action provides client-centered care (Oermann et al., 2018, p. 237). The observation of the team is important to impart to the learner prior to the activity and should be the focus of questioning afterwards; this is best exemplified in Option A. Options B, C, and D address learning about clinical skills and care activities and do not focus on the interprofessional team.

Test Blueprint: 1 B 6
Cognitive Code: Application

57. A learner participates in an interprofessional team meeting with a client and family to discuss end-of-life care. Which aspect of learning is being developed most?
A. Affective domain
B. Critical thinking
C. Psychomotor skills
D. Clinical reasoning

Correct Answer: A

Rationale: Professional nurses are expected to hold and act on certain values regarding client care, such as respect for the client's uniqueness, supporting client autonomy and right to choose, and the confidentiality of client information (Oermann et al., 2018, p. 24). End-of-life discussions are commonly client focused and outcomes depend on the values of all involved. These are the tenets of affective learning, which is Option A. Options B and D are components of the cognitive domain. Option C is a component of the psychomotor domain.

Test Blueprint: 1 B 6
Cognitive Code: Recall

58. Which learning activity helps foster critical thinking skills best?
A. Examining a client's chart for possible reasons for a drug interaction
B. Comforting a client who is experiencing a negative drug reaction
C. Administering an antidote to a client who has overdosed on a drug
D. Teaching a client about potential signs of a drug-drug interaction

Correct Answer: A

Rationale: Critical thinking is a process used to determine a course of action involving collecting appropriate data, analyzing the validity and utility of the information, evaluating multiple lines of reasoning, and coming to valid conclusions (Oermann et al., 2018, p. 20). Option A presents the learner with the opportunity to investigate and analyze what is happening to the client. Options B, C, and D are appropriate nursing interventions but are not representative of critical thinking activities.

Test Blueprint: 1 B 7
Cognitive Code: Application

59. Which activity fosters the development of critical thinking skills best?
    A. Having learners complete a chart with a list of commonly used medications on the unit
    B. Assigning learners to watch online videos based on specific client diagnoses
    C. Asking high-level care-related questions with each learner throughout the clinical day
    D. Developing a checklist for the learner to use when performing a dressing change

Correct Answer: C

Rationale: Learning to think critically requires active participation and engagement. Through interactions, such as the use of high-level Socratic questions, Option C, learners can convert information into knowledge and improve critical thinking skills (Phillips, 2016, p. 261). Options A, B, and D are teaching activities that are useful in helping learners acquire knowledge related to content; they are methods for transmitting and documenting information but do not guarantee high-level learning.

Test Blueprint: 1 B 7
Cognitive Code: Application

60. A clinical nurse educator is approached by a learner who notes that a client has a latex allergy documented in the chart but does not have any specific latex-free equipment or any other bedside indicators of latex allergy. Which action is most appropriate to encourage problem-solving abilities?
    A. Discuss the finding with the nurse manager and seek guidance about next actions to take.
    B. Instruct the learner to discuss this finding with the nurse manager and seek further direction.
    C. Praise the learner for finding the discrepancy and note it on the learner evaluation.
    D. Obtain appropriate signage for the client's bedside and call for a latex allergy cart.

Correct Answer: B

Rationale: Clinical learning activities provide rich sources of realistic practice problems to be solved (Oermann et al., 2018, p. 19). One way to strengthen problem-solving ability is to encourage interpersonal communication. Clinical learning opportunities to build collaborative relationships with other health care professionals are essential (Oermann et al., 2018, p. 22). In

Options A and D, the clinical nurse educator is solving the problem for the learner. Option C is not encouraging problem-solving. Only Option B promotes problem-solving by the learner.

Test Blueprint: 1 B 7
Cognitive Code: Application

61. Which clinical learning activity would allow a learner to demonstrate critical thinking and clinical reasoning skill best?
A. Narrative nursing note
B. Process recording
C. Nursing care plan
D. Concept map

Correct Answer: D

Rationale: Concept maps, Option D, evaluate learners' ability to document thinking processes and allow learners to create a diagram of client needs and nursing responses, including relationships among concepts. Concept maps can also evaluate learners' abilities to synthesize concepts in care of specific clients; thus, concept maps can allow learners to demonstrate clinical reasoning abilities (Bonnel, 2016, p. 450). Options A, B, and C require only lower-level cognitive skills and do not require higher-level thinking, such as critical thinking and clinical reasoning abilities. Option A assists the learners to organize collected assessment data. Option B focuses on interpersonal skills of the learner and allows for self-evaluation of communication skills. Option C does allow for learners to prioritize care needs based on an individual client; however, with the availability of numerous standardized care plans, critical thinking has been minimized. Option D allows learners to demonstrate their critical thinking and clinical reasoning as they create the concept map.

Test Blueprint: 1 B 7
Cognitive Code: Application

62. The clinical nurse educator is preparing orientation materials for preceptors. Including which information would best help preceptors assist learners to apply classroom learning to the clinical setting?
A. Contact information of the clinical educator
B. A list of expectations for the learner
C. A copy of weekly course content
D. Conflict resolution strategies

Correct Answer: C

Rationale: One disadvantage when using the preceptor model is the lack of integration of didactic learning and clinical practice (Oermann et al., 2018, p. 89). By including a copy of the weekly course content, as in Option C, the preceptor can facilitate the application of classroom information to the clinical setting. Options A, B, and D should also be included in the orientation materials but will not necessarily help assist the learner to apply classroom learning to the clinical setting.

Test Blueprint: 1 B 8
Cognitive Code: Application

63. A clinical nurse educator is teaching a preceptorship clinical course. Which task is most important for the nurse educator to complete first?
A. Clarifying educator, learner, and preceptor expectations and roles
B. Evaluating the learners compared to established clinical standards
C. Performing purposeful check-ins with the learners and the preceptors
D. Remaining accessible to all parties throughout the clinical course

Correct Answer: A

Rationale: Option A is a critical first task for educators to complete in preceptorships (Gubrud, 2016), especially since educators will not often be physically present at the clinical agency. Clarifying expectations and roles is essential to this teaching model's success. Options B, C, and D are all important tasks during preceptorship clinical courses (Gubrud, 2016); however, Option A should be completed by the nurse educator first. Clear expectations and roles will ensure that all parties know how to successfully implement the clinical course.

Test Blueprint: 1 B 8
Cognitive Code: Application

64. The clinical nurse educator is asked to discuss the dedicated education unit as a clinical teaching model. Which statement is most appropriate?
A. "The dedicated education unit is the optimal clinical experience for beginning learners."
B. "Dedicated education units require a partnership between clinical nurse educators and bedside clinicians."
C. "The dedicated education unit and traditional clinical teaching methods yield the same learning outcomes."
D. "One of the primary benefits of the dedicated education unit is the reduction in graduate nurse orientation time."

Correct Answer: B

Rationale: The dedicated education unit clinical teaching model is a strategy used to create an optimal teaching and learning environment in which staff nurses and clinical nurse educators work together in partnership to support safe learning and promote safe client care (Gaberson et al., 2015; Rusch, McCafferty, Schoening, Hercinger, & Manz, 2018). Options A, C, and D are not supported in the literature.

Test Blueprint: 1 B 8
Cognitive Code: Recall

65. Which scenario best describes a traditional model of clinical teaching?
A. A clinical educator guides learners to provide care for clients that are like those discussed in the classroom.
B. A staff nurse coaches learners when providing the shift report.
C. A staff nurse oversees learners administering medications for a jointly assigned client while the clinical nurse educator serves as a clinical coordinator.
D. A learner provides care to clients on a clinical unit the learner is assigned to throughout the nursing program.

Correct Answer: A

Rationale: In the traditional model of clinical teaching, as in Option A, the educator provides the instruction and evaluation for a small group of nursing learners and is on site during the clinical experience (Oermann et al., 2018, p. 87). Option B does not describe the traditional model of clinical teaching but more likely represents a preceptor or mentoring model. Option C describes a preceptor model of clinical teaching. Option D describes a collaborative cluster education model.

Test Blueprint: 1 B 8
Cognitive Code: Recall

66. Which scenario best describes a preceptor model of clinical education?
    A. A clinical educator guides learners to provide care for clients that are like those discussed in the classroom.
    B. Staff nurses partner with a single nursing program and work collaboratively with learners as a care delivery team.
    C. A staff nurse oversees a learner administer medications for a jointly assigned client while the clinical nurse educator serves as a clinical coordinator.
    D. A learner provides care to clients on a clinical unit the learner is assigned to throughout the nursing program.

Correct Answer: C

Rationale: In the preceptor model of clinical teaching, an expert nurse guides and supports learners and serves as a role model while clinical nurse educators serve as coordinators of the experience, often off-site during the clinical experience (Oermann et al., 2018, p. 89). Option C best describes a preceptor model of clinical teaching. Option A describes a traditional model of clinical nursing education. Option B represents a model using a dedicated education unit. Option D describes a collaborative cluster education model.

Test Blueprint: 1 B 8
Cognitive Code: Recall

67. Which scenario best describes clinical education using a dedicated education unit?
    A. A clinical educator guides learners to provide care for clients that are like those discussed in the classroom.
    B. Staff nurses partner with a single nursing program and work collaboratively with learners as a care delivery team.
    C. A staff nurse oversees a learner administer medications for a jointly assigned client while the clinical nurse educator serves as a clinical coordinator.
    D. A learner provides care to clients on a clinical unit the learner is assigned to throughout the nursing program.

Correct Answer: B

Rationale: In a model using a dedicated education unit, staff nurses, clinical nurse educators, and learners form a learning triad (Oermann et al., 2018, p. 90); Option B represents a model using a dedicated education unit. Option A describes a traditional model of clinical nursing education. Option C best describes a preceptor model of clinical teaching. Option D describes a collaborative cluster education model.

Test Blueprint: 1 B 8
Cognitive Code: Recall

68. Which activity performed during clinical orientation aligns best with Constructivist Learning Theory?
    A. Create individualized learning objectives that allow for active involvement during the clinical experience.
    B. Collaborate with peers to review charts of current clients and discuss possible interventions.
    C. Practice taking admission histories using the electronic medical record system on the unit and get feedback about performance.
    D. Reflect on prior experiences and explain what they think will be different about this unit.

Correct Answer: A

Rationale: Constructivist Learning Theory is the foundation of active learning. Learners are the leaders of their learning and the clinical nurse educator is the facilitator. As the expert, the clinical nurse educator will ultimately approve the learning outcomes; however, by making learners responsible for identifying the learning outcomes, the learners are in charge of learning (Brandon & All, 2010). Option A best represents Constructivist Learning Theory because it allows the learner to take an active role in creating the learning. Option B represents social learning concepts. Option C is the application of Behaviorist Theory. Option D, with a focus on reflection, describes cognitive learning concepts.

Test Blueprint: 1 B 9
Cognitive Code: Recall

69. Using Experiential Learning Theory, which activity would be most appropriate?
    A. Sharing common experiences to form a sense of community
    B. Allowing time to reflect on experiences and think about their observations
    C. Using new modes of learning to teach learners from diverse backgrounds
    D. Bracketing understanding of previous life experiences

Correct Answer: B

Rationale: Although learning styles vary with each learner, according to Experiential Learning Theory, new information is constantly being compared with what is known from a previous experience. How learners incorporate new knowledge and make sense of previous experiences is key to experiential learning, which is considered a requirement for adaptation and learning (Kolb & Kolb, 2005). The experiential model involves concrete experiences that serve as a basis for reflection, as in Option B. Options A, C, and D are not congruent with the experiential learning approaches since they do not involve the best active pedagogical strategies that engage the learners in constructing meaning from the experience.

Test Blueprint: 1 B 9
Cognitive Code: Analysis

70. The clinical educator states, "I noticed that you didn't check the client's blood pressure before giving the medication. That concerns me because that medication may cause a decrease in blood pressure. Can you tell me what you were thinking at that time?" Which debriefing method is demonstrated?
   A. Debriefing for Meaningful Learning
   B. Plus Delta
   C. Debriefing with Good Judgment
   D. Structured and Supported Debriefing

Correct Answer: C

Rationale: The educator is using advocacy and inquiry, which is part of the Debriefing with Good Judgment framework, Option C, for debriefing (Rudolph, Simon, Dufresne, & Raemer, 2006). Option A focuses on reflective thinking and Socratic questioning (Dreifuerst, 2012). Option B, Plus Delta, focuses on what went well and what could be better. The Structured and Supported Debriefing model, as in Option D, involves three phases of information: Gather, Analyze, and Summarize (O'Donnell et al., 2009).

Test Blueprint: 1 B 9
Cognitive Code: Recall

71. Which best demonstrates the use of Sociocultural Learning Theory in the clinical setting?
   A. Developing a skills return demonstration activity
   B. Asking learners to share their clinical experiences during postclinical conference
   C. Having learners role play a client interaction
   D. Creating a portfolio assignment documenting achievement of learning outcomes

Correct Answer: B

Rationale: Sociocultural Learning Theory allows learners to be responsible for their learning by communicating and collaborating with others. This theory includes reflection, sharing, and questioning as ways to learn from others (Candela, 2016, p. 215). Option B displays this theory best. Option A is an example of Behavioral Learning Theory that has a clear step-by-step learning experience, with behavior that can be observed and measured. Option C is an example of Social Learning Theory. Option D is an example of Adult Learning Theory.

Test Blueprint: 1 B 9
Cognitive Code: Recall

72. When suggesting course revisions based on evidence-based guidelines, which initial action is most appropriate?
   A. Discussing the new evidence-based guidelines and asking learners to share information with the classroom educator
   B. Presenting the proposed changes to the lead educator for the course
   C. Informing the learners the current content is outdated and should not be used
   D. Requesting a meeting with the nursing program director to discuss the proposed changes

Correct Answer: B

Rationale: The health care system is ever changing and this influences curriculum. Clinical teaching is performed within a curriculum that is planned and offered (Oermann et al., 2018, p. 3). While the clinical nurse educator wishes to share the suggestion for change, the means in which the suggestion is made is important. The use of a chain of command allows for the clinical nurse educator to discuss topics with the lead educator for the course, as in Option B. This should occur prior to speaking with the nursing program director, Option D. It is not appropriate for the clinical nurse educator to ask the learners to share the suggested revision with the course educator, Option A, nor is it appropriate to take the action in Option C.

Test Blueprint: 1 B 10
Cognitive Code: Application

73. In two consecutive academic terms, the clinical nurse educator finds that many learners have significant deficits in understanding a specific client disease process. Which action by the clinical educator would best address this issue?
   A. At the beginning of the term, inform learners to study the specific disease processes prior to beginning clinical learning.
   B. At the end of the course, give feedback to the nursing program director about the need for curriculum revisions.
   C. Contact the lead educator for the course to describe issues noted and create a collaborative plan to address the knowledge deficits.
   D. Provide learners with a list of resources related to the disease processes, including websites, videos, and study guides.

Correct Answer: C

Rationale: The clinical nurse educator should collaborate with the lead classroom educator to determine methods of instruction that would best meet learning objectives related to the disease process. Option C presents a strategy for collaborating in the planning and development of teaching strategies that align with learning outcomes of the classroom and clinical experiences (Oermann, De Gagne, & Phillips, 2018, p. 183). Options A, B, and D do not help identify learning needs nor create specific, collaborative educational interventions to address the issue.

Test Blueprint: 1 B 10
Cognitive Code: Analysis

74. A group of clinical nurse educators are providing a summary of learner clinical sites used during the most recent clinical rotations. Which assessment finding is most concerning?
   A. Only four learners were allowed in the pediatric unit at one time.
   B. Senior-level learners were assigned to a skilled nursing unit.
   C. The average length of stay on the cardiovascular unit was 3.5 days.
   D. Sites have medical learners on the unit at the same time.

Correct Answer: A

Rationale: Clinical placements are in high demand. Because of the increasingly specialized nature of many acute units, it is hard for learners to see the broad scope of client problems when there is a lack of diversity within the clinical setting (Gaberson & Oermann, 2007, p. 244). The limited number of learners allowed on the unit at one time, as in Option A, means that other learners may be completing an alternative activity, such as an observation experience, elsewhere. Option B is not a concern because senior-level learners can gain valuable experiences when caring for clients on a skilled nursing unit. The length of stay for clients, as in Option C, is not a concern. While there may be concerns about the medical learners performing skills and procedures of the nurse, as in Option D, these concerns should not limit the care that learners can provide. Forecasted concerns cannot be validated without more information.

Test Blueprint: 1 B 10
Cognitive Code: Analysis

75. During a postclinical conference discussion, learners refer to lecture notes and a slide presentation outlining the steps for completing a skill-based procedure. The clinical nurse educator knows that the procedure has updated evidence-based best practices. Which is the best action?
A. Notify the program administrator and report the discrepancy.
B. Contact the lead educator and discuss the changes in the literature.
C. Do nothing since the clinical nurse educator is not on the curriculum committee.
D. Tell the learners they were taught incorrect information and re-educate them immediately.

Correct Answer: B

Rationale: It is the responsibility of all educators to acknowledge current guidelines that may have changed based on new evidence. It is appropriate for the clinical nurse educator to question the information that is different from the practice standards and guidelines found in the literature (Gaberson et al., 2015). Option A is incorrect because it is important to follow the chain of command and discuss the situation with the theory educator responsible for the content. Option C implies that the clinical nurse educator does not have input into the curriculum without being on the committee. It also relegates the professional responsibility to ensure that current, safe, and competent practices are being maintained. Option D is not the best response at the current time. Changes to the content may result after the clinical nurse educator collaborates with the course educator and determines whether instructional changes are needed.

Test Blueprint: 1 B 10
Cognitive Code: Application

76. Which information should a clinical nurse educator know before authorizing learners' use of mobile devices on a clinical unit for client care?
A. Whether the unit has a firewall that may hinder access to the Internet
B. How many learners in the clinical group have social media accounts
C. Whether clients have granted permission for photographs to be taken
D. The nursing program policies for electronic device use

Correct Answer: D

Rationale: Technology misuse can have serious consequences for learners and clients. Nursing programs should develop and enforce specific policies regarding the use of electronic devices and social media (Oermann et al., 2018, p. 109). This is an ethical issue and clinical nurse educators must understand the guidelines prior to allowing mobile devices in the clinical setting. It is important for the educator to know nursing policies so that learner use of mobile devices in the client care area adheres to those policies, as suggested in Option D. Option A is a later consideration. Options B and C are not relevant since social media and client photographs should not be used.

Test Blueprint: 1 C 1
Cognitive Code: Application

77. Which statement is true regarding the Americans with Disabilities Act and nursing education?
    A. Learners with a disability are evaluated using different performance criteria than other learners.
    B. The clinical nurse educator is responsible for identifying accommodations needed for a learner with a disability.
    C. A nursing program must provide needed accommodations for a learner with a disability regardless of the cost.
    D. A learner with a disability must be able to perform all essential functions in the nursing role.

Correct Answer: D

Rationale: Learners must self-disclose disabilities and formally request needed accommodations under the Americans with Disabilities Act (ADA). Reasonable accommodations are required for the known disability of the learner and should be offered within the context of the program's resources (United States Equal Employment Opportunity Commission, 2008). However, learners must still be able to perform all essential functions of the nursing role and should be evaluated with the same performance criteria, making Option A incorrect (Southern Regional Education Board, n.d.). It is not the clinical nurse educator's responsibility to identify needed accommodations, as in Option B. Accommodations must be reasonable and may vary with size and resources available at the institution (Southern Regional Education Board, n.d.), thus making Option C incorrect.

Test Blueprint: 1 C 1
Cognitive Code: Application

78. Which is the primary reason for the clinical nurse educator to address ethical behavior in the nursing program of study?
    A. Ensuring client safety
    B. Preserving the image of the profession
    C. Facilitating all domains of learning
    D. Maintaining control of the clinical learning environment

Correct Answer: A

Rationale: Options B, C, and D are important; however, the clinical nurse educator ultimately has the responsibility to provide for client safety, thus making Option A the correct response. With recent literature suggesting that incivility in the workplace jeopardizes safety, it is important for the nurse educator to convey and model appropriate relationship skills between professionals for positive client outcomes (Houck & Colbert, 2017).

Test Blueprint: 1 C 1
Cognitive Code: Analysis

79. Which statement made by a clinical nurse educator likely warrants correction?
   A. "I am not liable because I selected learning activities aligned with this week's objectives."
   B. "Since I provided competent guidance, I am not liable."
   C. "The learner practiced the prerequisite skill in the skills laboratory, so I am not liable."
   D. "I am liable because the learner practiced under my license."

Correct Answer: D

Rationale: Clinical nurse educators should be familiar with the National Council of State Boards of Nursing Model Nurse Practice Act (2014). As such, educators are not liable for negligent acts performed by learners if they select appropriate learning activities based on objectives, Option A, learners have prerequisite knowledge skills and attitudes, Option C, and provided competent guidance, Option B (Oermann et al., 2018, pp. 110–111). Option D warrants correction because learners are liable for their own actions if they provide usual standard of care for their education and experience and seek guidance as needed (Oermann et al., 2018, p. 110).

Test Blueprint: 1 C 1
Cognitive Code: Analysis

80. A learner has accommodations for a vision deficit and demonstrates difficulty preparing medication in a syringe. Which action by the clinical nurse educator would likely pose a legal concern?
   A. Providing the learner with a magnifying glass to better see the syringe markings
   B. Asking the learner questions about how to give the medication to the client
   C. Asking disabilities services for a written copy of the recommended clinical accommodations
   D. Asking the course coordinator whether the learner has accommodations

Correct Answer: A

Rationale: Clinical nurse educators should not attempt to determine whether an accommodation is indicated, nor should they decide on the specific type of accommodation necessary (Oermann et al., 2018, p. 107). Options C and D both comply with the federal laws: the Americans with Disabilities Act (ADA) of 1990 and the ADA Amendment Act of 2008. Option B would be an appropriate question to ask any learner who is preparing medications. Only the disabilities service officer determines qualification of a disability and issues a written, formal description of the required clinical accommodations. Therefore, Option A poses a legal concern because the educator should not be making the assessment for specific accommodations nor deciding what accommodations are appropriate.

Test Blueprint: 1 C 1
Cognitive Code: Analysis

81. Which likely poses a legal concern?
   A. Keeping in confidence learner-disclosed personal information
   B. Removing learner identification from clinical folders that are used for learner records
   C. Discussing a learner's area of weakness with the next-semester clinical nurse educator
   D. Storing learner evaluations in a locked file in the campus office

Correct Answer: C

Rationale: Informing other educators about an individual learner's strengths or weaknesses, Option C, may provide prejudicial information and could be interpreted as unjust and violate the learner's right to privacy (Christensen, 2016, p. 39). Educators should not share personal or private information disclosed by a learner, as suggested in Option A, unless there is a compelling professional purpose or safety concern (Christensen, 2016, p. 39). Learner identification numbers and social security numbers should not be available to others in a public setting; removing the identifications, as suggested in Option B, would be an appropriate action. Learner records and evaluation notes must also be securely stored to protect learner privacy; thus, Option D is not a legal concern.

Test Blueprint: 1 C 1
Cognitive Code: Analysis

82. A new clinical nurse educator is upset after hearing that a learner performed a procedure without the required supervision of the clinical nurse educator or a licensed nurse. Which statement made by the new educator warrants follow-up?
   A. "The learner is liable for his/her own behaviors and decisions."
   B. "I sent the learner off the unit as soon as I heard about the situation."
   C. "There will likely be disciplinary action for failure to follow the rules."
   D. "I am going to be in trouble because the learner is practicing under my license."

Correct Answer: D

Rationale: Learners are liable for their own actions if they are performing according to the usual standard of care for their education and experience. It is not true that learners practice under the educator's license, as in Option D. Clinical nurse educators are not liable for acts performed by their learners if appropriate learning activities have been selected; learners have the knowledge, skills, and attitudes to complete the care; and competent guidance is provided by the clinical nurse educator (Gaberson & Oermann, 2007, p. 85). Options A, B, and C are correct statements and thus do not warrant follow-up. The learner should be removed from the situation until the situation can be reviewed based on agency and program policies. It is possible that there will be consequences for failure to follow the rules.

Test Blueprint: 1 C 1
Cognitive Code: Application

83. A clinical nurse educator is discussing professional nursing ethics with a learner. Which statement made by the learner likely indicates the need for further teaching?
    A. "I should assess a client's pain level before determining which dose of as-needed medication to administer."
    B. "I will ask the client if they would like family members to stay in the room when completing my assessment."
    C. "I am required to withhold cardiopulmonary resuscitation (CPR) for a client with a Do Not Resuscitate (DNR) order."
    D. "I did not assess the client's vital signs at the time they were ordered because the client was sleeping."

Correct Answer: D

Rationale: Deontology uses rules, rather than consequences, to determine whether something is right or wrong. Deontology includes taking or omitting actions based on moral significance (O'Connor, 2015, p. 401). Option D suggests that the learner decided not to follow the physician's orders to obtain the client's vital signs at a designated time. The learner believed that allowing the client to sleep was the "right" decision. Options A, B, and C would not result in an ethical dilemma.

Test Blueprint: 1 C 1
Cognitive Code: Application

84. Which action by the clinical nurse educator would be an ethical concern?
    A. Asking client permission before assigning a learner to provide care for the day
    B. Allowing the learner to catheterize the client even after repeated unsuccessful attempts
    C. Allowing the learner to obtain vital signs despite it taking twenty minutes to complete
    D. Suggesting that the learner use guided imagery as a nonpharmacological pain management strategy

Correct Answer: B

Rationale: The clinical nurse educator is responsible for ensuring that learning activities do not prevent achievement of service goals (Oermann et al., 2018, p. 100). Option B is the response that raises ethical concerns because repeated attempts at catheterization would cause risk to the client and unnecessarily increase operational expenses. Options A, C, and D do not present an ethical concern. The clinical nurse educator would respect client rights by asking permission to assign a learner in Option A, thereby upholding the ethical principle related to client autonomy. Option C, although not efficient delivery of care, does not pose an ethical concern. Option D is acceptable nursing practice and does not raise an ethical concern. The use of guided imagery considers client integrity and allows client care choices.

Test Blueprint: 1 C 1
Cognitive Code: Analysis

85. Which statement made by the clinical nurse educator would be appropriate to share with the clinical nurse educator teaching in the next semester?

A. "The learner has clinical experience working with continuous intravenous infusions, but not with intravenous push medications."

B. "The learner does not seek new learning opportunities as much as a senior learner should."

C. "The learner likes to talk a lot, but I guess his/her clients like that about him/her, so I haven't mentioned anything in his/her evaluation."

D. "I personally think the learner will make an excellent nurse and I see no problems with their performance thus far."

Correct Answer: A

Rationale: When sharing information about learners, clinical nurse educators should focus on factual statements about performance without adding personal judgments. Characterizing or labeling learners is rarely helpful, and such behavior violates ethical standards of privacy as well as respect for persons (Oermann et al., 2018, pp. 102–103). Options B, C, and D include the educator's personal opinion or bias. Only Option A presents factual information about learner performance.

Test Blueprint: 1 C 1
Cognitive Code: Analysis

86. Which action is unnecessary for the clinical nurse educator to do to avoid liability for negligent acts committed by a learner?

A. Having the charge nurse review and approve the client assignments

B. Ensuring that the learners have adequate supervision during client care

C. Providing client assignments that are consistent with the learning outcomes for the course

D. Assigning clients that are congruent with learner individual ability and level in the program

Correct Answer: A

Rationale: The clinical nurse educator should inform the staff which clients have been assigned to a learner; however, the charge nurse does not assume liability for the learners. If the clinical nurse educator provides adequate supervision, as in Option B, assigns clients that meet the learning outcomes of the course, as in Option C, and ensures that the individual learner has the skills and knowledge needed to care for the clients assigned, as in Option D, the clinical nurse educator is not liable for a learner's negligence (Oermann et al., 2018, p. 257).

Test Blueprint: 1 C 1
Cognitive Code: Application

87. The semester before graduate learners complete their advanced nursing practicum experience, a clinical nurse educator meets with learners to discuss the prior clinical experiences, as well as their current and future goals. Which best describes the purpose of gathering this information?
A. Determining whether the learner is in the correct graduate program
B. Identifying a clinical site placement, preceptor, and developing individualized goals
C. Ascertaining whether the learner is adequately prepared to complete the practicum experience
D. Deciding how the learner will be evaluated in the graduate course

Correct Answer: B

Rationale: Assessing learner abilities and needs prior to clinical learning experiences, such as a graduate-level practicum course, is important to helping ensure that learning outcomes are achieved (Shellenbarger, 2019). This assessment may be especially important in courses in which learners will have highly individualized experiences away from educators, such as those completing a mentored practicum experience. By discussing prior experiences and goals, Option B, the clinical nurse educator can identify the most appropriate placement and preceptor and begin to help learners identify goals for the experience. Creation of learning contracts, for example, often includes learner-created goals and objectives and are a good way to individualize learner experiences (Oermann & Gaberson, 2017). Options A and C do not represent the purpose of this meeting and likely do not support learner success. Option D is likely not the purpose of this meeting because, typically, although there might be some flexibility in exactly how and when assignments are completed, standard evaluations are also usually present (Oermann & Gaberson, 2017).

Test Blueprint: 1 C 2
Cognitive Code: Application

88. Which initial step by the clinical nurse educator is most appropriate when working with learners who are completing their community health clinical experience as part of their RN-BS/BSN program?
A. Assessing prior clinical experiences and learner goals
B. Delivering course materials to administrators and preceptors
C. Reviewing evaluation and grading criteria with learners
D. Discussing learner preferences for assignments with preceptors

Correct Answer: A

Rationale: Assessing learner abilities and needs prior to clinical learning, such as in this RN-BS/BSN community health clinical experience, is important to help ensure that learning outcomes are achieved (Shellenbarger, 2019). Since the educator is working with licensed nurses with previous experience, an appropriate initial step in preparing for the experience is to understand learner's prior experiences and goals for the rotation, as in Option A; this will help the achievement of learning outcomes. The other options may also be important and appropriate steps, but they are not the most appropriate initial step in preparing for the experience.

Test Blueprint: 1 C 2
Cognitive Code: Application

89. A novice clinical nurse educator teaching in a religious-based sectarian institution asks for feedback regarding the nurse educator's planned clinical learning activities. Which learning activity is likely the least appropriate?
   A. Developing a teaching plan outlining various birth control measures for teenage clients
   B. Requiring volunteer hours with homeless families during a community health experience
   C. Completing reflection journals during an international learning experience in China
   D. Allowing learners to pray with clients prior to surgery

Correct Answer: A

Rationale: In addition to providing active learning activities that promote learner engagement and higher-level thinking skills (Phillips, 2016), activities should also support the mission, goals, and values of the academic institution and the clinical agency (Shellenbarger, 2019). Option A is probably not appropriate because clinical nursing education should align with the mission, goals, and values of the academic institution and clinical agency. Given that this is a religious-based sectarian school, Option A may present a conflict with school beliefs. Options B, C, and D are all appropriate learning activities that likely support the academic institution and the clinical agency; thus, these are not the correct responses.

Test Blueprint: 1 C 3
Cognitive Code: Application

90. A nursing program does not permit learners to perform skills that involve central venous access devices. A clinical nurse educator hears a staff nurse telling a learner to flush a central venous line. Which response is most appropriate?
   A. "The learner can flush the central venous line, but only under my direct supervision."
   B. "That's a great learning opportunity for the learner, so please observe the learner for me."
   C. "The learner is not allowed to perform skills that include central venous access devices, but they may observe you."
   D. "I already informed you that the learners cannot perform that skill. Why are you asking them to do this skill?"

Correct Answer: C

Rationale: Clinical nurse educators must follow program policies, procedures, and practices. It is also necessary for the clinical nurse educator to build relationships with agency personnel. In this situation, the clinical nurse educator needs to have follow-up communication with the staff nurse to discuss program policies related to the care of central venous access devices, as in Option C (Gubrud, 2016, p. 285). Options A and B indicate that the clinical nurse educator is not following program policy. Option D does not demonstrate effective and professional communication with the staff nurse.

Test Blueprint: 1 C 4
Cognitive Code: Analysis

91. Which action by the clinical educator best enhances communication about clinical learning activities with nursing staff?
  A. Providing a handout to staff nurses that includes learning goals and expectations
  B. Sending an electronic copy of the course syllabus and clinical objectives to the nurse manager
  C. Posting a list of assignments and activities for the clinical day at the nursing station
  D. Telling learners to inform staff of the focus of the clinical experience

Correct Answer: A

Rationale: Details of the clinical learning activity, including when learners will be there, what their learning goals are, what they are expected to do, and how they can participate, as in Option A, must be communicated with staff (Oermann et al., 2018, p. 48). Option B provides information to the nurse manager but does not ensure dissemination of information with staff. While Option C includes learner activities for the day, it does not include learning goals and staff participation. Option D places the responsibility on the learners to communicate with staff rather than the clinical nurse educator directly communicating with the staff; this option may lead to miscommunication.

Test Blueprint: 1 C 4
Cognitive Code: Analysis

92. Which initial action should the clinical nurse educator take after receiving a call that a learner has an expired cardiopulmonary resuscitation (CPR) certification?
  A. Negotiate for the learner to finish the clinical day in simulation.
  B. Clarify the program and agency policy for learner requirements for clinical experiences.
  C. Allow the learner to participate in clinical experiences but only performing nurse assistant tasks.
  D. Send the learner to the postclinical conference room to watch clinical videos.

Correct Answer: B

Rationale: Learners and clinical nurse educators are required to follow program and clinical agency policies. When the violation is identified, proper intervention is required. Notification of the lack of a CPR certification will result in an investigation to determine an appropriate action based on program and agency policies (Bonnel, 2016, p. 459). Options A, C, and D are not the best initial responses to the current situation, as they may violate program and agency policy requirements.

Test Blueprint: 1 C 5
Cognitive Code: Application

93. A learner made a medication error by administering a medication via the wrong route. Which is the best response?

A. Document the error in the client's medical record and report it to the primary nurse.

B. Report the error to the unit nurse manager and document the error in the learner's evaluation.

C. Report the error to the primary nurse and physician and complete an incident report.

D. Report the error to the dean of nursing, primary nurse, and client's physician.

Correct Answer: C

Rationale: Countless efforts have been made to prevent medical errors from occurring; however, errors still occur. If an error occurs, it is important to teach learners to be honest and admit the error to both the clinical nurse educator and agency personnel so that interventions can be implemented to ensure client safety following the incident (Oermann et al., 2018, p. 28). Health care agencies have internal reporting systems for errors for quality improvement. Learners should not be punished for their mistakes, because it creates a culture of dishonesty. The goal is to learn from the mistakes and prevent them from happening in the future (Oermann et al., 2018, p. 28). Option C is correct because the other health care providers need to be informed of the error and an incident report needs to be completed. It is not a priority to notify the dean of nursing, as suggested in Option D. The error should be reported to the primary nurse and not the nurse manager, as suggested in Option B. The medication error should not be listed as an error on the client's medical record, as suggested in Option A; rather, an incident report should be completed.

Test Blueprint: 1 C 6
Cognitive Code: Application

94. A clinical nurse educator is observing a learner who is incorrectly setting up a sterile field. When the clinical nurse educator corrects and instructs the learner to start over, the learner states: "That is not the way the primary nurse showed me how to do it last week." Which is the best response?

A. "That is wrong. Set the field up the way I taught you and I will speak to the nurse."

B. "Continue the way you were doing it and we will look it up in your textbook after."

C. "Let's go together and review this procedure in the agency policy and procedure manual."

D. "Go look up the procedure in your textbook while I set up the sterile field in the meantime."

Correct Answer: C

Rationale: Learners often imitate the behaviors they observe, including omitting steps that the educator may believe are important to produce safe, effective outcomes. The educator should encourage learners to discuss the differences in practice habits, evaluate them in terms of evidence for practice, and identify more positive role models (Oermann et al., 2018, p. 28). Option C is guiding the learner to find evidence and consult agency policy without causing potential conflict with the primary nurse, as in Option A, harming the client, as in Option B, or doing the skill for the learner, as in Option D.

Test Blueprint: 1 C 6
Cognitive Code: Application

95. A learner has completed the 1100 vital signs and finger stick blood sugars. It is time for the clinical group to go to lunch. The learner reports that the results have not been entered because the computers were occupied. Which action by the clinical nurse educator is most appropriate?
   A. Send the other learners to the conference room to wait for the learner.
   B. Send the others to lunch and wait with the learner until a computer is available.
   C. Allow the learner to give the results to the nursing assistant who is currently on the computer.
   D. Tell the learner results can be entered as soon as the group returns from lunch.

Correct Answer: B

Rationale: The learner is responsible for documenting client assessment results in the medical record. Learners are being socialized to the role of a nurse through the acquisition of knowledge, behaviors, and values. It is the obligation of the clinical nurse educator to ensure that the documentation has been completed (Gaberson & Oermann, 2007, p. 52). It would be inappropriate to delay the lunch break for the other learners, as in Option A. It would not be appropriate to ask the nursing assistant to document the results, as in Option C. Option D delays data entry and may pose a care risk for the client, particularly if the results are abnormal.

Test Blueprint: 1 C 6
Cognitive Code: Analysis

96. Which learner behavior demonstrates academic dishonesty that should be addressed by the clinical nurse educator?
   A. Suggesting reference sources to another learner who is struggling with an assignment
   B. Paraphrasing and citing a source in a written clinical assignment
   C. Asking a nurse for assistance calculating a medication dose, but claiming to have done the calculation alone to the clinical nurse educator
   D. Recognizing an error in charting and seeking the clinical nurse educator's assistance in correcting the error

Correct Answer: C

Rationale: Examples of academic dishonesty include cheating, lying, and plagiarizing work. Asking for a staff member's assistance and then lying about it is a form of academic dishonesty, as in Option C (Oermann et al., 2018, p. 103). Suggesting sources to another learner, as in Option A, is helpful and not dishonest. Paraphrasing and citing sources, as in Option B, is an appropriate academic action and represents ethical behavior. Honestly admitting an error is not being dishonest, making Option D an appropriate ethical behavior.

Test Blueprint: 1 C 6
Cognitive Code: Recall

97. Which would likely be an ethical concern?
  A. Making learning objectives clear for staff and clients
  B. Befriending a learner on a personal social media account
  C. Developing policies related to uncivil behavior in the clinical setting
  D. Avoiding personal and social relationships with learners

Correct Answer: B

Rationale: Befriending learners on personal social media networking sites raises boundary issues (Oermann et al., 2018, p. 102). Option B is the correct choice since the use of social media may pose possible ethical concerns. It is essential for the clinical nurse educator to ensure that the learning objectives are clear to all parties involved, as suggested in Option A (Oermann et al., 2018, p. 100). Option C suggests that educators must establish clear policies related to incivility; this does not raise ethical concerns (Oermann et al., 2018, p. 101). Relationships with learners can be warm, friendly, and collegial without being social or personal in nature, as suggested by Option D; thus, this option does not raise an ethical concern (Oermann et al., 2018, p. 102).

Test Blueprint: 1 C 7
Cognitive Code: Analysis

References

Adelman-Mullally, T., Mulder, C. K., McCarter-Spalding, D. E., Hagler, D. A., Gaberson, K. B., Hanner, M. B., ... Young, P. K. (2013). The clinical nurse educator as leader. *Nurse Education in Practice*, 13(1), 29–34. doi:10.1016/j.nepr.2012.07.006

Akram, A. S., Mohamad, A., & Akram, S. (2018). The role of clinical instructor in bridging the gap between theory and practice in nursing education. *International Journal of Caring Sciences*, 11(2), 876–882.

Alexander, G. R. (2016). Multicultural education in nursing. In D. M. Billings & J. A. Halstead (Eds.), *Teaching in nursing: A guide for faculty* (5th ed., pp. 263–281). St. Louis, MO: Elsevier.

Bauce, K., Kridli, S. A., & Fitzpatrick, J. J. (2014). Cultural competence and psychological empowerment among acute care nurses. *Online Journal of Cultural Competence in Nursing and Healthcare*, 4(2), 27–38. doi:10.9730/ojccnh.org/v4n2a3

Bonnel, W. (2016). Clinical performance evaluation. In D. M. Billings & J. A. Halstead (Eds.), *Teaching in nursing: A guide for faculty* (5th ed., 443–462). St. Louis, MO: Elsevier.

Brandon, A., & All, A. (2010). Constructivism theory analysis and application to curricula. *Nursing Education Perspectives*, 31(2), 89–92.

Candela, L. (2016). Theoretical foundations of teaching and learning. In D. M. Billings & J. A. Halstead (Eds.), *Teaching in nursing: A guide for faculty* (5th ed., pp. 211–229). St. Louis, MO: Elsevier.

Christensen, L. S. (2016). The academic performance of students: Legal and ethical issues. In D. M. Billings & J. A. Halstead (Eds.), *Teaching in nursing: A guide for faculty* (5th ed., pp. 35–54). St. Louis, MO: Elsevier.

Dreifuerst, K. T. (2012). Using debriefing for meaningful learning to foster development of clinical reasoning in simulation. *Journal of Nursing Education*, 51(6), 326–333. doi:10.3928/01484834-20120409-02

Gaberson, K. B., & Oermann, M. H. (2007). *Clinical teaching strategies in nursing* (2nd ed.). New York, NY: Springer.

Gaberson, K. B., Oermann, M. H., & Shellenbarger, T. (2015). *Clinical teaching strategies in nursing* (4th ed.). New York, NY: Springer.

Gubrud, P. (2016). Teaching in the clinical setting. In D. M. Billings & J. A. Halstead (Eds.). *Teaching in nursing: A guide for faculty* (5th ed., pp. 282–303). St. Louis, MO: Elsevier.

Heise, B. A., & Gilpin, L. C. (2016). Nursing students' clinical experience with death: A pilot study. *Nursing Education Perspectives*, 37(2), 104–106.

Houck, N. M., & Colbert, A. M. (2017). Patient safety and workplace bullying: An integrative review. *Journal of Nursing Care Quality*, 32(2), 164–171.

International Nursing Association for Clinical Simulation and Learning Standards Committee (2016). INACSL standards of best practice: Simulation^SM simulation design. *Clinical Simulation in Nursing*, 12, S5–S12. doi:10.1016/j.ecns.2016.09.005

Interprofessional Education Collaborative Expert Panel. (2011). *Core competencies for interprofessional collaborative practice: Report of an expert panel*. Washington, DC: Interprofessional Education Collaborative. Retrieved from https://www.aacom.org/docs/default-source/insideome/ccrpt05-10-11.pdf?sfvrsn=77937f97_2

Kolb, A. Y., & Kolb, D. A. (2005). Learning styles and learning spaces: Enhancing experiential learning in higher education. *Academy of Management Learning & Education*, 4(2), 193–212.

Luparell, S. (2015). Facilitate learner development and socialization. In L. Caputi (Ed.), *NLN certified nurse educator review book: The official NLN guide to the CNE exam.* Washington, DC: National League of Nursing.

National Council of State Boards of Nursing Model Nurse Practice Act (2014). *NCSBN model act.* Retrieved from https://www.ncsbn.org/3867.htm

O'Connor, A. (2015). *Clinical instruction and evaluation: A teaching resource.* (3rd ed.). Burlington, MA: Jones and Bartlett.

O'Donnell, J., Rodgers, D., Lee, W., Edelson, D., Haag, J., Hamilton, M., … Meeks, R. (2009). *Structured and supported debriefing.* Dallas, TX: American Heart Association.

Oermann, M. H. (1997). Evaluating critical thinking in clinical practice. *Nurse Educator, 22*(5), 25–28.

Oermann, M., De Gagne, J. C., & Phillips, B. C. (2018). *Teaching in nursing and role of the educator: The complete guide to best practice in teaching, evaluation, and curriculum development* (2nd ed.). New York, NY: Springer.

Oermann, M. H., & Gaberson, K. B. (2009). *Evaluation and testing in nursing education* (3rd ed). New York, NY: Springer.

Oermann, M. H., & Gaberson, K. B. (2017). *Evaluation and testing in nursing education* (5th ed.). New York, NY: Springer.

Oermann, M. H., Shellenbarger, T., & Gaberson, K. B. (2018). *Clinical teaching strategies in nursing* (5th ed.). New York, NY: Springer.

Paul, R., & Elder, L. (2008). Critical thinking: The art of Socratic questioning, part III. *Journal of Developmental Education, 31*(3), 34–35.

Phillips, J. M. (2016). Strategies to promote student engagement and active learning. In D. M. Billings & J. A. Halstead (Eds.), *Teaching in nursing: A guide for faculty* (5th ed., pp. 245–262). St. Louis, MO: Elsevier.

Popkess, A. M., & Frey, J. L. (2016). Strategies to support diverse learning needs of students. In D. M. Billings & J. A. Halstead (Eds.), *Teaching in nursing: A guide for faculty* (5th ed., pp. 15–34). St. Louis, MO: Elsevier.

Rudolph, J. W., Simon, R., Dufresne, R. L., & Raemer, D. B. (2006). There's no such thing as "nonjudgmental" debriefing: A theory and method for debriefing with good judgment. *Simulation in Healthcare: The Journal of the Society for Medical Simulation, 1*(1), 49–55.

Rusch, L. M., McCafferty, K., Schoening, A. M., Hercinger, M., & Manz, J. (2018). Impact of the dedicated education unit teaching model on the perceived competencies and professional attributes of nursing students. *Nurse Education in Practice, 33,* 90–93.

Shellenbarger, T. (2019). Function within the education and health care environments. In T. Shellenbarger (Ed.), *Clinical nurse educator competencies: Creating an evidence-based practice for academic clinical nurse educators.* Washington, DC: National League for Nursing.

Southern Regional Education Board. (n.d.). *The Americans with Disabilities Act: Implications for nursing education.* Retrieved from https://www.sreb.org/publication/americans-disabilities-act

United States Equal Employment Opportunity Commission. (2008). *Facts about the Americans with Disabilities Act.* Retrieved from http://www.eeoc.gov/facts/fs-ada.html

4

Facilitate Learning in the Health Care Environment

1. The clinical nurse educator plans to use peer learning as a teaching strategy during postclinical conference to review evidence-based nursing care when managing an indwelling urinary catheter. Which statement best describes how to implement peer learning?

   A. "Separate into two groups. Each group will make a list of evidence-based nursing actions to reduce catheter-associated urinary tract infections. Each correct response gets one point. The group with the most points wins."

   B. "In groups of two or three learners, talk together for the next five minutes to create a list of evidence-based nursing actions to reduce catheter-associated urinary tract infections."

   C. "Since you have pre-read the chapter in the course textbook about indwelling urinary catheters before coming to the clinical site today, each of you will tell the group one thing you learned."

   D. "On a piece of paper, each of you will diagram the different factors leading to catheter-associated urinary tract infections as well as preventive nursing actions."

Correct Answer: B

Rationale: Peer learning is a reciprocal learning activity whereby learners in small groups share mutually beneficial knowledge, ideas, and experiences (Phillips, 2016). Option B represents peer learning since learners are sharing their knowledge with each other. Option A describes team-based learning with a gaming approach. Option C demonstrates a flipped classroom model. Option D describes a solitary concept mapping strategy. Although Options A, C, and D are appropriate teaching-learning strategies, they are not the best representation of peer learning.

Test Blueprint: 2 A
Cognitive Code: Application

2. During a clinical conference, a learner verbalized frustration and disapproval when discussing the client's history of illicit drug use. Which learning activity would best facilitate development of the learner's self-awareness while connecting the clinical experience to an affective learning outcome?
   A. Reflective journaling
   B. Reading assignments
   C. Skill demonstration
   D. Portfolio

Correct Answer: A

Rationale: Option A is correct because the affective domain relates to the development of values, attitudes, and beliefs consistent with standards of professional nursing practice (Oermann & Gaberson, 2017). Through reflection, learners detail personal learning experiences and connect them to learning outcomes (Phillips, 2016). Learners can discover their own beliefs and values when writing. The other learning activities found in Options B, C, and D would not be the best learning activity since they do not require consideration of self-awareness.

Test Blueprint: 2 A
Cognitive Code: Analysis

3. A clinical nurse educator is organizing a service learning experience. Which is the most appropriate initial action to help design this experience?
   A. Planning time for learner reflections of the experience through individual or group work
   B. Developing a list of community settings and agencies appropriate for the learning experience
   C. Allowing learners to turn in documentation of volunteer hours in lieu of participating in the learning experience
   D. Interacting with members of the community to evaluate outcomes of the learning experience

Correct Answer: B

Rationale: To prepare for any clinical experience, the educator needs to do some preparatory work, such as developing a list of community settings and agencies that would be appropriate for this learning experience, as in Option B. Option A could be a valuable part of formative evaluations (Oermann & Gaberson, 2017) but is not the most appropriate initial action. Option C is inappropriate because volunteer hours are different from service learning; service learning experiences allow learners to gain a deeper understanding of course content, citizenship, and the nursing profession (Oermann, Shellenbarger, & Gaberson, 2018, pp. 159–161). Volunteer hours are thus not an appropriate substitute for this experience. Option D may be an important evaluation action (Oermann & Gaberson, 2017) but is not the most appropriate initial action.

Test Blueprint: 2 A
Cognitive Code: Application

4. Which action would best prepare a learner to give an end-of-shift report to an oncoming nurse?
   A. Encouraging the learner to observe a nurse give an end-of shift report
   B. Providing an opportunity for the learner to practice giving an end-of-shift report during clinical conference time
   C. Allowing the learner to practice giving an end-of-shift report and providing performance feedback
   D. Showing a video during post-conference to prepare the learner to give an end-of-shift report the next clinical learning day

Correct Answer: C

Rationale: The clinical nurse educator can provide opportunities to enhance learners' ability to communicate to other health care professionals. These opportunities can reinforce the learners' communication skills and they will receive feedback in a supportive environment to develop their skills (Johnson & Blakely, 2019). Feedback and reflection can allow learners to expand and develop their skills while recognizing their limits and challenges. Options A, B, and D, while helpful, do not incorporate learning, practice, and feedback opportunities that can enhance learner performance.

Test Blueprint: 2 A
Cognitive Code: Application

5. During a clinical conference, the clinical nurse educator demonstrates the proper way to give an end-of-shift report to learners. Then, the clinical nurse educator provides a client scenario to each learner, affording the opportunity to practice reporting skills with another learner. Which action is most appropriate next?
   A. Listening to each practice session and then providing performance feedback
   B. Encouraging learners to discuss their feelings in a postclinical experience journal
   C. Allowing learners to practice and responding to questions at the end of the practice session
   D. Reinforcing the importance of paying attention to the clinical nurse educator's expectations

Correct Answer: A

Rationale: By listening to each group of learners, the clinical nurse educator is gaining an opportunity to listen to learners' questions, needs, and concerns in a nonthreatening way and offering immediate feedback; Option A promotes learning from classmates and can allow for the learner to practice and receive feedback about performance. It may also help learners identify what client information is vital in the end-of-shift report (Johnson & Blakely, 2019). Option B focuses only on feelings about the experience and is inadequate for skill development. Option C allows for practice but does not provide learners with feedback that can help improve performance. Option D focuses only on the clinical nurse educator's expectations and not on enhancing skill development.

Test Blueprint: 2 A
Cognitive Code: Analysis

6. Which environment would be most appropriate for holding a clinical conference discussion at the end of the clinical day?
   A. Nurses lounge on the unit
   B. Round table in the corner of the cafeteria
   C. Large conference room with seats arranged in rows like a classroom
   D. Room with chairs arranged in a semi-circle or U shape

Correct Answer: D

Rationale: Face-to-face discussions are often conducted during clinical conferences. A room structured in a semi-circle or U shaped format best facilitates discussion among the group members, as it allows for face-to-face conversations. Option A is not appropriate to promote discussion, as there may be interruptions and distractions. Additionally, learners may not feel free to discuss their experiences in a public area such as the nurses lounge. The seating arrangement in Option C does not facilitate group discussion. Option B is not appropriate as confidential information could be heard in a public setting such as the cafeteria (Gardner & Suplee, 2010).

Test Blueprint: 2 A
Cognitive Code: Application

7. A new clinical nurse educator is being mentored by a colleague. Which observed behavior performed during a postclinical conference should be addressed by the colleague?
   A. Asking learners to openly share one area they would like to improve
   B. Requesting that learners provide constructive peer feedback to one another
   C. Providing learners time to analyze the clinical experiences that occurred that day
   D. Presenting learners new content outside what was presented in the classroom

Correct Answer: D

Rationale: Postclinical conferences are not intended as time for classroom instruction in which the educator lectures and presents new content, thus making Option D the correct response (Oermann et al., 2018, p. 198). Options A, B, and C are incorrect because they demonstrate actions that are appropriate for the clinical nurse educator to use during a postclinical conference.

Test Blueprint: 2 A
Cognitive Code: Analysis

8. Which learning activity best supports the goal of meeting diverse learner needs?
   A. Learner-selected method for presenting a client scenario
   B. Role play practicing crucial conversations
   C. Round table discussion at postclinical conference
   D. Short written reflective assignment

Correct Answer: A

Rationale: Option A allows learners to choose their method for presenting a client scenario; this activity allows learners to be creative and select the presentation method that will most engage and meet their diverse learning needs (Phillips, 2016; Popkess & Frey, 2016). Options B, C, and D are all appropriate activities for engaging learners (Phillips, 2016), though they are not the best representation of meeting diverse learner needs since they are preestablished.

Test Blueprint: 2 A
Cognitive Code: Analysis

9. To understand discharge teaching from a client's perspective, which learning activity would be most effective?
   A. Case study
   B. Role play
   C. Reflective journaling
   D. One-minute paper

Correct Answer: B

Rationale: Role play is an effective strategy to expose learners to another perspective (DeYoung, 2015). Experiencing a situation from a different perspective, as in Option B, may change the learner's attitude and behavior. Options A, C, and D are learning activities that could be used to help understand discharge teaching but do not provide the best approach to understanding the client's perspective.

Test Blueprint: 2 A
Cognitive Code: Application

10. The clinical nurse educator is designing a simulation to teach administration of subcutaneous injections. Which type of simulation equipment would be most appropriate?
    A. An orange
    B. An injection pad
    C. A full-body mannequin
    D. A computerized mannequin

Correct Answer: B

Rationale: When teaching a basic technical skill, it is most appropriate to use low-fidelity simulation equipment, as in Option B (Reedy, 2015). A full-body mannequin and high-fidelity simulators, such as Options C and D, may be overwhelming to the novice learner who needs to focus on development of a technical skill. Option A, an orange, does not provide the most realistic learning opportunity for the learner.

Test Blueprint: 2 A
Cognitive Code: Analysis

11. Which simulation modality would be the best choice for learners to practice therapeutic communication with clients?
    A. Standardized patient
    B. Task trainer
    C. High-fidelity mannequin
    D. Computer-based simulation

Correct Answer: A

Rationale: Option A is correct because standardized patients provide the best opportunity for the most lifelike client scenario. Option B is best for practicing in a skills scenario. Options C and D do not provide the best options for a communication scenario because they do not present the best realistic interactions (International Nursing Association for Clinical Simulation and Learning Standards Committee, 2016b).

Test Blueprint: 2 A
Cognitive Code: Analysis

12. Which action will best help motivate learners in the clinical setting?
    A. Selecting clients who will need many procedures
    B. Allowing learners to have some input into client assignments
    C. Allowing learners to attend observational experiences off the unit
    D. Selecting clients with the same diagnosis as the topics that are being covered in theory class

Correct Answer: B

Rationale: Allowing learners to have some autonomy and input into client assignments, as suggested in Option B, may engage the learner (Gubrud, 2016). Performing procedures, Option A, or participating in observational experiences, Option C, may not be motivating to all learners. Selecting a client with a diagnosis similar to what is covered in theory class, as in Option D, may provide application of the lecture content, but it might not be as motivating as giving the learner a choice in the experience.

Test Blueprint: 2 A
Cognitive Code: Application

13. The clinical nurse educator notes that a learner is having difficulty using the situation, background, assessment, and recommendation (SBAR) technique when communicating with the health care provider. Which strategy would be most effective in improving the learner's use of the SBAR technique?
    A. Provide a review of the SBAR technique in postclinical conference.
    B. Have the learner write the report before calling the provider.
    C. Pair the learner with a peer who has strong communication skills and can coach the learner.
    D. Refer the learner to the learning lab to practice giving a report with a clinical nurse educator.

Correct Answer: D

Rationale: Options A, B, and C may be beneficial for improving the learner's understanding of the SBAR technique; however, providing a low-stakes environment for the learner to practice the SBAR technique with a clinical nurse educator, as in Option D, will more likely improve the learner's performance of the skill (Lanz & Wood, 2018).

Test Blueprint: 2 A
Cognitive Code: Application

14. Which question most likely represents best practices for debriefing after a simulation scenario?
   A. "Did you think that scenario went well?"
   B. "How did you feel as the nurse?"
   C. "Why did you give that medication during the scenario?"
   D. "I think that scenario went well, did you?"

Correct Answer: B

Rationale: Debriefing during simulation should include open-ended questions asked in a nonjudgmental environment that promote active learner participation (Jeffries, Swoboda, & Akintade, 2016, p. 315). Also, debriefing should not involve lecturing about the correct way of providing care. Instead, it should allow learners to reflect on the experience, as in Option B. Options A and D are closed-ended questions; therefore, they are not appropriate during debriefing. Option C is an open-ended question but could be perceived as judgmental.

Test Blueprint: 2 A
Cognitive Code: Application

15. A clinical nurse educator asks a colleague for guidance regarding which teaching strategy best promotes the learner's reflection on classroom learning and connections with clinical experiences. The colleague would most likely suggest which teaching strategy?
   A. Journaling
   B. Role play
   C. Gaming
   D. Socratic questioning

Correct Answer: A

Rationale: The use of journaling as a teaching strategy encourages learners to relate knowledge gained in the classroom to clinical learning experiences through reflection on practice, making Option A correct (Oermann et al., 2018, p. 244). Option B, role play, is incorrect because it requires learners to improvise behaviors that demonstrate expected outcomes (Bradshaw & Lowenstein, 2017). Option C, gaming, and Option D, Socratic questioning, are incorrect because they do not promote reflection best. They are effective strategies to help learners identify areas they need to further study (Bradshaw & Lowenstein, 2017).

Test Blueprint: 2 A
Cognitive Code: Application

16. Which best enhances learner engagement?
   A. Writing anecdotal notes and giving learners evaluative feedback during scheduled meetings
   B. Providing performance expectations in the syllabus and reviewing with learners at the beginning of the course
   C. Allowing learners to provide client care uninterrupted
   D. Encouraging learners to work together and collaborate with others

Correct Answer: D

Rationale: Principles that facilitate learning and engagement include collaboration (Phillips, 2016, p. 245). Option D is the best option to engage learners and allow them to work collaboratively with others. Feedback, as in Option A, should be given in a timely manner but does not necessarily enhance learner engagement. Providing performance expectations, as in Option B, does not ensure learner engagement. Allowing learners to provide client care uninterrupted, as in Option C, is not an appropriate action because it does not ensure client safety.

Test Blueprint: 2 A
Cognitive Code: Application

17. Which is most appropriate for a clinical nurse educator planning to expand the use of clinical questioning?
    A. Including most clinical questioning during preconference when all learners are available
    B. Creating several open-ended questions, such as "how will you prioritize your care today?"
    C. Using clinical questioning for summative evaluation of learners
    D. Using clinical questioning with the two weakest learners in the clinical group

Correct Answer: B

Rationale: Clinical questioning should promote critical thinking (Herman, 2016, pp. 177–178), as suggested by the open-ended question posed in Option B. Clinical questioning should be used throughout the clinical experience and not just during preclinical conferencing, as suggested in Option A. Questioning should be used throughout the clinical experience and should not be the focus of summative evaluation, as in Option C. Clinical nurse educators should use questioning with all learners and not just poorly performing learners; therefore, Option D is incorrect.

Test Blueprint: 2 A
Cognitive Code: Application

18. A pediatric clinical site has a limited number of clients. How should the clinical nurse educator best maximize the learners' clinical experience?
    A. Consider other clinical sites, such as a school or childcare setting.
    B. Provide a room for learners to complete pediatric case studies throughout the clinical day.
    C. Pair the learners to care for an uncomplicated pediatric client.
    D. Assign learners to the adjacent critical care unit.

Correct Answer: A

Rationale: Other settings such as childcare agencies and schools may offer other clinical sites that promote learning and meet course objectives (Oermann et al., 2018, pp. 40–41). Option A allows for the exploration of these other sites. Option B is incorrect because case studies may be beneficial for short periods of clinical learning but should not be used as the primary clinical learning approach since they do not allow learners to practice skills and interact with clients. Pairing learners with an uncomplicated client may limit learning and prevent learners from providing independent care, as in Option C. Critical care experience, as in Option D, is beyond the scope of learning for a pediatric clinical experience and does not align with the focus of a pediatric course.

Test Blueprint: 2 A
Cognitive Code: Analysis

19. A clinical nurse educator structures a laboratory experience for learners. One of the topics includes injection practice for adults and neonates. Which best represents what needs to be included in this lab experience?
    A. Include a medication order and various injection supplies.
    B. Require learners to perform the skill exactly as demonstrated.
    C. Demonstrate the skill for the learners and let them practice on each other.
    D. Use laboratory time for instruction related to the theoretical component of the skill.

    Correct Answer: A

    Rationale: Providing a variety of supplies enables the learners to choose appropriately, as in Option A (O'Connor, 2015, p. 150). Option B is incorrect because there may be multiple ways the learners may handle the equipment and prepare the medication. The clinical nurse educator should allow learners to manipulate the equipment and find an approach that works for them; the clinical nurse educator will need to ensure that general principles are followed rather than adhering to exact approaches. Thus, adherence to rigid steps, as suggested in Option B, does not allow the learner to adjust the psychomotor activity. Option C is incorrect as it would be a safety concern. Laboratory time should be used for skill practice, making Option D incorrect.

    Test Blueprint: 2 A
    Cognitive Code: Application

20. Which statement would best promote critical thinking in a case study based on a child experiencing dehydration?
    A. "Tell me about the assessment findings for a child experiencing dehydration."
    B. "Describe the possible approaches that could be used to care for this child."
    C. "Identify intravenous fluids that this child may need."
    D. "List laboratory data needed to determine dehydration."

    Correct Answer: B

    Rationale: Critical thinking development involves consideration of multiple perspectives and approaches to care (Oermann et al., 2018, p. 174), as in Option B; this option requires learners to consider multiple approaches to care. Options A, C, and D require lower-level thinking based on recall of information learned.

    Test Blueprint: 2 A
    Cognitive Code: Analysis

21. A clinical nurse educator identifies a learner having difficulty assessing a client's level of orientation. Which teaching-learning strategy would best address the learner's needs?
A. Questioning
B. Demonstration
C. Role play
D. Case study

Correct Answer: B

Rationale: The use of demonstration, Option B, as a teaching strategy first involves the educator visibly showing a learner a process; the learner is then provided the opportunity to ask questions and participate in a supervised practice session. Performing the steps of the assessment after observing a demonstration provides the best opportunity for learning this skill (Phillips, 2016, pp. 252–253). Option C is incorrect because role play requires learners to improvise behaviors that demonstrate expected outcomes but may not assist the learner in gaining the needed information to perform the skill appropriately (Bradshaw & Lowenstein, 2017). The use of questioning, Option A, is appropriate to help the learner identify areas that need further study but may not improve skill psychomotor performance (Bradshaw & Lowenstein, 2017). The use of a case study, Option D, supports the learner completing an analysis of a clinical situation within the context of what was learned in the classroom setting but focuses on cognitive knowledge, not skill demonstration (Phillips, 2016, pp. 255–256).

Test Blueprint: 2 A
Cognitive Code: Application

22. The clinical nurse educator should initiate which initial action when preparing to use the teaching strategy of discussion?
A. Determine how the discussion will be structured.
B. Decide on which topics the discussion will address.
C. Identify the outcomes to be achieved in the discussion.
D. Draft sample questions that will be used in the discussion.

Correct Answer: C

Rationale: When preparing to use discussion, the clinical nurse educator should first identify the outcomes and goals to be achieved, as in Option C (Oermann et al., 2018, p. 189). Options A, B, and D are planning steps that occur after the purpose of the activity is established.

Test Blueprint: 2 A
Cognitive Code: Application

23. Which active learning activity would best facilitate learning about conflict management?
A. Observation of a nurse manager
B. Completing NCLEX-style questions
C. Clinical simulation
D. Concept map assignment

Correct Answer: C

Rationale: Clinical nurse educators play an important role in training learners on conflict resolution methods. Simulation scenarios will assist clinical nurse educators in teaching these techniques, which will help learners develop positive conflict management strategies (Labrague & McEnroe, 2017). Therefore, Option C is correct. Options A, B, and D would not be best to facilitate active learning about conflict management strategies. Observation, Option A, does not guarantee that a learner would have an opportunity to observe appropriate conflict management strategies implemented in practice. NCLEX-style questions, Option B, do not provide opportunities for active engagement with concepts of conflict management. A concept map assignment, Option D, does not ensure that learners are actively engaged in learning related to conflict management.

Test Blueprint: 2 A
Cognitive Code: Application

24. Which teaching-learning strategy would be most beneficial for an English-as-second-language (ESL) learner?
    A. Organize team-based learning activities that partner ESL and native English-speaking learners.
    B. Mandate individual tutoring sessions for the ESL learners so that they can learn clinical terminology.
    C. Suggest that ESL learners complete their clinical assignments both written and orally.
    D. Require ESL learners to take additional English language classes before starting clinical courses.

    Correct Answer: A

    Rationale: Difficulties experienced by ESL learners are frequently the result of language issues. Pairing ESL learners with native English-speaking learners who can coach them in proper use and understanding of English helps improve overall language proficiency (Oermann et al., 2018). Imposing additional requirements on ESL learners, as in Options B, C, and D, may not be the most beneficial approach for their learning and could present other concerns.

    Test Blueprint: 2 A
    Cognitive Code: Application

25. Which learning activity would best foster learners' self-reflection and enable them to examine their feelings about the clinical experience?
    A. Concept mapping
    B. Think-pair-share
    C. Socratic questioning
    D. Journaling

    Correct Answer: D

    Rationale: Self-reflection allows for a greater internalization of the clinical experience for the learner. The learner is provided time to articulate one's thoughts (Bonnel, 2012). Option D, journaling, provides learners with the direct opportunity to articulate their thoughts and reflect on their clinical experiences, making this the correct response. Options A, B, and C promote cognitive learning but do not focus on self-reflection.

Test Blueprint: 2 A
Cognitive Code: Application

26. Which initial action by the clinical nurse educator is most appropriate when discovering that a learner has a learning disability?
    A. Revising all the assignments for the clinical course
    B. Giving the learner some additional time when completing clinical exams
    C. Referring the learner to campus disability services
    D. Administering a learning style inventory questionnaire

Correct Answer: C

Rationale: The campus disability services office specializes in assisting learners with various disabilities—including physical, psychological, learning, neurological, medical, vision, hearing, and temporary impairments—to achieve their academic goals. The learner should be evaluated by disability services, as suggested in Option C, prior to implementing any potential accommodations by the clinical nurse educator (Christensen, 2010). Options A, B, and D may not be appropriate for this learner with the disability and are not the best initial actions.

Test Blueprint: 2 A
Cognitive Code: Application

27. Which learning strategy is most appropriate for the nurse educator to use when teaching a group of adult learners?
    A. Minimizing learner engagement and participation in learning activities
    B. Avoiding the use of teaching strategies that foster reflective practice
    C. Providing highly structured learning activities that limit individualized learning
    D. Developing learning experiences that build on previous experiences

Correct Answer: D

Rationale: Options A, B, and C are strategies that would not be beneficial with adult learners because adult learners gravitate to more self-directed learning with less structure to meet their learning outcomes (Candela, 2012). Past experiences play a key role in adult learning; therefore, Option D is the best strategy to use with adult learners and is the correct option.

Test Blueprint: 2 B
Cognitive Code: Application

28. For learners with a preference for kinesthetic learning, which strategy is most appropriate?
    A. Providing hands-on activities while learning about injections
    B. Allowing digital recordings of postclinical conferences
    C. Providing handouts that require the learner to fill them in
    D. Incorporating periods of time during the clinical day for learners to review policies

Correct Answer: A

Rationale: Kinesthetic learners advance their learning when the clinical nurse educator provides opportunities to touch materials or practice skills with equipment (Oermann et al., 2018). Options B, C, and D do not provide the tactile experiences needed for kinesthetic learning.

Test Blueprint: 2 B
Cognitive Code: Application

29. The clinical nurse educator is using role modeling as a teaching strategy during a dressing change with a client. Which outcome demonstrates effective role modeling?
    A. Learners observe the techniques of a wound dressing change.
    B. Learners critique dressing changes conducted by other learners in a skills lab practice session.
    C. Learners use the techniques observed in future wound dressing changes with clients.
    D. Learners ask questions about wound care in a post-conference.

Correct Answer: C

Rationale: Role modeling serves as a teaching strategy in the clinical setting to assist learners by observation of tasks, interventions, or critical thinking skills; in return, learners can demonstrate those actions (Adelman-Mullally et al., 2013). Therefore, Option C is correct. Option A states that the learners will observe techniques but does not state that they will use the same techniques in future wound dressing changes. Option B requires knowledge of wound care performance but may be unrelated to the role modeling. Option D states that the learners will observe and ask questions in the post-conference but does not indicate that role modeling has been effective in enhancing learning.

Test Blueprint: 2 B
Cognitive Code: Analysis

30. Incorporating active teaching strategies is best supported by which educational theory?
    A. Behaviorism
    B. Essentialism
    C. Humanism
    D. Constructivism

Correct Answer: D

Rationale: The use of active teaching strategies requires learners to engage with content and respond to the learning experience (Scheckel, 2016, pp. 165–166). The educational theory of Constructivism assumes that learners build knowledge through active engagement in seeking the meaning of new experiences, as indicated in Option D (Candela, 2016, p. 214). Option A, Behaviorism, is incorrect because it uses behavior modification to guide learning. Essentialism, Option B, involves a belief that things have a set of characteristics that make them what they are. Humanism, Option C, is incorrect because it focuses on role modeling for learning. Constructivism, Option D, uses the learner's previous experiences to construct meaning in the learning situation.

Test Blueprint: 2 B
Cognitive Code: Recall

31. Which statement aligns best with Adult Learning Theory?
A. "Encourage adult learners to use previous experience and apply new knowledge to problem-solve."
B. "Adult learners are usually proficient with client care because they can draw on their past experiences."
C. "Offer a variety of auditory, visual, and kinesthetic approaches to address the different learning styles of adults."
D. "Provide a comfortable and stress-free learning environment because adult learners do best when relaxed."

Correct Answer: A

Rationale: Adult Learning Theory describes adult learners as using experience from the past and knowledge learned to problem-solve through situations (Candela, 2016, p. 216). Option A best reflects teaching that is derived from adult learners' experiences and needs. Option B may not be true of all adult learners and, even though they may have past experiences, there is no guarantee that adult learners are proficient with client care. Option C discusses different learning styles but is not the primary focus of Adult Learning Theory. Option D indicates Brain-Based Learning Theory.

Test Blueprint: 2 B
Cognitive Code: Recall

32. A clinical nurse educator asks a colleague to provide feedback regarding their discussion facilitation during a preclinical conference. Which behavior likely warrants correction?
A. Correcting learners' errors in thinking while they are responding to questions
B. Making notes on a piece of paper while learners' respond to questions asked
C. Posing a question to the group as a whole
D. Reinforcing learners' responses

Correct Answer: A

Rationale: Correcting learners' errors in thinking while they are responding to questions may result in the learner feeling belittled or ridiculed, making Option A the correct response (Oermann et al., 2018, p. 190). Options B, C, and D are incorrect because they demonstrate actions that are appropriate when facilitating a discussion.

Test Blueprint: 2 B
Cognitive Code: Analysis

33. A clinical nurse educator identifies the need to implement teaching strategies that would support development of learners' beliefs that they can successfully administer intermuscular injections. Which educational theory best addresses this belief?
A. Situated Learning Theory
B. Social Cognitive Theory
C. Experiential Learning Theory
D. Adult Learning Theory

Correct Answer: B

Rationale: The behavior the clinical nurse educator is targeting is self-efficacy. Self-efficacy is one's perception of the ability to succeed at completing the identified task. The behavior is one of the concepts of interest in Social Cognitive Theory, as suggested by Option B (Bandura, 1991). Options A, C, and D are incorrect because they focus on other aspects of learning, such as experiences or apprenticeships to guide learning.

Test Blueprint: 2 B
Cognitive Code: Recall

34. When interviewing for a position, a clinical nurse educator states, "I feel I connect best with the learners when I share how I felt the first time I completed a particular nursing skill." This clinical nurse educator most likely supports the beliefs associated with which teaching strategy?
    A. Lecture
    B. Discussion
    C. Narrative pedagogy
    D. Role play

Correct Answer: C

Rationale: Narrative pedagogy, Option C, involves the sharing of personally lived experiences. The use of personal stories for learning thus aligns with Option C (Candela, 2016, pp. 222–223). Lecture, Option A, is incorrect because it is a strategy utilized to present content. Use of discussion, Option B, is incorrect because it supports the exchanging of ideas (Candela, 2016, pp. 248–249). Role play, Option D, is incorrect because it requires learners to improvise behaviors that demonstrate expected outcomes (Bradshaw & Lowenstein, 2017).

Test Blueprint: 2 B
Cognitive Code: Recall

35. Which environment best provides learners with the optimal debriefing experience following a simulation scenario?
    A. At the bedside immediately after the simulation scenario ends
    B. In a lecture hall that has audiovisual equipment available for PowerPoint projection
    C. During the theory class the next day when all learners are present
    D. In a conference room with a round table, chairs, and a whiteboard

Correct Answer: D

Rationale: Debriefing supports a constructivist theory of education allowing for learner reflection and assimilation (Dreifuerst, 2012). A discussion that occurs as close to the simulation experience as possible in a setting that is conducive to learning allows for confidentiality and open communication is ideal (International Nursing Association for Clinical Simulation and Learning Standards Committee, 2016a). Option A is more conducive for providing feedback to correct individual learner mistakes and does not allow for reflection. Option B is not optimal because debriefing is not a time to reteach learners using presentation technology. Additionally, a lecture hall does not promote discussion and an exchange of information expected with debriefing. Option C does not provide debriefing in a timely manner.

The setting described in Option D allows for an open exchange of information and discussion that is part of best practices of debriefing.

Test Blueprint: 2 B
Cognitive Code: Application

36. Which is the best example of a Socratic question that could be used during simulation debriefing?
    A. "Did you remember to check the allergy band before giving the medication?"
    B. "Was client safety your first thought when you entered the room?"
    C. "How did you feel when you saw the client was crying?"
    D. "After you checked the client's blood pressure, what was your next priority and why?"

Correct Answer: D

Rationale: Option D requires learners to reflect on and analyze simulation performance (Dreifuerst, 2012; International Nursing Association for Clinical Simulation and Learning Standards Committee, 2016a). Options A and B are yes/no questions and may not allow for further response. Option C allows for expression of emotions but does not allow for an analysis of performance.

Test Blueprint: 2 B
Cognitive Code: Application

37. Which active learning strategy would best prepare a learner for simulation learning?
    A. Assigning readings about the simulation topic that must be completed before the simulation
    B. Providing a report about the simulated client at the start of the simulation
    C. Allowing learners to develop a plan of care before entering the simulation room
    D. Showing a video that demonstrates the care needed by the simulated client

Correct Answer: C

Rationale: Preparation activities should promote learner simulation success (International Nursing Association for Clinical Simulation and Learning Standards Committee, 2016b). Option C is an active learning strategy that will allow learners to plan care for the client. Options A and D are passive learning activities. Option B provides information to the learner and does not require active engagement by the learner.

Test Blueprint: 2 B
Cognitive Code: Analysis

38. Which learning outcome is written at the highest level of Bloom's taxonomy?
    A. Distinguish between normal and abnormal breath sounds.
    B. Define the terms *rhonchi* and *crackles*.
    C. Develop a plan of care for the client in respiratory distress.
    D. Appraise the care provided by health care team members.

Correct Answer: C

Rationale: Option C is written at the highest level of Bloom's taxonomy, which requires learners to create or produce original work (Scheckel, 2016). Option D is a learning objective written at the evaluation level of Bloom's taxonomy. Option A is written at the analysis level. Option B is written at the lowest level of Bloom's taxonomy, only requiring learners to remember information.

Test Blueprint: 2 B
Cognitive Code: Analysis

39. Which initial action is most appropriate when selecting a new technology teaching tool?
    A. Assessing the learners' comfort level with using technology
    B. Exploring barriers at the clinical site that may impede use of the technology
    C. Personally trying out the technology to assess for usability and comfort with use
    D. Identifying the behaviors that learners will be expected to demonstrate when using the technology

Correct Answer: D

Rationale: When choosing a new technology tool, the clinical nurse educator should first identify the types of interactions that will be required of learners to support achieving the learning objectives, making Option D correct (Oermann et al., 2018, p. 160). Options A, B, and C are incorrect because they are planning steps that occur after expected behaviors are identified.

Test Blueprint: 2 C
Cognitive Code: Application

40. While planning the implementation of a simulation scenario, a clinical nurse educator is deciding which level of fidelity to choose. The scenario involves fundamental skills in which learners must communicate with the client while collecting information for a health history. Which simulator is most appropriate for this situation?
    A. Low-fidelity simulator
    B. Moderate-fidelity simulator
    C. High-fidelity simulator
    D. Standardized patient

Correct Answer: D

Rationale: Standardized patients can provide experiences for learners related to communication (Oermann et al., 2018, p. 138). Therefore, this is the best selection of a simulator for this scenario. Low-fidelity simulators, as in Option A, allow for practice of skills and do not provide a high level of realism. Moderate-fidelity simulators, as in Option B, allow for assessment but lack interactive features. High-fidelity simulators, as in Option C, produce the most lifelike scenarios. However, since the scenario requires therapeutic communication and requires little hands-on skills, the standardized patient is the most appropriate.

Test Blueprint: 2 C
Cognitive Code: Application

41. Which best demonstrates effective debriefing following a simulation?
  A. Engaging only the simulation participants during the debriefing discussion
  B. Using questions such as "did the nurse communicate effectively with the client?" to promote discussion among the clinical group members
  C. Providing theoretical information in a lecture format throughout the debriefing session
  D. Reviewing simulation objectives and confidentiality with all learners prior to the start of the debriefing

Correct Answer: D

Rationale: During debriefing, the clinical nurse educator should first review objectives and establish a trusting relationship (Oermann et al., 2018, pp. 147–148), as in Option D. Debriefing should engage all learners and not just the participants in the simulation, as suggested in Option A. In Option A, the clinical nurse educator does not engage both participants and observers during the debriefing. Debriefing should not use close-ended questions, as in Option B, but rather the educator should use questions during the debriefing that support open-ended responses. The clinical nurse educator is a facilitator and should refrain from lecturing during debriefing, as suggested in Option C.

Test Blueprint: 2 C
Cognitive Code: Application

42. When implementing an electronic health record experience, which activity would provide the learner with the highest level of cognitive learning?
  A. Documenting vital signs and recording intake and output
  B. Searching the records for client demographic information
  C. Reviewing medication administration and physician orders
  D. Developing a written report based on findings from the electronic health record

Correct Answer: D

Rationale: Electronic health records in the academic and clinical setting provide learning opportunities for learners (Oermann et al., 2018, pp. 161–162). Option D provides learners with a higher-level thinking activity, as it involves not only gathering data from the electronic health record but also analyzing the data to create the written report. Option B involves searching the electronic health record and Option C involves a review of data; however, these do not require high-level thinking. Documentation, as suggested in Option A, engages the learner in the use of the electronic health record but does not involve high-level thinking.

Test Blueprint: 2 C
Cognitive Code: Application

43. During a simulation, a learner does not ask the client about allergies and administers a medication that causes an allergic reaction. Which is the best initial response?
A. Deliver cues to the learner about a possible allergy during the scenario.
B. Privately discuss the learner error with the learner prior to group debriefing.
C. Stop the scenario as soon as the incorrect medication was administered.
D. Continue with the scenario and ignore that this medication was given.

Correct Answer: A

Rationale: The simulation facilitator provides cues to draw attention to specific items during the scenario (International Nursing Association for Clinical Simulation and Learning Standards Committee, 2016b), as in Option A. Errors may occur during a simulation experience, but the educator can provide cues to assist the learner to identify the errors. During debriefing, all learners observing and participating in a simulation scenario can reflect on what occurred. Option B allows for a discussion of the events but is not the best initial action and does not provide an opportunity for the learner to self-identify the error. Stopping the scenario, as in Option C, does not give the learner a chance to identify and correct errors. Letting the learner continue with the simulation and ignoring the medication error, as in Option D, represents a safety concern.

Test Blueprint: 2 C
Cognitive Code: Analysis

44. A clinical nurse educator is developing an activity using an online learning management system. Which prompt used for an online discussion best engages learners in reflection?
A. "What medications did your client need today?"
B. "What are the reasons that your client's discharge was delayed?"
C. "What assessment findings were abnormal?"
D. "What client teaching did you do today?"

Correct Answer: B

Rationale: Active engagement of the learner through an online discussion to promote reflection requires open-ended prompts that help the learner identify what is important in a specific situation (Oermann et al., 2018, p. 167), as in Option B. Options A, C, and D do not prompt the learner to evaluate the situation and identify what is important; they require learner recall of information only.

Test Blueprint: 2 C
Cognitive Code: Application

45. Which clinical nurse educator action demonstrates adherence to best practices of debriefing?
A. Using the same debriefing questions for all clinical groups
B. Periodically observing other experienced educators conducting debriefing
C. Participating in continuing education about simulation
D. Attending workshops focused on clinical evaluation tools and item writing

Correct Answer: C

Rationale: When facilitating debriefing, the educator must be competent (International Nursing Association for Clinical Simulation and Learning Standards Committee, 2016a). This competence can be ensured by participation in educational activities, as suggested in Option C. While observing experienced educators conducting debriefings, as in Option B, may be beneficial, there is no guarantee that the educators are performing the debriefing competently and accurately. Education should be focused on debriefing and not just on general educational concepts, as in Option D. Debriefing should be tailored to the clinical group; therefore, Option A is incorrect since the educator is not tailoring the debriefing.

Test Blueprint: 2 C
Cognitive Code: Application

46. Which is the priority action when beginning a high-fidelity simulation scenario with a group of learners?
   A. Provide briefing about the background of the simulated client.
   B. Offer an orientation to the simulated client room.
   C. Review what happened in the scenario.
   D. Orient learners to the client electronic health record.

Correct Answer: A

Rationale: When implementing a simulation scenario, the educator should first review background information about the client, such as relevant client health history, as in Option A (Oermann et al., 2018, p. 144). Options B and D are incorrect because they should be done after background information is provided. Option C is incorrect because it represents debriefing, which occurs at the end of the scenario.

Test Blueprint: 2 C
Cognitive Code: Application

47. Which statement made by a clinical nurse educator colleague would be most concerning?
   A. "I am being trained on the new handheld documentation system next week."
   B. "I check all learners' documentation using the electronic health record."
   C. "I have not received training for using the electronic health record."
   D. "I need to learn more about ways high-fidelity simulation can support learning."

Correct Answer: C

Rationale: In Option C, the nurse educator does not have proficiency with the electronic health record, which is an integral part of using technology skillfully to support learning in the clinical setting (Killingsworth, 2019). Therefore, a colleague may be concerned if an educator does not know how to use the electronic health record to carry out teaching-learning responsibilities. Option A is an appropriate statement since the technology is new and the educator is being trained regarding its use. Option B is an appropriate and skillful use of technology in clinical learning. Option D is an appropriate educator development topic.

Test Blueprint: 2 C
Cognitive Code: Analysis

48. A clinical nurse educator is preparing to teach learners the correct technique for administering subcutaneous injections. The selection of which simulator demonstrates the clinical nurse educator's understanding of the best approach for skill teaching?
A. Low-fidelity simulator
B. Moderate-fidelity simulator
C. High-fidelity simulator
D. Standardized patient

Correct Answer: A

Rationale: An important planning consideration when preparing to use a simulated learning experience involves selecting the appropriate level of fidelity (Oermann et al., 2018, p. 140). Administering a subcutaneous injection would be considered a basic skill; low-fidelity simulators offer opportunities for basic procedural skills practice, making Option A correct (Oermann et al., 2018, p. 137). Options B, C, and D are incorrect because they involve higher fidelity than is necessary when teaching basic nursing skills.

Test Blueprint: 2 C
Cognitive Code: Application

49. When developing a simulation scenario using best practices in simulation education, it is most important for the clinical nurse educator to consider which principle?
A. Simulation experiences are purposefully designed to meet identified objectives and optimize achievement of expected outcomes.
B. The goal of simulated experiences is to perfect skill performance and ensure consistent safe client outcomes.
C. Simulation experiences should be used to evaluate learner performance and align with course grades.
D. The more realistic the simulated environment, the better the learning outcome will be for learners.

Correct Answer: A

Rationale: Option A is correct because all simulation experiences should be planned with learning objectives and outcomes (International Nursing Association for Clinical Simulation and Learning Standards Committee, 2016b). Option B is incorrect because the purpose of simulation is not to perfect skills but to enhance skill improvement. Simulation can be used for both learning and evaluation and not just for high-stakes evaluation and grading, as in Option C. Although providing a realistic simulation may help learning, there is no guarantee that it will lead to better learning outcomes, making Option D incorrect.

Test Blueprint: 2 C
Cognitive Code: Application

50. Which would be the best rationale for pilot testing a simulation with a small group of learners before implementing the scenario with a group of clinical learners?
   A. Determining if learners will like the simulation experience
   B. Practicing with simulation equipment and troubleshooting if it does not work
   C. Determining the number of educators needed for simulation implementation
   D. Identifying and correcting any confusing or missing elements of the simulation

Correct Answer: D

Rationale: Option D is correct because pilot testing ensures that the simulation is effective and learning objectives can be met. During a trial run of the scenario, educators can correct any underdeveloped areas of the simulation (International Nursing Association for Clinical Simulation and Learning Standards Committee, 2016b). While it is desirable that learners like the simulation experience, Option A, that should not be a reason for pilot testing the simulation. Options B and C can be accomplished without facilitating the simulation with a group of learners.

Test Blueprint: 2 C
Cognitive Code: Application

51. The clinical nurse educator wants to give learners the opportunity to practice sterile technique during catheter insertion. Which simulation modality would be the best choice?
   A. Standardized patient
   B. Task trainer
   C. High-fidelity mannequin
   D. Computer-based simulation

Correct Answer: B

Rationale: A task trainer, Option B, is the best option for psychomotor skill practice and demonstration. Standardized patients, Option A, provide the best opportunity for the most lifelike client scenario but would be inappropriate for an invasive procedure such as a catheterization. Options C and D involve a higher level of fidelity and are not needed for basic psychomotor skill practice and demonstration (International Nursing Association for Clinical Simulation and Learning Standards Committee, 2016b).

Test Blueprint: 2 C
Cognitive Code: Analysis

52. A clinical nurse educator is preparing to teach learners skills needed to care for a client who is experiencing a myocardial infarction. The selection of which simulator demonstrates the clinical nurse educator's understanding of the best approach for skills teaching?
   A. Low-fidelity simulator
   B. Moderate-fidelity simulator
   C. High-fidelity simulator
   D. Standardized patient

Correct Answer: C

Rationale: An important planning consideration when preparing to use a simulated learning experience involves selecting the appropriate level of fidelity (Oermann et al., 2018, p. 140). Providing care for a client who is actively experiencing a myocardial infarction would be considered a complex situation in which the learner would need to appropriately interpret subjective and objective data. High-fidelity simulators, Option C, produce the most lifelike simulated learning experience, thus this option is the most appropriate simulator for this scenario (Oermann et al., 2018, p. 137). A low-fidelity simulator, Option A, and a moderate-fidelity simulator, Option B, are incorrect because they do not adequately portray the complexity of the client situation. A standardized patient, Option D, is incorrect because the standardized patient would be unable to portray the physiologic changes associated with a client experiencing a myocardial infarction. Additionally, learners would be unable to perform interventions on the standardized patient.

Test Blueprint: 2 C
Cognitive Code: Application

53. A clinical nurse educator is preparing to teach learners effective therapeutic communication skills. The selection of which simulator type demonstrates the clinical nurse educator's understanding of the best approach for teaching these skills?
    A. Low-fidelity simulator
    B. Moderate-fidelity simulator
    C. High-fidelity simulator
    D. Standardized patient

Correct Answer: D

Rationale: An important planning consideration when preparing to use a simulated learning experience involves selecting the appropriate level of fidelity (Oermann et al., 2018, p. 140). The use of a standardized patient, Option D, provides a unique learning opportunity for learners to refine their communication skills (Oermann et al., 2018, p. 138) and further develop skills associated with both cognitive, psychomotor, and affective domains of learning, making Option D correct. Options A, B, and C are not the most appropriate level of simulation for this scenario because they do not provide the realism or spontaneous interactive communication needed for this scenario.

Test Blueprint: 2 C
Cognitive Code: Application

54. According to the National Council of State Boards of Nursing (NCSBN) simulation study, laboratory simulations can be substituted for clinical experiences in which situation?
    A. When at least one clinical nurse educator is trained in simulation pedagogy
    B. When there are not enough clinical sites to meet the learning outcomes of the course
    C. When there are not enough clinical nurse educators to supervise the learners
    D. When the simulation is conducted under the same conditions as the simulations in the study

Correct Answer: D

Rationale: According to the NCSBN study results (Hayden, Smiley, Alexander, Kardong-Edgren, & Jeffries, 2014), the conditions of the simulation must match the conditions of the study to substitute simulation for traditional clinical experiences. The conditions are as follows: clinical nurse educator members who are teaching simulation must be trained using evidence-based simulation strategies, a realistic environment is created in the simulation, there are enough clinical nurse educators to run the simulations, and the debrief is conducted using a theory-based technique. Options A, B, and C were not supported in the NCSBN study.

Test Blueprint: 2 C
Cognitive Code: Recall

55. A clinical nurse educator is preparing to debrief learners after a simulation. Which best describes the Plus-Delta method of debriefing?
    A. Asking the learners to describe what they did during the simulation, why they did it, and ways to improve their performance in future simulations
    B. Asking the learners to reflect on their own expertise in caring for clients with chest tubes and critique their performance during the simulation
    C. Creating a two-column chart and asking the learners to list what went well during the simulation and what actions they would change if they had an opportunity to repeat the simulation
    D. Asking each learner to quietly document what happened in the simulation from their individual perspectives

Correct Answer: C

Rationale: The two-column chart option describes the process of using the Plus-Delta method of debriefing. In this method, learners discuss what went well and what actions should be changed in the simulation. Option A describes the Gather-Analyze-Summarize method. Option B describes the Debriefing for Meaningful Learning method. Option D describes the method of debriefing using emotion, experience counts, communication, higher-order thinking, accentuate the positive, time, and structure, or EE-CHATS (Dreifuerst, Horton-Deutsch, & Henao, 2014).

Test Blueprint: 2 C
Cognitive Code: Recall

56. Which action would best help a learner view a simulated clinical experience as realistic?
    A. Stage the simulation room with props and moulage for mannequins.
    B. Include family members or other participants in the simulation.
    C. Purchase simulated clinical scenarios from reputable companies.
    D. Select clinical experiences that require use of a high-fidelity simulator.

Correct Answer: B

Rationale: Learners benefit the most from simulated experiences that are viewed as realistic (Oermann et al., 2018, pp. 139–140). Including family members and other participants in the simulation, as in Option B, enhances the psychological fidelity of the experiences and helps establish realism, making Option B correct (International Nursing Association for Clinical Simulation and Learning Standards Committee, 2016b). Staging the simulation room, as in Option A, is helpful in establishing a realistic simulated experience but not as important as including the family members and other participants in the simulation. Option C, purchasing scenarios from a reputable company, does not aid in establishing realism. Use of a high-fidelity simulator, as in Option D, does not guarantee the establishment of a realistic environment.

Test Blueprint: 2 C
Cognitive Code: Application

57. Which initial action should the clinical nurse educator take when developing a simulated clinical learning experience?
A. Determine how the simulated learning experience will be structured.
B. Decide which skills the simulated learning experience will address.
C. Identify the purpose of the simulated learning experience.
D. Draft sample questions that will be used in the debriefing session.

Correct Answer: C

Rationale: When preparing to develop a simulated clinical learning experience, the clinical nurse educator should first identify the purpose of the simulated experience (International Nursing Association for Clinical Simulation and Learning Standards Committee, 2016b). The clinical nurse educator should then use the purpose of the simulated experience, Option C, to design and structure the appropriate scenario. Options A, B, and D are incorrect because they are planning steps that occur after the purpose is identified.

Test Blueprint: 2 C
Cognitive Code: Application

58. The clinical nurse educator wants to support the professional socialization of learners. Which social networking tool is most appropriate?
A. Facebook
B. Twitter
C. LinkedIn
D. Instagram

Correct Answer: C

Rationale: LinkedIn is a social media platform that supports building a professional identity and engaging or networking with other professionals. Some recent studies suggest that most respondents prefer the use of LinkedIn for professional connections and discipline knowledge sharing (Halevi, Liu, & Yoon, 2018). Options A, B, and D are social media sites that are considered personal, with a focus on conveying lifestyle information.

Test Blueprint: 2 C
Cognitive Code: Analysis

59. Which question best helps the learner develop critical thinking and clinical reasoning skills?
   A. "When does the premature newborn need a Vitamin K injection?"
   B. "How will you administer the Vitamin K injection?"
   C. "What is the correct needle to use when administering a Vitamin K injection?"
   D. "Why administer a Vitamin K injection to a premature newborn?"

Correct Answer: D

Rationale: Clinical reasoning uses cognition and metacognition to analyze and evaluate client information (Oermann et al., 2018). Asking why the learner would need to administer Vitamin K to the premature newborn, as in Option D, is a broader question that involves more than just recall; this question requires the learner to consider and analyze the client situation. Options A, B, and C require only lower-level cognitive skills and do not require higher-level thinking and clinical reasoning.

Test Blueprint: 2 D
Cognitive Code: Application

60. Which question helps learners develop clinical reasoning abilities best?
   A. "Which of your client's lab results are abnormal?"
   B. "What questions will you ask the oncoming shift based on your chart review?"
   C. "What medications are due to be given during our shift and when?"
   D. "What was the reason for your client's admission?"

Correct Answer: B

Rationale: Clinical reasoning is the process of gathering and thinking about client information, analyzing the options, and evaluating alternatives (Gubrud, 2016). It requires cognitive and metacognitive processes (Berman, Snyder, & Frandsen, 2016). Option B gives the learner the opportunity to prioritize and make decisions based on collected relevant data. When learners are guided to go beyond answering questions and are asked to contemplate what questions to ask, this will make them better able to reason through changing clinical situations and engage in critical, creative, and scientific reasoning (Benner, Sutphen, Leonard, & Day, 2010). The other options simply ask the learner to recall collected data.

Test Blueprint: 2 D
Cognitive Code: Application

61. Which question best helps learners develop clinical reasoning?
   A. "What is the most likely complication to anticipate today with this client?"
   B. "Does the client have an order for a regular diet?"
   C. "Is your client's pain well controlled today?"
   D. "What is the underlying pathophysiology of your client's diagnosis?"

Correct Answer: A

Rationale: Clinical reasoning is the process of gathering and thinking about client information, analyzing the options, and evaluating alternatives (Gubrud, 2016). Benner et al. (2010) describe the components of clinical reasoning to include setting priorities, developing rationales, learning how to act, clinical reasoning-in-transition, and responding to changes in the client's condition. Option A best reflects this clinical reasoning. Options B, C, and D do not include those components of clinical reasoning and would likely result in factual responses.

Test Blueprint: 2 D
Cognitive Code: Application

62. Which statement or question best guides learner reflection during a simulation debriefing session?
    A. "Was there anything you missed on report or was there other information that you needed so you could act more effectively?"
    B. "You missed some really key information that would have changed the outcome of the simulation. Start by telling us what went wrong during report."
    C. "Tell me why you prioritized your care the way you did instead of how I have taught you to do assessments in the clinical laboratory."
    D. "Talk about all the areas where you made mistakes and how you plan to fix your errors in the future."

Correct Answer: A

Rationale: "Because debriefing can be critical for learning, teachers need to carefully plan and consider the methods, format, and approach used while also ensuring that they can effectively facilitate this activity" (Oermann et al., 2018, p. 200). Effective methods for simulation debriefing involve leveraging therapeutic communication techniques to ask for learner feedback and reflection. Option A uses a probing open-ended question to help learners engage in reflective conversations and identify areas for improvement. Option B focuses on the errors that the learner made and does so without allowing the learner to initially reflect on the experience. Option C places blame on the learner and Option D focuses primarily on mistakes identified.

Test Blueprint: 2 D
Cognitive Code: Application

63. Which question by the clinical nurse educator regarding urinary output requires the learner to think critically?
    A. "Have you thought about the client's urinary output?"
    B. "Did you make sure to measure output?"
    C. "What is the output in milliliters?"
    D. "Why do you think measuring output is so important for this client?"

Correct Answer: D

Rationale: Clinical nurse educators can effectively guide clinical learning activities by asking thought-provoking questions without learners feeling that they are being interrogated. The ability to think critically is integral to providing safe and quality care; this skill can be encouraged through questioning in the clinical setting (Oermann et al., 2018, p. 82). Options A and B require only yes/no responses from the learner and do not promote critical thinking. Option C requires only recall of information by the learner. Option D requires the learner to consider the concept and think critically about the topic.

Test Blueprint: 2 D
Cognitive Code: Analysis

64. Which is the best action to take when a client who was assigned to a learner suddenly deteriorates and needs resuscitative measures?
   A. Debriefing the learners involved in resuscitation, allowing them to reflect on the experience
   B. Evaluating learner performance during the emergent situation
   C. Asking the learner to care for another client so other members of the health care team can assume care for the deteriorating client
   D. Assembling all clinical learners on the unit to watch the resuscitative efforts

Correct Answer: A

Rationale: Debriefing following a clinical experience provides an opportunity for the learners to identify areas of improvement (Gubrud, 2016, p. 290). Option A allows learners to reflect on the experience. Option B should not be a priority during these emergent situations and the learner may not have an active role during a critical situation. Asking the learner to care for other clients, as in Option C, does not allow the learner to benefit from observing and engaging in the care for the client assigned. Option D would be intrusive for the client, may get in the way of those responding to the emergency, and would leave the learners' clients uncared for during the observation.

Test Blueprint: 2 D
Cognitive Code: Application

65. Which question would best encourage higher-level thinking?
   A. "What are the clinical manifestations of asthma?"
   B. "What nursing intervention is associated with respiratory distress?"
   C. "What discharge teaching is needed for a client who was recently diagnosed with sickle cell anemia?"
   D. "How do the findings of your school-aged client compare to those of a toddler?"

Correct Answer: D

Rationale: Higher-level questions help learners develop critical thinking (Oermann et al., 2018, pp. 193–197). Option D is correct because it requires the learner to analyze and compare, which are higher-level thinking skills. Option A is a lower-level question that involves thinking only at the knowledge level. Options B and C demonstrate comprehension, which also require lower-level thinking.

Test Blueprint: 2 D
Cognitive Code: Application

66. When discussing discontinuing a Foley catheter with a learner, which statement best promotes critical thinking?
   A. "Tell me how the nurse determines when the Foley catheter can be discontinued."
   B. "Record total intake and output for the past eight hours before discontinuing the catheter."
   C. "Describe the urine that is currently in the Foley catheter bag."
   D. "Explain perineal care for a client following Foley catheter removal."

Correct Answer: A

Rationale: When critically thinking, the learner has to examine the situation and make decisions (O'Connor, 2015, p. 248). Option A requires the learner to critically consider the situation and make evaluative judgments, an important part of critical thinking. Options B, C, and D are incorrect because the statements focus only on recall or observation rather than critically analyzing the situation.

Test Blueprint: 2 D
Cognitive Code: Application

67. A clinical nurse educator is planning a postclinical conference with learners. Which teaching-learning strategy is most appropriate to enhance cognitive skill development?
    A. Meet with each learner individually to discuss clinical performance related to cognitive skill development.
    B. Provide time to complete a clinical assessment form during postclinical conference.
    C. Initiate a discussion regarding identification of obstacles to solve a problem.
    D. Pose a statement, such as "describe a fetal heart rate deceleration."

Correct Answer: C

Rationale: Development of cognitive skills during postclinical conferences can be facilitated by asking questions or making statements that promote higher-level thinking (Oermann et al., 2018, p. 192), as suggested in Option C. Option A is an evaluation of each individual learner and is not reflective of cognitive skill development. Completion of the assessment form, as in Option B, does not necessarily enhance cognitive skill development. Recall of information is lower-level thinking, making Option D incorrect.

Test Blueprint: 2 D
Cognitive Code: Analysis

68. Following an observational experience, the clinical nurse educator asks learners to complete a written journal entry. Which statement regarding journaling is most appropriate?
    A. "Use closed-ended prompts to guide learners' writing."
    B. "Record events that occurred during the experience."
    C. "Include details about the clinical assignment."
    D. "Describe reflections about the experience."

Correct Answer: D

Rationale: When providing a journal response, learners should describe their reflections on the experience (O'Connor, 2015, p. 253), as suggested in Option D. Options A, B, and C are incorrect because the purpose of the journal entry is to promote reflection and enhance thinking; these options do not promote reflection. Closed-ended prompts limit the learner, as in Option A, and recording events and specific details, as in Options B and C, may not encourage higher-level reflective thinking.

Test Blueprint: 2 D
Cognitive Code: Application

69. A learner is caring for a client with end-stage renal disease. Which question best supports learner development of clinical reasoning skills?
A. "What are the treatment options for end-stage renal disease?"
B. "What is the most important problem for this client?"
C. "What is the client's plan of care for this shift?"
D. "What was the client's creatinine level last week?"

Correct Answer: B

Rationale: Option B asks the learner to not only identify the main client problems, but also asks the learner to prioritize the client issues. This question will encourage critical thinking and clinical reasoning skills (Oermann, 1997; Paul & Elder, 2008). Options A, C, and D may be important questions to ask but do not necessarily facilitate development of clinical reasoning skills themselves and may likely result in simple factual responses by the learner.

Test Blueprint: 2 D
Cognitive Code: Analysis

70. Which question or statement is the best example of Socratic questioning?
A. "Tell me about your client."
B. "What did you do well today?"
C. "How did you know that to be true?"
D. "How did you feel when you were performing that procedure?"

Correct Answer: C

Rationale: "How did you know that to be true" is an example of a prompt to probe the reasons for a learner's action (Oermann et al., 2018, p. 200). Without a follow-up question, Options A and B may engage the learners but do not necessarily stimulate critical thinking, as Socratic questioning aims to do. Option D does engage learners in the affective domain but does not necessarily stimulate critical thinking.

Test Blueprint: 2 D
Cognitive Code: Analysis

71. Which question would be least helpful in encouraging critical thinking?
A. "Why do you think the client is still experiencing pain?"
B. "What other interventions might be helpful for this client who is anxious about the upcoming surgery?"
C. "What would happen if you gave the client this medication at this time?"
D. "How did you feel when the health care provider explained the diagnosis to the client?"

Correct Answer: D

Rationale: Option D is asking a question that assesses the affective domain, but it is not related to encouraging critical thinking. Options A, B, and C are questions that should elicit reflection and problem-solving from the learner. Reflection and problem-solving are elements of critical thinking (Forneris & Fey, 2018).

Test Blueprint: 2 D
Cognitive Code: Analysis

72. A clinical nurse educator is coaching a learner during an indwelling urinary catheter insertion. Which statement by the clinical nurse educator is most appropriate?

A. "Make sure to remember to put the lubricant on the end of the catheter."
B. "What are you doing? Don't forget about the lubricant on the catheter."
C. "Tell me what else you should do before you proceed to insert the catheter."
D. "You cannot proceed until you lubricate the end of the catheter."

Correct Answer: C

Rationale: Effective clinical teaching requires clinical nurse educators to develop clinical reasoning abilities in their learners (Gubrud, 2016, p. 289). Also, it is important to correct mistakes of the learners without belittling them (Gubrud, 2016, p. 291). Option A is incorrect because it tells the learner what to do without allowing the learner to reflect on what should be done next. Option B is incorrect because it belittles the learner. Option D is incorrect because it directs the learner's actions without allowing the learner to think independently. Option C is correct because it promotes clinical reasoning while also demonstrating support and respect for the learner.

Test Blueprint: 2 D
Cognitive Code: Analysis

73. A clinical nurse educator is observing a learner who is preparing to administer a beta blocker medication. The client's blood pressure prior to administration is 90/50 mmHg. Which question by the clinical nurse educator would best facilitate critical thinking?

A. "Do you think that you should hold this medication?"
B. "What are the side effects of this medication?"
C. "Which two values should you monitor prior to administering this medication?"
D. "What are your next actions considering this client data?"

Correct Answer: D

Rationale: When questioning learners, questions should allow the learners to think beyond what is evident and should promote critical thinking (Oermann et al., 2018, pp. 82–83). Additionally, questions should be open-ended to facilitate critical thinking. Option D is an open-ended question that helps develop critical thinking skills. Options A, B, and C are closed-ended questions that do not promote critical thinking.

Test Blueprint: 2 D
Cognitive Code: Analysis

74. Which post-conference discussion would best help develop critical thinking skills?

A. Debating views about the ethical issue of medicating prior to client death
B. Discussing what was learned during client care during the clinical day
C. Explaining findings regarding an assigned case study
D. Providing instruction on a topic that was presented in theory class that week

Correct Answer: A

Rationale: Postclinical conferences are held at the end of the clinical learning activity and should facilitate critical thinking. They are not for lecturing or intended as a substitute for classroom instruction (Oermann et al., 2018, p. 198). Option B is incorrect because, although it allows for learner reflection, it does not necessarily stimulate critical thinking. Option C may facilitate some critical thinking; however, it offers instruction rather than stimulating learners to think critically or connect learning to the clinical experience. Option D in incorrect because it includes lecturing without learner participation. Option A best facilitates critical thinking.

Test Blueprint: 2 D
Cognitive Code: Application

75. A learner asks the clinical nurse educator a question regarding a medication's mechanism of action. Which action would best promote critical thinking skills?
    A. Responding to the learner's question regarding the medication mechanism of action
    B. Showing the learner how to look up the question in the online drug guide
    C. Having the learner look up the mechanism of action and present it during a clinical conference
    D. Telling the learner that the online reference is a good resource for that information

Correct Answer: C

Rationale: Proper clinical teaching skills involve encouraging critical thinking of the nursing learner and allowing learners to think independently (Oermann et al., 2018, p. 85). Option C is correct because it allows the learner to think critically and learn about the concept while sharing it with the clinical group. Options A, B, and D do not necessarily promote critical thinking.

Test Blueprint: 2 D
Cognitive Code: Application

76. A new clinical nurse educator asks a colleague, "How do I encourage learners to evaluate their own learning to identify their knowledge gaps?" Which learner attribute is the clinical nurse educator most likely describing?
    A. Autonomy
    B. Metacognition
    C. Self-confidence
    D. Curiosity

Correct Answer: B

Rationale: The behavior the clinical nurse educator is describing is metacognition. Metacognition is commonly referred to as thinking about thinking. Metacognition, Option B, is viewed as an active process in which learners participate in the monitoring of their own thinking, and the modifying of their approach to learning, making Option B correct (Sullivan, 2016, p. 112). Options A, C, and D do not address the concept the educator is discussing.

Test Blueprint: 2 D
Cognitive Code: Recall

77. Which teaching-learning strategy would develop clinical reasoning abilities best?
   A. Debate
   B. Group discussion
   C. Lecture
   D. Case presentations

Correct Answer: A

Rationale: Using debate as a teaching strategy, Option A, provides an opportunity for learners to complete an in-depth analysis of a complex issue. Debates require learners to listen to their peers and analyze the different perspectives shared to develop a rationale they will use to defend a position they are taking regarding the issue, thus enhancing clinical reasoning abilities and making Option A correct (Oermann et al., 2018, p. 198). Lecture, Option C, is incorrect because it is a strategy used to present content. Option B, group discussion, does supports the exchanging of ideas and facilitates comprehension; however, it may not guarantee that learners are developing clinical reasoning skills (Candela, 2016, p. 248). Learners may not be analyzing options or evaluating alternatives, which are important components of clinical reasoning (Popkess & Frey, 2016, p. 27). Case presentations, Option D, is incorrect because it allows for a discussion of content but does not ensure analysis of an issue.

Test Blueprint: 2 D
Cognitive Code: Application

78. Before using a new technology in the clinical environment, which step helps ensure a culture of safety best?
   A. Educating learners on specific policies regarding appropriate online conduct
   B. Identifying the learner needs that will be addressed with using the technology
   C. Exploring barriers at the clinical site that may impede use of the technology
   D. Assessing the learners' comfort level with technology

Correct Answer: A

Rationale: When preparing to use a technology teaching tool, the educator should first discuss with learners appropriate online conduct, as in Option A (Oermann et al., 2018, p. 98). Having this discussion helps create a culture of safety and prevents potential harm to clients and serious consequences for nursing learners, nursing programs, and health care agencies due to online misconduct (Oermann et al., 2018, pp. 98–99). Options B, C, and D are incorrect because, although they are considerations for technology use, they are not related to ensuring a culture of safety.

Test Blueprint: 2 E
Cognitive Code: Application

79. The clinical nurse educator is incorporating which Quality and Safety Education for Nurses (QSEN) competency when encouraging learners to recognize client preferences, values, and needs when providing care?
A. Patient-centered care
B. Safety
C. Collaboration
D. Quality improvement

Correct Answer: A

Rationale: Option A, the patient-centered care QSEN competency, addresses the multiple cultural, ethical, cost-effectiveness, safety, and physiologic dimensions of patient-centered care (Cronenwett et al., 2007). Options B, C, and D represent other QSEN competencies.

Test Blueprint: 2 E
Cognitive Code: Recall

80. The clinical nurse educator is incorporating which Quality and Safety Education for Nurses (QSEN) competency when encouraging learners to work with interprofessional health care providers and demonstrate open communication, mutual respect, and shared decision-making?
A. Patient-centered care
B. Teamwork and collaboration
C. Quality improvement
D. Safety

Correct Answer: B

Rationale: Option B, the teamwork and collaboration QSEN competency, involves the fostering of interprofessional team communication and mutual respect (Cronenwett et al., 2007). Options A, C, and D represent other QSEN competencies.

Test Blueprint: 2 E
Cognitive Code: Recall

81. The clinical nurse educator is incorporating which Quality and Safety Education for Nurses (QSEN) competency when asking learners to locate current research to support their client care?
A. Evidence-based practice
B. Patient-centered care
C. Quality improvement
D. Safety

Correct Answer: A

Rationale: Evidence-based practice, Option A, represents the QSEN competency that involves the integration of best current evidence with clinical expertise (Cronenwett et al., 2007). Options B, C, and D represent other QSEN competencies.

Test Blueprint: 2 E
Cognitive Code: Recall

82. The clinical nursing educator facilitates learning of which Quality and Safety Education for Nurses (QSEN) competency when asking learners to search an electronic database to locate research articles pertaining to client care?
A. Informatics
B. Quality improvement
C. Teamwork and collaboration
D. Safety

Correct Answer: A

Rationale: Option A, the QSEN informatics competency, uses information and technology to communicate, manage knowledge, mitigate error, and support decision-making (Cronenwett et al., 2007). Options B, C, and D represent other QSEN competencies.

Test Blueprint: 2 E
Cognitive Code: Recall

83. The clinical nurse educator understands that the learner is exhibiting which Quality and Safety for Nurses (QSEN) competency when discussing a client's cultural needs for health care?
A. Evidence-based practice
B. Quality improvement
C. Patient-centered care
D. Teamwork and collaboration

Correct Answer: C

Rationale: Option C, the QSEN patient-centered care competency, recognizes the client or the designee as the source of control and full partner in providing compassionate and coordinated care based on respect for client preferences, values, and needs (Cronenwett et al., 2007). Options A, B, and D represent other QSEN competencies.

Test Blueprint: 2 E
Cognitive Code: Recall

84. Which action would best help learners meet the clinical learning outcome: *Learners will provide client-centered care to all assigned clients in the health care setting*?
A. Reviewing how agency technology can help monitor client health status
B. Demonstrating how to find peer-reviewed, scholarly journal articles
C. Discussing how people from different cultures perceive and manage pain
D. Describing how the nurse can be a change agent by suggesting practice updates

Correct Answer: C

Rationale: Option C is a suggested activity to meet the knowledge, skills, and attitudes listed in the Quality and Safety Education for Nurses (QSEN) patient-centered care competency (QSEN, 2019). Option A links to the informatics competency and Options B and D correlate with the evidence-based practice competency (QSEN, 2019).

Test Blueprint: 2 E
Cognitive Code: Analysis

85. Which learning activity best fosters learners' development of clinical decision-making?
   A. Reading a section of the American Nurses Association Scope and Standards of Practice
   B. Checking daily laboratory reports for an assigned client
   C. Performing a complete head-to-toe physical assessment on an assigned client
   D. Participating in client rounds with the physician, nurse, client, and family

Correct Answer: D

Rationale: In nursing, clinical decision-making is mutual and participatory with clients and staff members so that the decisions are more likely to be accepted (Oermann et al., 2018, pp. 21–22). Only Option D includes more than just the learner in the clinical decision-making process.

Test Blueprint: 2 E
Cognitive Code: Application

86. Which action will best help learners meet the clinical learning outcome supportive of evidence-based practice: *Learners will identify interventions to care for client needs in the clinical setting*?
   A. Discussing how agency technology can help monitor client health status
   B. Discussing who has the authority to make decisions for pediatric clients
   C. Discussing how different cultures perceive and manage pain
   D. Discussing how the nurse can be a change agent if practice needs to be updated

Correct Answer: D

Rationale: Option D is a suggested learning activity to meet the knowledge, skills, and attitudes competencies listed in the Quality and Safety Education for Nurses (QSEN) evidence-based practice competency (QSEN, 2019). Option A is linked to the informatics competency and Options B and C best correlate with the patient-centered care competency (QSEN, 2019).

Test Blueprint: 2 E
Cognitive Code: Analysis

87. Which clinical activity best enhances learners' skills related to safety?
   A. Discussing the concept of safety after observing a medication error
   B. Assigning the learner to read an article related to client safety
   C. Attending a lecture related to client safety
   D. Participating in a simulation related to safety with other learners

Correct Answer: D

Rationale: Safety efforts minimize client and provider harm (QSEN, 2019); therefore, Option D is correct because it engages learners in realistic practice that promotes safety. The active teaching-learning strategy of simulation allows learners to demonstrate skills related to safety. Prevention of errors should be a priority. Therefore, letting an error occur in the clinical setting and then discussing it with learners, as in Option A, poses harm to the client. Options B and C do provide safety learning but are not active learning strategies that provide practice opportunities for learning and thus would not be the best activities.

Test Blueprint: 2 E
Cognitive Code: Application

88. On the first day of a new clinical rotation, a senior-level learner is assigned to the task of cleaning a tracheostomy site. The learner reports having performed this skill many times before. Which is the most appropriate response?
    A. Go with the learner the first time the learner performs the task.
    B. Ask the learner to describe the steps for cleaning the tracheostomy site.
    C. Send the learner with the nursing staff to perform the tracheostomy cleaning.
    D. Ask the learner for documentation of completing the skill in a previous rotation.

Correct Answer: A

Rationale: Even though the learner reports that the skill has been performed previously, as in Option A, the clinical nurse educator is responsible for assessing learners' prior knowledge. The clinical nurse educator should observe the learner the first time a procedure is performed during a clinical rotation (Niederriter, Eyth, & Thoman, 2017). Options B and D do not ensure that the learner can perform the skill safely and appropriately. It is not the staff responsibility to evaluate learners and ensure their safe practice; therefore, Option C is incorrect.

Test Blueprint: 2 E
Cognitive Code: Analysis

89. A clinical nurse educator is observing a learner performing a dressing change. The learner performs the procedure out of order but not in a manner that will lead to client harm. Which is the most appropriate response?
    A. Step in and complete the dressing change for the learner.
    B. Stop the learner immediately and ask the learner to repeat the procedure.
    C. Say nothing since the learner's technique will not lead to client harm.
    D. Allow the learner to complete the dressing change and then review the proper technique.

Correct Answer: D

Rationale: The learner should be allowed to continue the procedure provided there is no harm to the client and appropriate principles are followed. After the procedure, the clinical nurse educator should talk with the learner about the learner's techniques and review the standard procedure, as in Option D. There can be multiple approaches to a dressing change procedure. As long as the learner's approach does not harm the client and adheres to principles of asepsis and standard nursing care, the learner can proceed with the dressing change (O'Connor, 2015). Options A and B are not necessary since appropriate care was provided. Option C does not allow the learner to review the procedure with the clinical nurse educator.

Test Blueprint: 2 E
Cognitive Code: Application

90. The clinical nurse educator and a learner approach a physician about a medication that was prescribed for the wrong client. Which is the next best action?
    A. Report the error using the agency's medication safety reporting system.
    B. Report the physician to the nursing supervisor.
    C. Continue with medication pass of the other medications.
    D. Do not report the situation since it did not impact the client.

    Correct Answer: A

    Rationale: One of the Quality and Safety Education for Nurses (QSEN) competencies for learners is safety. This competency suggests that there are skills that learners should possess related to safety. One of these skills is to use safety reporting systems for near misses and medication errors (QSEN, 2019). Although this error did not impact the client, it is considered a near miss and therefore should be reported, making Option A correct. Option B is incorrect because reporting the physician who performed the error does not necessarily allow the error to be prevented in the future. Options C and D are incorrect because they do not include reporting the error.

    Test Blueprint: 2 E
    Cognitive Code: Application

91. Which activity is the most effective way to teach learners about safety related to medication errors?
    A. Have all learners participate in a simulation in which medication errors occur.
    B. Discuss common medication errors during postclinical conference.
    C. Have learners submit a written assignment in which they discuss a medication error they observed.
    D. Have a learner discuss a personal encounter with a near-miss medication error in a postclinical conference

    Correct Answer: A

    Rationale: Simulation is an effective teaching-learning method for providing novice and experienced practitioners with learning opportunities related to safety and medication errors (Alden & Durham, 2017, p. 246). Option A is correct because it allows all learners to participate in learning activities and helps ensure that they are knowledgeable about safe medication administration. Options B, C, and D provide experiences to learn about safety but do not allow learners to have the opportunity to apply knowledge; therefore, these options are not the most effective teaching-learning approaches.

    Test Blueprint: 2 E
    Cognitive Code: Application

92. Which statement made by the clinical nurse educator best supports a culture of safety?
    A. "Client restraints need an order renewed every 24 hours."
    B. "Reporting errors and near misses is important to identifying system issues."
    C. "We need to be careful when administering high-risk medications."
    D. "You should check your monitor alarm limits every four hours."

    Correct Answer: B

Rationale: Option B denotes the clinical nurse educator's understanding of an integral part of the culture of safety, that is, reporting of errors and near misses to help identify and improve issues, not to blame individuals (American Nurses Association, 2019). Options A and D may be important to client safety but will depend on a variety of factors, including client acuity levels, unit and/or institutional policies, and device types; these options do not encompass a culture of safety so much as they outline individual safety measures. Option C, although important to client safety, is nonspecific and does not fully encompass the culture of safety.

Test Blueprint: 2 E
Cognitive Code: Analysis

93. Which teaching-learning approach would best create a positive learning environment for learners starting a new clinical rotation?
    A. Loosely structuring the first day of clinical learning experiences for new learners
    B. Planning a scavenger hunt on the new clinical unit prior to the first day of client care
    C. Using a preclinical conference to identify areas of weakness each learner should improve
    D. Assigning readings about agency-specific policies and procedures

Correct Answer: B

Rationale: Learners frequently perceive starting a new clinical rotation as a stressful event. Planning specific activities that allow learners to become familiar and comfortable with the clinical learning environment, such as the scavenger hunt offered in Option B, will help alleviate anxiety (Oermann et al., 2018, p. 69). Options A, C, and D are incorrect because they would not prepare learners for a new clinical rotation nor support a positive learning environment.

Test Blueprint: 2 F
Cognitive Code: Analysis

94. A new clinical nurse educator is frustrated because two learners in the clinical group are not performing at the expected level and are consuming a lot of the educator's time. Which is the best initial response by an experienced educator?
    A. "Did you share your observations with the lab educator? You can require additional lab learning time for practice activities."
    B. "You seem frustrated. Have you talked to the learners about your concerns?"
    C. "I don't understand the rush. We have many more weeks to get everything done."
    D. "Perhaps it would be best to transfer those two learners to another clinical group."

Correct Answer: B

Rationale: Nurse educators' commitment to learner success is crucial. At-risk learners need additional resources to support learning. Talking to the learners about the concerns, Option B, will allow the clinical nurse educator to assess the learners' needs. The clinical nurse educator also has the obligation to serve as an advocate for learners (O'Connor, 2015; Popkess & Frey, 2016, p. 22). Option A is not the best response initially; the first intervention should be to discuss the concerns with the learners and ascertain whether other barriers may be present. Options C and D do not demonstrate a clinical nurse educator's responsibility to support learner success and commitment to the program.

Test Blueprint: 2 F
Cognitive Code: Application

95. Which behavior by the clinical nurse educator would warrant intervention?
    A. Assisting learners with the prioritization of tasks
    B. Providing critical feedback to a learner at the nurses' station
    C. Giving learners their cell phone number for emergencies
    D. Providing the nursing staff with clinical course objectives

Correct Answer: B

Rationale: Feedback that is critical should be provided in a private and confidential setting. This feedback should not be delivered in a public forum—this is unprofessional behavior, making Option B inappropriate and the correct response as it warrants intervention (Bonnel, 2012, p. 498). Options A, C, and D are all appropriate behaviors and do not warrant correction.

Test Blueprint: 2 F
Cognitive Code: Application

96. A learner confides that another learner makes comments that are discriminatory. Which is the best initial response by the clinical nurse educator?
    A. Tell the learner to ignore the comments.
    B. Discuss the issue with the entire clinical group.
    C. Ask the learner to explain why the learner feels that the statements are discriminatory.
    D. Talk to the learner who made the comments.

Correct Answer: C

Rationale: Clinical nurse educators must provide a climate of mutual trust and respect (Oermann et al., 2018, p. 8). Option C allows the nurse educator to explore the comments and make evaluative decisions about how to proceed after hearing the learner's perspective. The clinical nurse educator is not being supportive by dismissing the learner's concerns, as in Option A. Discussing this issue with the entire group of learners, as in Option B, violates privacy and trust. Talking to the other learner, as in Option D, may be necessary; however, this should not be the initial response by the educator.

Test Blueprint: 2 F
Cognitive Code: Application

97. A learner reports having a negative interaction with a staff nurse on the clinical unit. Which is the best initial response by the clinical nurse educator?

A. "I'm sorry that you experienced this interaction. That usually does not happen."

B. "That situation was nothing compared to what can happen between staff members in practice."

C. "Tell me specifically what happened so we can determine what to do next."

D. "I will assign you to a different client so you can work with another staff nurse and have a better day."

Correct Answer: C

Rationale: Learning occurs through experience. Clinical nurse educators facilitate learning in the clinical setting (Oermann et al., 2018, p. 6). Option C provides the opportunity for the learner to describe the interaction and for the clinical nurse educator to gather more information; the clinical nurse educator can then discuss the situation and devise appropriate approaches with the learner. Options A and D do not address the problem and are not helpful in ensuring a positive learning environment. Option B implies a negative view of the practice environment, which should not be shared with learners; it also does nothing to help resolve the issue the learner confronted.

Test Blueprint: 2 F
Cognitive Code: Application

98. The clinical nurse educator notices that one of the learners is falling asleep during a postclinical conference discussion. Which is the best initial response by the clinical nurse educator?

A. Do nothing since this is the first time the learner fell asleep.

B. Stop the activity and ask to speak privately with the learner.

C. Point out to the other learners that someone is asleep.

D. Call on the learner to respond to a question related to the activity.

Correct Answer: D

Rationale: When a learner is distracting to others, it is important to address the issue (O'Connor, 2015); Option D engages the learner and attempts to prevent further distraction. Option A is incorrect because the behavior may continue throughout the course and this learner is not demonstrating appropriate professional behaviors. Options B and C publicly identify that there is a concern and are not the best ways to approach this situation.

Test Blueprint: 2 F
Cognitive Code: Application

99. The clinical nurse educator assigns a learner to a client with a complicated social history. The learner explains to the clinical nurse educator that the assigned client's social history conflicts with the learner's personal beliefs. Which is the best action for the clinical nurse educator?
   A. Inform the learner that a nonjudgmental approach is needed when providing client care.
   B. Allow the learner to change the client assignment since there is a conflict.
   C. Discuss the conflict with the charge nurse and ask for the agency policy regarding client assignments.
   D. Review the nursing program handbook regarding conflict of interest.

Correct Answer: A

Rationale: All learners should be treated fairly and be held to the same standards (Christensen, 2016, p. 39). Option A helps learners recognize that nonjudgmental care is an important professional practice component. Options B, C, and D may not indicate fair treatment and are not the best actions.

Test Blueprint: 2 F
Cognitive Code: Application

100. The clinical nurse educator notices that one learner does not actively participate and contribute to discussions during postclinical conference. Which is the best next action?
   A. Ask the learner to lead the next conference discussion.
   B. Call on the learner first during the next conference.
   C. Ask the learner to provide a written reflection about the clinical day.
   D. Talk to the learner privately about why the learner does not participate in conference discussions.

Correct Answer: D

Rationale: It is important to understand the reason that the learner in not participating in the discussion. Options A and B are strategies that may make some learners uncomfortable and thus are not the best next action. Option C might offer a different strategy; however, the reason the learner is not participating has not been identified. Only Option D allows the clinical nurse educator to explore the problem in a caring and positive way and understand the reasons that the learner is not participating before further actions are taken (O'Connor, 2015).

Test Blueprint: 2 F
Cognitive Code: Application

101. Which statement or question best demonstrates caring behaviors?
   A. "I understand you have things going on but you need to pay attention."
   B. "You have a blank stare, what questions do you have?"
   C. "You look very tired, are you prepared for your clinical experience today?"
   D. "You need to leave your problems at home, the client needs you."

Correct Answer: B

Rationale: Option B describes a question asked by a clinical nurse educator and is directed to a potentially confused learner. Instead of being accusatory, the educator notes the observed behavior, that is, a blank stare, and encourages the learner to ask questions in a nonthreatening manner (Killingsworth, 2019). In Options A and D, although the educator seems to acknowledge that the learner may be struggling in some way, the educator is accusatorily stating things, such as the learner "need[s] to pay attention." In Option C, the educator acknowledges that the learner may be tired; however, the educator also jumps immediately to suggesting that the learner may not be prepared for the clinical experience, which could be perceived as threatening by the learner.

Test Blueprint: 2 F
Cognitive Code: Application

102. A staff nurse preceptor informs the clinical nurse educator that the learner was rude during the day. Which is the best next action?
   A. Make an appointment with the learner the next day to discuss the issue.
   B. Tell the preceptor that the learner has been having a bad day.
   C. Pull the learner aside, tell the learner what the preceptor observed, and ask what happened.
   D. Ask the learner what happened at the end of the clinical day.

Correct Answer: C

Rationale: Feedback about learner performance should be provided at the time of learning or immediately after, as in Option C (Oermann et al., 2018, p. 259). Option C is also nonaccusatory and attempts to gain the learner's perspective. Options A and D are incorrect because they delay addressing the issue. Option B is incorrect because it does not address the problem and is also dismissive of the preceptor's concern; this could result in the preceptor not sharing other current and/or future concerns with the educator.

Test Blueprint: 2 F
Cognitive Code: Application

103. Which is the primary benefit of the dedicated education unit (DEU) model for clinical learning?
   A. Learners have opportunities to establish professional connections with nurse mentors on the unit.
   B. Learners can assume higher levels of autonomy by the end of the experience.
   C. Learners develop an improved personal relationship between themselves and the nurses on the unit.
   D. Clinical unit nurse mentors are more likely to pursue clinical specialty certifications.

Correct Answer: A

Rationale: Results of studies of DEUs suggest that learners on DEUs have consistent interactions with the unit staff, leading to closer bonds with the nurse mentors, as suggested in Option A (Rhodes, Meyers, & Underhill, 2012). Although the learners report a quality experience on a DEU, there is no evidence that learners are more autonomous because of time on the DEU, as suggested in Option B. Learners may develop professional relationships with nurses on the clinical unit, but there is no evidence to support their development of a personal relationship, as in Option C. Nurse mentors may be more likely to return for further education, but that is not the primary benefit for clinical learning, as in Option D.

Test Blueprint: 2 G
Cognitive Code: Recall

104. When meeting a new group of clinical learners, which initial action is most appropriate?
    A. Having learners complete a group introduction activity
    B. Sharing an outline of clinical course content
    C. Reviewing the assignments and explaining grading policies
    D. Describing clinical rules and agency policies

    Correct Answer: A

    Rationale: The clinical nurse educator should begin the experience by building relationships (Stokes & Kost, 2012). Team-building activities, as in Option A, will help learners develop relationships that can be beneficial during the clinical learning experience. Options B, C, and D are activities that may follow the introductory relationship-building activity.

    Test Blueprint: 2 G
    Cognitive Code: Application

105. Which best establishes trust between learners and clinical nurse educators?
    A. Discussing learner concerns with colleagues
    B. Encouraging learners to ask questions
    C. Relying on initial impressions when evaluating learner performance
    D. Sharing learners' mistakes during clinical conferences

    Correct Answer: B

    Rationale: Relational integrity is established through trusting relationships between clinical nurse educators and their learners. This trust is gained through learner empowerment, coaching, encouragement, and active listening, as in Option B (Adelman-Mullally et al., 2013, p. 32). Options A and D do not demonstrate a trusting relationship and inappropriately share information about a learner with others. Option C is incorrect because the clinical nurse educator should remain open to the learner performance and not judge a learner based on initial impressions.

    Test Blueprint: 2 G
    Cognitive Code: Application

106. Which would be the best example of collegial working relationships with clinical agency staff?
    A. Asking the unit manager at the clinical agency whether there is availability for learning experiences
    B. Providing the nursing staff with information about the course learning objectives and expectations
    C. Explaining that the learners will leave the clinical unit early when the nurse-to-client ratio is high
    D. Including only administrative and educational staff at the agency in planning clinical learning activities

    Correct Answer: B

Rationale: Providing specific information to nursing staff assists in cultivating collegial work relationships (Oermann et al., 2018, p. 48); therefore, Option B promotes a collaborative approach to clinical teaching and learning. Most nursing programs have a designated individual organizing clinical placements, not the specific clinical nurse educator or unit manager, making Option A incorrect. There is no reason to leave the clinical unit earlier than planned if the nurse-to-client ratio is high, as in Option C. Including nursing staff, those working directly with the learners, would be important to include in the planning process; Option D is incorrect because nursing staff are not included in the planning.

Test Blueprint: 2 G
Cognitive Code: Application

107. A clinical nurse educator observes a learner asking a question to a staff nurse. In response to the question, the staff nurse rolls their eyes at the learner. Which is the best response?
    A. Immediately confront the staff member.
    B. Instruct the learner to ignore the behavior.
    C. Remove the learners from the clinical unit.
    D. Hold a debriefing session with the learner.

    Correct Answer: D

    Rationale: Educators can hold debriefing sessions, listen to learners' perceptions, and make concerted efforts to balance learners' feelings and thoughts by using appropriate strategies to soften, yet not deny, the reality of the culture (Gubrud, 2016, p. 284). Options A, B, and C do not address listening to learner feelings and perceptions.

    Test Blueprint: 2 G
    Cognitive Code: Application

108. A staff nurse informs the clinical nurse educator about a problem with a learner. Which is the best initial response?
    A. Address the problem with the learner at the end of the clinical day.
    B. Discuss the problem with the learner and report back to the nurse.
    C. Review the problem with the clinical group during the post-conference discussion
    D. Ask the nurse to address the problem with learner.

    Correct Answer: B

    Rationale: The problem may impact quality and safety of client care, so it is important to discuss the issue with the learner. Informing the nurse about the issue resolution will guarantee that the nurse knows the concern was addressed (O'Connor, 2015, p. 376), as suggested in Option B. The problem may impact the client, thus it should be addressed immediately, making Option A incorrect. Learner issues should be kept confidential, making Option C inappropriate. The clinical nurse educator is responsible for the learner and should address the problem and not delegate this to the nurse, as in Option D.

    Test Blueprint: 2 G
    Cognitive Code: Application

109. A clinical nurse educator is reviewing charts with a learner at a nursing home clinical experience when they are approached by a staff member. The staff member is concerned about their client; the client choked earlier in the day and still has a hoarse voice. Which initial response is most appropriate?

A. "That does sound challenging. I am sorry you are having a rough day. We are busy with client care too."

B. "I am sure they are fine. Why don't you ask the doctor to order some throat numbing medication?"

C. "Tell me more about the client and the incident so I can help. This is a great learning opportunity for us."

D. "Well, did you get the problem resolved or will I need to drop everything from my busy schedule to come and help?"

Correct Answer: C

Rationale: Clinical nurse educators should demonstrate enthusiasm for teaching, learning, and nursing to help inspire and motivate learners (Killingsworth, 2019). In this scenario, a nursing home staff member has asked the clinical nurse educator for help with a client concern, turning to the educator for the educator's expertise. The educator, who is simply reviewing charts with a learner, should take the time to enthusiastically help the staff member reason through the issue, as in Option C, which will likely also inspire and motivate the learner. This action shows passion for teaching, learning, and nursing. Options A and B sound dismissive and are not helpful. Option D is accusatory. Moreover, Options A, B, and D do not demonstrate enthusiasm for teaching, learning, or nursing.

Test Blueprint: 2 H
Cognitive Code: Analysis

110. Learners are completing a one-day rotation in a health department as part of their community health clinical experience. Which statement made by the clinical nurse educator is least appropriate?

A. "A lot of your role today will be giving vaccines, so prepare for repetitive and mindless work."

B. "Make sure that all clients are aware of the services available to them at the health department."

C. "During your day today, see if you can determine what health issues are facing this community."

D. "Data monitoring is important to the role of a public health nurse."

Correct Answer: A

Rationale: Clinical nurse educators should demonstrate enthusiasm for teaching, learning, and nursing to help inspire and motivate learners (Killingsworth, 2019). In this scenario, the educator is discussing public health nursing. In Option A, although the learners may give vaccines during their rotation day, stating that this is "mindless work" is inappropriate and demeans the important role of the public health nurse; thus, this is an inappropriate statement and the correct response. Options B, C, and D are all appropriate statements, representing accurate and important roles of the public health nurse (American Public Health Association, 2013).

Test Blueprint: 2 H
Cognitive Code: Analysis

111. A clinical nurse educator has visited a clinical site to meet with a graduate learner who is completing the advanced nursing practicum experience. When meeting with the learner privately, the learner verbalizes frustration with "all this writing and paperwork" and states, "this is just busywork. It's not going to help me be a better nurse." Which is the most appropriate response?

A. "I know it's a lot. Stick with it and it'll be worth it when you complete the program and finish your degree."

B. "Well, why did you enter this program? Are you sure you want this degree? There will be lots of paperwork to do after you graduate."

C. "This is the nurse's responsibility to complete this important paperwork. How do you feel about doing all this paperwork?"

D. "I hear your frustration. Graduate school can be very challenging, but it can also be very exciting. Tell me more about your frustrations."

Correct Answer: D

Rationale: Clinical nurse educators should demonstrate enthusiasm for teaching, learning, and nursing to help inspire and motivate learners (Killingsworth, 2019). In this scenario, a graduate learner is frustrated with course assignments, which require a lot of writing. In Option D, the clinical nurse educator acknowledges the learner's feelings, but also verbalizes the excitement of learning new things. Additionally, the educator opens the door for more conversation by asking the learner to "tell [them] more," which could help the educator demonstrate enthusiasm and motivate the learner to enjoy learning and nursing. Option A is dismissive and does not help inspire the learner. Option B sounds accusatory and dismissive. Option C is inappropriate because the learner's feelings have already been stated, that is, that the work is "just busywork."

Test Blueprint: 2 H
Cognitive Code: Analysis

References

Adelman-Mullally, T., Mulder, C. K., McCarter-Spalding, D. E., Hagler, D. A., Gaberson, K. B., Hanner, M. B., ... Young, P. K. (2013). The clinical nurse educator as leader. *Nurse Education in Practice*, 13(1), 29–34. doi:10.1016/j.nepr.2012.07.006

Alden, K. R., & Durham, C. F. (2017). Integrating quality and safety competencies in simulation. In G. Sherwood & J. Barnsteiner (Eds.), *Quality and safety in nursing: A competency approach to improving outcomes* (2nd ed., pp. 233–252). Hoboken, NJ: Wiley & Sons.

American Nurses Association. (2019). Culture of safety. Retrieved from https://www.nursingworld.org/practice-policy/work-environment/health-safety/culture-of-safety/

American Public Health Association. (2013). *The definition and practice of public health nursing: A statement of the public health nursing section*. Washington, DC: Author.

Bandura, A. (1991). Social cognitive theory of self-regulation. *Organizational Behavior and Human Decision Processes, 50*, 248–287.

Benner, P., Sutphen, M., Leonard, V., & Day, L. (2010). *Educating nurses: A call for radical transformation*. San Francisco, CA: Jossey-Bass.

Berman, A., Snyder, S., & Frandsen, G. (2016). *Kozier & Erb's fundamentals of nursing: Concepts, process, and practice* (10th ed.). Boston, MA: Pearson.

Bonnel, W. (2012). Clinical performance evaluation. In D. M. Billings & J. A. Halstead (Eds.), *Teaching in nursing: A guide for faculty* (4th ed., pp. 485–502). St. Louis, MO: Elsevier.

Bradshaw, M., & Lowenstein, A. (2017). *Innovative teaching strategies in nursing and related health professions* (7th ed.). Burlington, MA: Jones and Bartlett Learning.

Candela, L. (2012). From teaching to learning: Theoretical foundations. In D. M. Billings & J. A. Halstead (Eds.), *Teaching in nursing: A guide for faculty* (4th ed., pp. 202–243). St. Louis, MO: Elsevier.

Candela, L. (2016). Theoretical foundations of teaching and learning. In D. M. Billings & J. A. Halstead (Eds.), *Teaching in nursing: A guide for faculty* (5th ed., pp. 211–229). St. Louis, MO: Elsevier.

Christensen, L. (2010). The law and disabilities: How the ADA affects nursing education. In L. Caputi (Ed.), *Teaching nursing: The art and science* (pp. 144–156). Glen Ellyn, IL: College of DuPage Press.

Christensen, L. (2016). The academic performance of students: Legal and ethical issues. In D. M. Billings & J. A. Halstead (Eds.), *Teaching in nursing: A guide for faculty* (5th ed., pp. 35–54). St. Louis, MO: Elsevier.

Cronenwett, L., Sherwood, G., Barnsteiner, J., Disch, J., Johnson, J., Mitchell, P., & Warren, J. (2007). Quality and safety education for nurses. *Nursing Outlook, 55*(3), 122–131.

DeYoung, S. (2015). *Teaching strategies for nurse educators* (3rd ed.). Upper Saddle River, NJ: Prentice Hall.

Dreifuerst, K. T. (2012). Using debriefing for meaningful learning to foster development of clinical reasoning in simulation. *Journal of Nursing Education, 51*(6), 326–333. doi:10.3928/01484834-20120409-02

Dreifuerst K., Horton-Deutsch, S., & Henao, H. (2014). Meaningful debriefing and other approaches. In P. Jefferies (Ed.), *Clinical simulations in nursing education: Advanced concepts, and trends* (pp. 44–57). Philadelphia, PA: Wolters Kluwer.

Forneris, S. G., & Fey, M. (2018). *Critical conversations: The NLN guide for teaching thinking.* Washington, DC: National League for Nursing.

Gardner, M. R., & Suplee, P. D. (2010). *Handbook of clinical teaching in nursing and health sciences.* Sudbury, MA: Jones and Bartlett.

Gubrud, P. (2016). Teaching in the clinical setting. In D. M. Billings & J. A. Halstead (Eds.), *Teaching in nursing: A guide for faculty* (5th ed., pp. 282–303). St. Louis, MO: Elsevier.

Halevi, G., Liu, A. C., & Yoon, J. H. (2018). Social media utilization by healthcare leaders. *Journal of Scientific Innovation in Medicine, 1*(1) 3–9.

Hayden, J., Smiley, R., Alexander, M. A., Kardong-Edgren, S., & Jeffries, P. (2014). The NCSBN national simulation study: A longitudinal, randomized, controlled study replacing clinical hours with simulation in prelicensure nursing education. *Journal of Nursing Regulation, 5*(2 Suppl), S3–S40.

Herman, J. W. (2016). *Creative teaching strategies for the nurse educator* (2nd ed.). Philadelphia, PA: F. A. Davis.

International Nursing Association for Clinical Simulation and Learning Standards Committee (2016a). INACSL standards of best practice: Simulation^{SM} debriefing. *Clinical Simulation in Nursing, 12,* S21–S25. doi:10.1016/j.ecns.2016.09.008

International Nursing Association for Clinical Simulation and Learning Standards Committee. (2016b). INACSL standards of best practice: Simulation ^{SM} design. *Clinical Simulation in Nursing, 12,* S5–S12.

Jeffries, P. R., Swoboda, S. M., & Akintade, B. (2016). Teaching and learning using simulations. In D. M. Billings & J. A. Halstead (Eds.), *Teaching in nursing: A guide for faculty* (5th ed., pp. 159–185). St. Louis, MO: Elsevier.

Johnson, C., & Blakely, K. (2019). Enhancing advanced practice nursing students' verbal patient report skills. *Journal of Nursing Education, 58*(1), 62. doi:10.3928/01484834-20190103-12

Killingsworth, E. (2019). Facilitate learning in the health care environment. In T. Shellenbarger (Ed.), *Clinical nurse educator competencies: Creating an evidence-based practice for academic clinical nurse educators* (pp. 21–38). Washington, DC: National League for Nursing.

Labrague, L. J., & McEnroe, P. D. M. (2017). An integrative review on conflict management styles among nursing students: Implications for nurse education. *Nurse Education Today, 59*, 45–52. doi:10.1016/j.nedt.2017.09.001

Lanz, A. S., & Wood, F. G. (2018). Communicating patient status: Comparison of teaching strategies in prelicensure nursing education. *Nurse Educator, 43*(3), 162–165.

Niederriter, J. E., Eyth, D., & Thoman, J. (2017). Nursing students' perceptions on characteristics of an effective clinical instructor. *Sage Open Nursing.* doi:10.1177/237796081665571

O'Connor, A. B. (2015). *Clinical instruction and evaluation: A teaching resource* (3rd ed.). Burlington, MA: Jones and Bartlett.

Oermann, M. H. (1997). Evaluating critical thinking in clinical practice. *Nurse Educator, 22*(5), 25–28.

Oermann, M. H., & Gaberson, K. B. (2017). *Evaluation and testing in nursing education* (5th ed.). New York, NY: Springer.

Oermann, M. H., Shellenbarger, T., & Gaberson, K. (2018). *Clinical teaching strategies in nursing* (5th ed.). New York, NY: Springer.

Paul, R., & Elder, L. (2008). Critical thinking: The art of Socratic questioning, part III. *Journal of Developmental Education, 31*(3), 34–35.

Phillips, J. M. (2016). Strategies to promote student engagement and active learning. In D. M. Billings & J. A. Halstead (Eds.), *Teaching in nursing: A guide for faculty* (5th ed., pp. 245–262). St. Louis, MO: Elsevier.

Popkess, A. M., & Frey, J. L. (2016). Strategies to support diverse learning needs of students. In D. M. Billings & J. A. Halstead (Eds.), *Teaching in nursing: A guide for faculty* (5th ed., pp. 15–34). St. Louis, MO: Elsevier.

Quality and Safety Education for Nurses Institute. (2019). QSEN competencies. Retrieved from http://qsen.org/competencies/pre-licensure-ksas/

Reedy, G. B. (2015). Using cognitive load theory to inform simulation design and practice. *Clinical Simulation in Nursing, 11*(8), 355–360.

Rhodes, M. L., Meyers, C. C., & Underhill, M. L. (2012). Evaluating outcomes of a dedicated education unit in a baccalaureate nursing program. *Journal of Professional Nursing, 28*(4), 223–230. doi:10.1016/j.profnurs.2011.11.019

Scheckel, M. (2016). Designing courses and learning experiences. In D. M. Billings & J. A. Halstead (Eds.), *Teaching in nursing: A guide for faculty* (5th ed., pp. 159–185). St. Louis, MO: Elsevier.

Stokes, L. G., & Kost, G. C. (2012). Teaching in the clinical setting. In D. M. Billings & J. A. Halstead (Eds.), *Teaching in nursing: A guide for faculty* (4th ed., pp. 311–334). St. Louis, MO: Elsevier.

Sullivan, D. T. (2016). An introduction to curriculum development. In D. M. Billings & J. A. Halstead (Eds.), *Teaching in nursing: A guide for faculty* (5th ed., pp. 89–117). St. Louis, MO: Elsevier.

5

Demonstrate Effective Interpersonal Communication and Collaborative Interprofessional Relationships

1. Upon arriving to the clinical unit, the clinical nurse educator is approached with a list of clients to assign to learners. The charge nurse states that the clients are "high-maintenance and high-acuity" and assigning learners to their care will help staff on the unit. Which is the best response?
   A. "Thank you for helping me assign the learners. You know the clients best, so I will use these assignments with learners today."
   B. "Thanks, but I am responsible for selecting clients for learners to provide care and I have my own process for this decision-making."
   C. "Thank you—can we review the list together? I want to make sure these assignments consider our learning outcomes, learning needs, and client needs."
   D. "Thanks, but I usually just get the list of clients and their diagnoses so that my learners can just choose who they would like."

Correct Answer: C

Rationale: There are many options for creating learning assignments; the clinical nurse educator should use a flexible yet robust process when selecting care opportunities. Option C uses the help offered from the nursing staff member who has provided care to these clients. In working with this staff member, the educator can best determine how learning needs and client needs can be met. Options A, B, and D all miss a key component that should be considered by the educator, such as learning objectives; needs of clients; availability and variety of learning opportunities; and the needs, interests, and abilities of learners (Oermann, Shellenbarger, & Gaberson, 2018, pp. 152–155).

Test Blueprint: 3 A
Cognitive Code: Analysis

2. Which strategy best promotes collaboration and teamwork?
   A. Have learners observe interactions that occur on the unit.
   B. Assign a written case study that involves learner collaboration.
   C. When a collaboration experience arises on the clinical unit, have learners participate.
   D. Establish a working relationship with agency staff to plan learning experiences.

Correct Answer: D

Rationale: Clinical nurse educators play an intricate role in facilitating interpersonal relationships on the clinical unit. Clinical nurse educators should plan for experiences by establishing trusting relationships with agency staff, which creates collaboration opportunities between learners and health care personnel (Fressola & Patterson, 2017, p. 121). Therefore, Option D is the correct response. Option A allows only for observation and does not provide the best opportunity for learning this concept. Option B relies on independent learning and learner collaboration and does not provide practice or guidance in development of collaboration or teamwork skills. Option C does not foster collaborative experiences; instead, learners must wait for opportunities to arise.

Test Blueprint: 3 A
Cognitive Code: Application

3. A learner is caring for a client whose respiratory status has declined in the last hour. Which statement made to the learner best supports appropriate communication within the health care team?
   A. "I think we need a new plan of care and daily goal for this client."
   B. "There needs to be more communication from the respiratory therapist to prevent this."
   C. "We should suggest a brief provider meeting to discuss the plan of care."
   D. "We will notify the respiratory therapist regarding the client's status."

Correct Answer: C

Rationale: Option C encourages frequent, respectful, and open communication with all members of the health care team (Lundeen, 2019) by involving all members in a meeting to discuss the plan of care after the change in client status. Option A may be true, but the statement itself does not encourage team communication, as it is occurring only between the nurse educator and the learner. Option B is accusatory and is not respectful of the respiratory health care team member. Option D encourages communication with one member of the team but involves one-way communication.

Test Blueprint: 3 A
Cognitive Code: Analysis

4. A clinical nurse educator wants to enhance interprofessional learning through assignments in a nursing clinical course. Which assignment or activity best helps learners understand the value of collaboration?
   A. Writing a one-page paper on the interprofessional education competencies and the importance for nursing
   B. Developing a learning module on interprofessional education competencies and having the learners discuss this information in their reflective journals
   C. Assigning learners to observe a clinical situation with various health care professionals and having them complete a reflective journal
   D. Observing a certified nursing assistant work with a client to perform activities of daily living (ADLs)

Correct Answer: C

Rationale: Interprofessional collaboration and coordination of care is vital for nursing and health care. Option C provides learners with opportunities to understand the importance of collaboration in the clinical environment. The reflective writing activity can provide the learner with support and additional knowledge to recognize the interprofessional competencies and behaviors (Vogelsang & Bergen, 2018). The experience of observing a situation and then reflecting on it allows the learner to grow in confidence to collaborate and work in an interprofessional team. Options A, B, and D do not provide opportunities to explore the value of collaboration but rather focus only on knowledge associated with collaboration.

Test Blueprint: 3 A
Cognitive Code: Application

5. A learner expresses uncertainty about the appropriate diet for a client with heart failure. Which best supports a shared learning environment?
   A. Reviewing the heart failure diet in postclinical conference
   B. Arranging for the learner to meet with a nutritionist
   C. Assigning the learner to look up the diet on the agency's client education Intranet site
   D. Locating the heart failure diet video for the learner to review

Correct Answer: B

Rationale: A shared learning environment provides opportunities for learners to gain knowledge from additional health care professionals. Option B allows for the learner to gain new insight into the heart failure diet by working with a nutritionist to better understand the diet; a shared learning environment also allows for the learner to learn more about the roles and responsibilities of the nutritionist. This is an essential component of interprofessional competency for collaborative practice, including recognizing one's limitations in skills, knowledge, and abilities (Oermann et al., 2018, p. 220). Options A, C, and D do not promote shared learning since they are isolated activities.

Test Blueprint: 3 B
Cognitive Code: Application

6. Which action best demonstrates development and maintenance of collegial working relationships with clinical agency personnel?
   A. When making learner assignments, ask staff for brief suggestions about which clients on the unit may be appropriate to assign to learners.
   B. Allow the charge nurse to make learner assignments since the charge nurse will be the most knowledgeable about client acuity.
   C. Share information with the nursing staff about learners' progress thus far in the course, including clinical performance evaluations.
   D. Encourage learners to avoid the charge nurse since the charge nurse is busy with management activities on the unit.

Correct Answer: A

Rationale: Developing collegial working relationships with clinical agency personnel can promote a positive learning environment (National League for Nursing, 2012). Option A is correct in that this simple act of communication is one way to build a trusting, supportive relationship with the staff on the unit. Nursing staff can be very helpful in guiding decision-making about learner assignments and can offer suggestions about which clients will align with learning needs (Gubrud, 2016). Option B is incorrect since the clinical nurse educators should oversee making learner assignments. Option C violates the Family Educational Rights and Privacy Act (FERPA). Option D is incorrect; learners should know who the charge nurse is in case assignments need to be revised or they need assistance when educators are not available (Gubrud, 2016); learners should not avoid the charge nurse.

Test Blueprint: 3 B
Cognitive Code: Application

7. Which action will most likely cause learner distrust?
   A. Reviewing the clinical evaluation tool during orientation
   B. Waiting until the end of the clinical rotation to provide feedback to learners
   C. Sharing an experience when the clinical nurse educator made a medication error
   D. Telling learners that during the shift they will be questioned about client care

Correct Answer: B

Rationale: Waiting until the end of a course to provide feedback, as suggested in Option B, may make the learner uneasy and does not provide time for the learner to modify performance, thereby contributing to distrust (Niederriter, Eyth, & Thoman, 2017). Feedback should be provided frequently. When a clinical nurse educator shares one's past mistakes, as in Option C, it may help learners to connect with the clinical nurse educator. Reviewing the evaluation tool during orientation, as in Option A, and letting learners know that they will be questioned about their client and plan of care, as in Option D, communicates expectations clearly, favorably impacting trust in the clinical environment.

Test Blueprint: 3 B
Cognitive Code: Application

8. Which action by the clinical nurse educator best demonstrates teamwork and collaboration?
   A. Answering a client's call bell
   B. Assigning learners to as many clients as possible
   C. Volunteering for learners to complete all client baths
   D. Offering to administer medications for a nurse who is especially busy

Correct Answer: A

Rationale: The clinical nurse educator should seek opportunities to collaborate with members of the health care team. Option A allows the clinical nurse educator to assist the team, thus promoting teamwork. Options B and D are not appropriate because they are beyond the clinical nurse educator's role on the unit. Option C is not appropriate because learning assignments should match learning outcomes; clinical assignments should be selected according to the learning objectives (Oermann et al., 2018, p. 122).

Test Blueprint: 3 B
Cognitive Code: Application

9. Which learner action best demonstrates effective delegation skills?
   A. Asking another learner for help turning a client
   B. Asking the nursing aide to record client intake and output
   C. Trading tasks with another learner in the clinical group
   D. Taking a client's temperature at the request of the primary nurse

Correct Answer: B

Rationale: Nurses need to know both the theory and skill of delegation: what to delegate, to whom, and under what circumstances (Oermann et al., 2018, p. 23). Option B is an appropriate learner action demonstrating effective delegation skills. Options A and C do not involve delegation. In Option D, the learner is not the person delegating tasks.

Test Blueprint: 3 C
Cognitive Code: Application

10. Which self-directed learning activity best helps learners refine interprofessional communication skills and collaborative abilities?
   A. Using an instructional medium that depicts client scenarios and models care of multiple clients
   B. Listening to audio files about overcoming communication barriers as a member of the interprofessional health care team
   C. Viewing a recorded simulation with peer nursing learners that focuses on the electronic health record and medication administration system
   D. Practicing with a virtual simulation session that involves reporting clinical findings to advanced practice providers

Correct Answer: D

Rationale: Self-directed learning activities—such as instructional media, audio files, simulation, computer-aided instruction, and virtual reality—may be used by the clinical nurse educator to meet outcomes of the course. These activities should be consistent with expected outcomes of the clinical course and competencies and chosen to meet specific learning needs (Oermann et al., 2018, p. 172), in this case, to improve interprofessional communication skills. Option D is the only self-directed learning activity that meets the learning goal of improving interprofessional communication; it allows the learner to practice the collaboration and communication skills.

Test Blueprint: 3 C
Cognitive Code: Application

11. Which learning activity best develops teamwork skills?
   A. Participating in a simulation to engage in interprofessional skills
   B. Shadowing and observing a leader to identify leadership skills
   C. Writing a paper to discuss various health care roles
   D. Role-modeling teamwork behaviors for learners to observe

Correct Answer: A

Rationale: Clinical nurse educators must not only possess the clinical skills necessary to be a nurse but also need to be able to assist learners in comprehending nursing concepts and implementing professional skills, such as teamwork skills. Learning activities can assist learners in achieving the objectives and outcomes for each course (Fressola & Patterson, 2017). The clinical nurse educator can best prepare nursing learners for a teamwork environment through practice, such as during a simulation; therefore, Option A is the correct response. Options B, C, and D could also be activities to prepare learners for a teamwork environment; however, they do not allow for active engagement in the skill development.

Test Blueprint: 3 C
Cognitive Code: Analysis

12. After interprofessional rounding with learners, which activity would be best to foster development?
    A. Reviewing the different roles of the health care team
    B. Evaluating the learners' performance using a summative approach
    C. Critiquing the composition of the health care team members
    D. Debriefing with learners to reflect on the experience

    Correct Answer: D

    Rationale: Following this activity, it is imperative that the clinical nurse educator debrief with the learners to discuss their experience (Oermann et al., 2018). Therefore, Option D would be the best choice. Option A would be an appropriate activity before the interprofessional rounding occurs. Option C does not require the learner to gain knowledge about rounding activities; rather, it requires only a critique of team composition and not actions. The question does not ask about the evaluation approach needed but is asking about the learning activity; therefore, Option B would be incorrect.

    Test Blueprint: 3 C
    Cognitive Code: Analysis

13. Which learning activity would best help learners develop interprofessional collaboration and team-building skills?
    A. Administering medications during a simulation scenario
    B. Observing a unit huddle with the nurse manager and staff
    C. Completing a reflective journal about care provided to the client
    D. Participating in interdisciplinary care conference for the learner's assigned client

    Correct Answer: D

    Rationale: Learners should have opportunities to develop an understanding of interprofessional and collaborative care. Option D is correct because members of the health care team will participate in an interdisciplinary care conference related to the learner's assigned client. Options A and C do not expose the learner to other members of the health care team. Option B includes only nursing staff and not other members of the health care team (Oermann et al., 2018).

    Test Blueprint: 3 C
    Cognitive Code: Application

14. Which learning activity would best assist the learner to understand interprofessional roles in the clinical setting?
 A. Journal reflection on the health care team roles
 B. Medication review assignment that identifies pharmacist roles
 C. Self-learning module addressing interprofessional roles
 D. Role-play activity where learners assume roles of the health care team

Correct Answer: D

Rationale: Role play is an effective approach in which individuals can assume the roles of others (Phillips, 2016, p. 251). Although Options A, B, and C allow the learner to address the roles of the health care team, role play actively engages the learner in the experience and can include opportunity for debriefing and further discussions, thus making Option D correct (Phillips, 2016, p. 251).

Test Blueprint: 3 C
Cognitive Code: Application

15. Which simulation scenario would provide the best opportunity to develop interprofessional collaboration skills in the clinical setting?
 A. Client recovering from an acute myocardial infarction, needing the learner to call the pharmacist regarding the client's medications
 B. Client recovering from a cerebral vascular accident (CVA) who is being prepared for discharge
 C. Client admitted with uncontrolled atrial fibrillation that requires the learner to call the physician for orders for care
 D. Client admitted with pneumonia who is receiving respiratory treatments

Correct Answer: B

Rationale: The clinical nurse educator should create learning opportunities to collaborate with other members of the health care team (National League for Nursing, 2018). Options A, C, and D may require interactions with other health care team members, but they do not provide opportunities to discuss the client's care and collaborate with another professionals in care decision-making. Option B allows the learner to include multiple disciplines when preparing the client for discharge.

Test Blueprint: 3 C
Cognitive Code: Application

16. Which clinical learning activity best encourages interprofessional collaboration and relationships?
 A. Asking a respiratory therapist to administer an as-needed breathing treatment
 B. Providing a nursing change-of-shift report
 C. Developing a client turn schedule with the nursing assistant
 D. Participation in interprofessional rounds with debriefing

Correct Answer: D

Rationale: Option D is a recommended teaching-learning activity for interprofessional education, including developing interprofessional collaboration and relationships (Speakman, 2016). Option A may be an important client care task with another health care discipline but does not represent collaboration and development of interprofessional relationships. Although valuable learning activities, Options B and C are not interprofessional in that they involve only nursing professionals.

Test Blueprint: 3 C
Cognitive Code: Application

17. A newly diagnosed diabetic client is struggling to administer insulin. The clinical nurse educator suggests that the learner consider options to support confidence in the client. Which learner action best demonstrates that learning occurred?
    A. The learner reviews the steps with the client and provides handouts.
    B. The learner works with a medical learner to develop and implement a teaching plan for the client and asks the client to restate the information after the teaching.
    C. The learner plays a DVD to the client prior to reviewing the steps and then asks whether the client has any questions.
    D. The learner asks the client whether the spouse would consider administering the insulin for the client.

    Correct Answer: B

    Rationale: Interprofessional teams can work together to implement the teach-back method for clients and aid in interprofessional collaboration and promote client learning (Oermann et al., 2018, p. 228). Option B shows that learning occurred since the learner sought help from a medical learner in formulating a plan to enhance the client's understanding to administer insulin by using the teach-back method. Using handouts, DVDs, or involving others in care does not show that the learning that has occurred; therefore, Options A, C, and D are not the best response.

    Test Blueprint: 3 C
    Cognitive Code: Analysis

18. The clinical nurse educator is working alongside learners on a medical-surgical floor when the interprofessional team starts rounding. Which action would best promote collaborative practice?
    A. Discuss with learners the importance of being part of collaborative practice.
    B. Seek out the nurse manager to see whether learners can observe the interprofessional team round on the next clinical day.
    C. Encourage learners to stay out of the way so that the interprofessional team members can complete their rounds quickly.
    D. Encourage learners to actively listen and participate when the team rounds on their clients.

    Correct Answer: D

    Rationale: The clinical nurse educator should promote opportunities for learners to collaborate with members of the interprofessional team so that they can learn from the various professionals of the health care team. Option D reinforces the importance of collaborative practice through participation in interprofessional rounding. Interprofessional rounding occurs on almost every floor daily and can provide an avenue to correlate bedside rounding with various health care professionals (Oermann et al., 2018, p. 226). Option A does not allow for participation in interprofessional practice and collaboration. The clinical nurse educator would not need to seek manager approval, Option B, to allow learners to engage in this activity. Suggesting that learners stay away from the interprofessional team, as in Option C, denies learners the opportunity to engage in this vital learning experience.

Test Blueprint: 3 C
Cognitive Code: Application

19. A learner was caring for a client who had a cardiac arrest. Learners from respiratory therapy and pharmacy were also present during the code. How could the clinical nurse educator best support all of the learners?
    A. Ask the learners whether the clinical nurse educator could contact their educators.
    B. Ask whether all of the learners would like to go to the conference room to discuss the code.
    C. Inform the learners that the code is over and they can go back to their departments.
    D. Encourage the nursing learner to lead a discussion about the code.

Correct Answer: B

Rationale: Since several learners from various disciplines were present for the code, the clinical nurse educator shows respect for all of the learners by offering to debrief with them about the code. A collaborative debriefing session would allow for every learner to learn from the observations of the others, helping lay the foundation for collaborative practice. The clinical nurse educator thus creates an opportunity for various learners to learn about and reflect on being part of a team (Oermann et al., 2018, p. 223). Option B is the best way to incorporate this collaborative practice. Options A and C ignore the need to debrief and discuss the events. Option D does not allow for an equal opportunity for all learners and assumes that the nursing learner can lead a discussion about a code though potentially not prepared to do so.

Test Blueprint: 3 C
Cognitive Code: Application

20. Which action best enhances collaboration?
    A. Providing resources and information about the various health care professionals in the agency for the learner to review
    B. Reaching out to other schools of nursing to see whether they have a unit preference for clinical experiences
    C. Arranging for a postclinical experience cooperative learning activity with other schools of nursing about psychiatric mental health disorders
    D. Assigning the learners to various observation experiences in the agency throughout the clinical rotation

Correct Answer: C

Rationale: The clinical nurse educator should foster multiple opportunities to collaborate with other members of the health care team. Option C allows for an opportunity to learn, collaborate, and work together to enhance learning. A cooperative learning activity can help with shared learning and interactions for learners and clinical nurse educators (Waldron, Washington, & Montague, 2016). The cooperative learning activity can also provide a safe environment for learning and allow the learner to grow in communication and working collaboratively. Option A does not actively engage the learner in collaborative activities. Option B—although it uses communication with other nursing schools—does not enhance collaboration, as there is no joint discussion or problem-solving. While Option D does expose learners to various areas throughout the agency, it does not necessarily involve collaboration.

Test Blueprint: 3 C
Cognitive Code: Application

21. When arriving at a code, the lead physician tells a learner to move out of the way so that someone who knows what to do can start chest compressions. Which is the best response?
    A. Ask the learner to step outside of the room until the code has been resolved.
    B. Inform the physician that this is a time for learning and the learner can stay in the room.
    C. Instruct the learner to relieve the individual doing chest compressions after three cycles.
    D. Suggest to staff that the learner can assist in chest compressions to relieve them.

Correct Answer: D

Rationale: Working collaboratively within a code situation can be very stressful. However, the clinical nurse educator can inform staff of the learner's abilities to assist in the code situation; this helps to establish the learner's role in the situation (Oermann et al., 2018, p. 219). Option D allows for the physician and code team to recognize that the learner is able to help and work within the team. Option A discounts the learner's knowledge and skills. During an emergency, it is not the time to engage in a verbal discussion and make demands about learner opportunities; thus, Option B is not the best response. Option C does not demonstrate effective collaborative and teamwork skills; rather, it puts the learner in an uncomfortable position during an already stressful situation.

Test Blueprint: 3 D
Cognitive Code: Analysis

22. Which learner behavior is considered uncivil and warrants intervention?
    A. Participating in group assignments during clinical learning activities
    B. Asking to turn in a clinical assignment late because of a personal emergency
    C. Not raising a hand to answer questions during postclinical conference
    D. Loudly debating with the clinical nurse educator about a test item

Correct Answer: D

Rationale: Incivility is considered speech or action that is rude or disrespectful (Luparell, 2011). Option A represents appropriate behavior because the learner is cooperating and engaging in group activities. Option B, while inconvenient, does not demonstrate uncivil behavior—the learner requested the extension due to an emergent issue. Postclinical conferences may involve informal discussion among the group and may not require learners to raise their hands when they want to contribute, making Option C an appropriate behavior. Loudly debating with a clinical nurse educator, as in Option D, does not demonstrate professional respect and illustrates incivility.

Test Blueprint: 3 D
Cognitive Code: Application

23. Which learner behavior would require the clinical nurse educator to intervene immediately?
    A. Borrowing a stethoscope from a staff member
    B. Using a cell phone while on the clinical unit
    C. Engaging in a personal conversation with another leaner during postclinical conference
    D. Making a verbal threat to another learner

    Correct Answer: D

    Rationale: An act of incivility is a form of disrespect to others (Oermann et al., 2018, p. 100). Options B, C, and D display incivility behaviors that should be addressed; however, the question seeks the behavior needing to be addressed immediately. Therefore, Option D is the correct response since it is a serious concern that demands immediate attention. Option A suggests that the learner may be unprepared for the clinical experience but it is not an uncivil behavior, nor does it demand immediate intervention by the clinical nurse educator.

    Test Blueprint: 3 D
    Cognitive Code: Analysis

24. Which is the most effective approach for the clinical nurse educator to manage incivility on a new clinical unit?
    A. Discuss behavioral expectations prior to the first day on the clinical unit.
    B. Address incivility incidences in a timely manner.
    C. Provide remediation following an incivility incident.
    D. Give a written warning to a learner after an incivility incident.

    Correct Answer: A

    Rationale: The most effective way to address incivility is through prevention (Oermann et al., 2018, p. 101). Therefore, discussing behavioral expectations at the beginning of a new clinical course is the most effective strategy, making Option A the correct response. Option B states to manage incivility in a timely manner. This is not a specific approach that would manage incivility effectively. Options C and D are strategies that can occur based on the institution's policies. The key aspect involves prevention, which eliminates Options B, C, and D.

    Test Blueprint: 3 D
    Cognitive Code: Application

25. How can a clinical nurse educator best foster a culture of civility when managing a clinical group?
   A. Establish a chain of command in the group with the clinical nurse educator at the top and learners at the bottom.
   B. Assign learners to watch a video about incivility and have them turn in an essay summarizing main points.
   C. Create and communicate clear guidelines for expectations regarding preparation, behavior, and attendance.
   D. Empathize with learners regarding their stressors and allow them to decide what they want to accomplish daily.

Correct Answer: C

Rationale: The most effective approach to managing incivility focuses on prevention (Oermann et al., 2018, p. 112). Prevention is rooted in communicating clear expectations. Option C reflects this while the other options are overly harsh and do not foster a culture of civility.

Test Blueprint: 3 D
Cognitive Code: Application

26. During a group debriefing session after a simulation scenario, two learners are having a separate conversation that is disrupting the group discussion. Which is the most appropriate initial response by the clinical nurse educator?
   A. "Do you have a question about the scenario?"
   B. "Don't you know that talking while others are talking is rude?"
   C. "That's enough. Stop talking."
   D. "Can you recall what your classmate just said?"

Correct Answer: A

Rationale: Debriefing after simulation should be presented in a nonjudgmental environment (Jeffries, Swoboda, & Akintade, 2016, p. 315). Option A is the only response that addresses the issue without sounding judgmental. Options B, C, and D are incorrect because they are judgmental and could be perceived as threatening; these options are not conducive to a supportive learning environment.

Test Blueprint: 3 D
Cognitive Code: Application

27. A staff nurse begins to use profanity and complains about a client's family when providing a report to a learner and educator. Which is the best response?
   A. Agree with the staff nurse and later explain that the nurse's language was inappropriate.
   B. Ignore the staff nurse's language and address it only if the learner asks.
   C. Ask the staff nurse to stop using profanity while giving a report.
   D. Report the staff nurse to the nurse manager after leaving for the day.

Correct Answer: C

Rationale: The clinical nurse educator serves as a role model to learners. In this situation, the clinical nurse educator needs to address the inappropriate behavior. Option C allows the clinical nurse educator to role model appropriate communication skills. Options A, B, and D do not role model appropriate behavior. The situation should also be discussed with the learners (Gardner & Suplee, 2010, p. 10).

Test Blueprint: 3 E
Cognitive Code: Analysis

28. A group of learners witnesses a medication error on a clinical unit, describing the nurse's actions as incompetent and lazy. When discussing the error with the learners, which response is best?
   A. "When errors occur, we must first ensure the client's safety, followed by an investigation of the cause of the errors."
   B. "What do you think went wrong and what should the nurse manager do about this?"
   C. "The staff nurse was unskilled and unprofessional today, and you should never act in such a manner."
   D. "We are not to discuss what happened today. As guests in the agency, it is not our responsibility to get involved."

Correct Answer: A

Rationale: Clinical nurse educators should display positive role modeling in attempting to direct learners to perform similar acts. If a medication error occurs, acknowledging the error and promoting reflection, safety, and quality improvement efforts is a display of positive role modeling versus acting or responding in a punitive manner (Adelman-Mullally et al., 2013). Therefore, Option A is correct. Option B presents questions to the learners; however, it may not be the best choice for a first response because client safety should be the priority. Option C would be considered a negative response in which the clinical nurse educator would be acting as a negative role model. Option D avoids a valuable learning experience and reflection and ignores professional responsibility.

Test Blueprint: 3 E
Cognitive Code: Application

29. The clinical nurse educator is developing a clinical conference concerning the use of therapeutic communication and wants the learners to provide examples of a nonjudgmental attitude. Which statement best displays a nonjudgmental attitude?
   A. "Clients with addictions never want to get better. They are here seeking more drugs."
   B. "All elderly clients have dementia and will not be able to live alone since they are confused."
   C. "Clients readmitted with congestive heart failure may need assistance when managing their salt intake."
   D. "Clients who are discharged against medical advice do not want to get better. There is nothing we can do if a client makes this decision."

Correct Answer: C

Rationale: A nonjudgmental statement does not reflect a person's opinions, personal views, or values (Folh, 2016). A nonjudgmental attitude is displayed in Option C. Options A, B, and D display a judgmental attitude of specific client populations.

Test Blueprint: 3 E
Cognitive Code: Analysis

30. A learner meets a client and family member for the first time at the beginning of the shift. The family member appears uncomfortable and starts anxiously moving about in the chair. Which is the best initial response?
A. Ignore the client's family member and encourage the learner to continue.
B. Ask the client's family member whether there are any questions or concerns.
C. Remind the family member that the learner is there to care for the family member and to assist the nurse.
D. Encourage the family member to step outside until the assessment is completed.

Correct Answer: B

Rationale: Communication is vital when working with clients and their family members. Option B addresses the family member's nonverbal behavior and allows the family members to ask questions. Asking the family members if they have questions allows them to feel a sense of empowerment and allows an opportunity for the learner and clinical nurse educator to listen to their concerns (Chan, 2017). This approach creates an environment that supports effective communication, builds rapport between the learner and the client's family member, and shows respect. Options A, C, and D do not involve the family member in the care nor engage the family member as a concerned part of the health care team.

Test Blueprint: 3 E
Cognitive Code: Analysis

31. Which clinical nurse educator action best demonstrates appropriate role modeling?
A. Administering medications for a client when their nurse is off the unit for a staff development training
B. Providing feedback to staff nurses that encourages them for doing a good job
C. Giving learners space to initiate conversations with clients to encourage independence
D. Holding the hand of an anxious preoperative client while the learner completes the preoperative checklist

Correct Answer: D

Rationale: Clinical nurse educators should model professional behaviors for the learners. Option D highlights an opportunity for the clinical nurse educator to offer compassion and interact with a client who needs additional support prior to surgery. The provision of holistic care and interaction by the clinical nurse educator can help establish professional behaviors of respect (Gibbs & Kulig, 2017). Role modeling is necessary for learners to observe from the clinical nurse educator to reinforce professional behaviors. It would be inappropriate for the clinical nurse educator to assume the staff nurse role and administer medications while staff are off the unit, thus making Option

A incorrect. Providing staff feedback and encouragement may help build positive relationships; however, since the feedback in Option B is nonspecific, it is not a good example of role modeling. Option C does provide learners with a learning opportunity, but does not demonstrate role modeling by the clinical nurse educator.

Test Blueprint: 3 E
Cognitive Code: Application

32. The clinical nurse educator finds out that a learner incorrectly documented client vital signs in the electronic health record. Although the error has been corrected, the charge nurse states that it almost led to significant changes in the client's plan of care. Which is the best initial action for the clinical nurse educator?
    A. Immediately remove the learner from the clinical unit, document the error on the clinical evaluation tool, and send the learner home.
    B. Call the client's physician to apologize for the error and discuss how the learner will be reprimanded.
    C. Bring the learner to a private location to discuss the documentation error, providing opportunities for reflection, formative feedback, and development of an improvement plan.
    D. Discuss the error in clinical conference with all learners and inform learners that medications will no longer be given while at this agency.

Correct Answer: C

Rationale: Clinical teaching requires an educator who relates effectively to learners and role models important professional behaviors, including respect through honest and direct communication. Option C provides an opportunity for effective clinical evaluation in which the educator is giving performance feedback to the learner with suggestions on improving performance in a safe and collaborative manner (Oermann et al., 2018, pp. 325–327). Option A implements punitive action without creating an environment in which the learner can share an account of the issue. Options B and D are not respectful of the learner, they do not support the learner through approachable or caring behaviors, and they may violate the learner's privacy.

Test Blueprint: 3 E
Cognitive Code: Analysis

33. During a clinical conference, learners begin complaining about their classroom educator and ask the clinical nurse educator to review a classroom assignment. Which is the best response by the nurse educator?
    A. "Yes, I'll review the assignment with you and can give you writing tips since I have a lot of experience with these topics."
    B. "It's great that you have a rubric to help you understand assignment's expectations. Why don't you make an appointment with your classroom educator to review your questions?"
    C. "Everyone complains about this educator's grading and I don't know why our nursing program hasn't done anything about it yet."
    D. "Let me take a look at the rubric and I will talk with the educator about your grading and assignment concerns."

Correct Answer: B

Rationale: Effective clinical nurse educators demonstrate professionalism in interactions with peers and colleagues, helping learners engage in behaviors that encourage ownership of learning. Option B demonstrates clinical teaching skill by guiding learning and use of resources for learning (Oermann et al., 2018, p. 107). Options A, C, and D undermine the evaluation rights of the classroom educator and may demonstrate educator-to-educator incivility.

Test Blueprint: 3 E
Cognitive Code: Application

34. A client on the clinical unit calls the clinical nurse educator into the client's room. The client is visibly upset and asks for the assigned learner to be removed from the client's care. Which is the best initial action?
    A. Remove the learner from the client's care and quickly reassign the learner to another client.
    B. Call the learner into the room to facilitate a conversation between the learner and client.
    C. Tell the client how learning assignments are made and offer to supervise all interactions.
    D. Calmly inform the client of the right to request the learner be removed from the client's care.

Correct Answer: D

Rationale: According to Oermann et al. (2018), "patients should receive adequate information about the presence of learners in the settings where they are receiving care before giving their informed consent to participate in clinical learning activities" (p. 126). Option D considers the rights and needs of the client when planning clinical learning activities; Options A, B, and C fail to both assess and address needs of the learner and client.

Test Blueprint: 3 E
Cognitive Code: Analysis

35. Learners express concern to the clinical nurse educator during postclinical conference that unit staff nurses are not using evidence-based care in their practice. Which is the best response?
    A. "I'm sure you saw some things that are incorrect—that happens in the real world because you just don't have time to do *everything* right."
    B. "Tell me more about the differences in practice habits you observed today in comparison to the theory or principle that you have learned."
    C. "I'll address it with their manager to help them start providing care the correct way."
    D. "That nurse may not be using the right practices, so I will make sure you are paired with a better role model next time."

Correct Answer: B

Rationale: Although role models have a powerful influence over learners' behavior and attitudes, the clinical educator should be careful not to label methods as correct and all other ways as incorrect based on the educator's opinion (Oermann et al., 2018, p. 33). Option B encourages learners to discuss the differences in practice habits that they have observed and evaluate them in terms of theory or principles (Gardner & Suplee, 2010, pp. 9–10). Options A, C, and D do not encourage learner reflection nor do these options represent respectful communication.

Test Blueprint: 3 E
Cognitive Code: Analysis

36. Which activity would best communicate learning expectations to a learner who will participate in a community-based clinical experience?
   A. Conducting a pre-experience meeting with the learner to verbally communicate learning expectations
   B. Reviewing specific learning objectives and providing written learner performance expectations for the community setting prior to the experience
   C. Asking staff in the community setting to review their expectations with the learner at the beginning of the experience
   D. Providing learners with a written summary of care in the community setting and sharing a list of learning resources

Correct Answer: B

Rationale: Learners who complete learning activities in unfamiliar environments, such as the community setting, report confusion, insecurity, isolation, and feeling unprepared (Leh, 2011). Option B uses both written and verbal communication techniques to provide the learner with a structured learning activity, providing time for the learner to reflect and ask questions. Options A, C, and D use only one communication modality that may not suit the learner's preferred learning style and do not use open-communication techniques or allow adequate time to build an environment of trust with the learner.

Test Blueprint: 3 F
Cognitive Code: Application

37. Which best establishes open communications with learners on the first day of a clinical learning experience?
   A. Inform learners that the clinical nurse educator has strict policies and expectations.
   B. Review expectations with learners and offer opportunities for learners to discuss concerns.
   C. Encourage learners to write concerns in their reflective journal for review by the clinical nurse educator.
   D. Discuss the importance of checking email daily since this is the official means of communication.

Correct Answer: B

Rationale: The clinical nurse educator should allow the learners to express their concerns after the clinical nurse educator reviews their expectations. Option B gives the learners the opportunity to ask questions and establishes a working relationship with the clinical nurse educator. The first day of the clinical experience is vital for the clinical nurse educator to review the roles and expectations with the learners while discussing the lines of communication (Oermann et al., 2018, p. 71). Options A, C, and D do not allow for learners to learn about the specific expectations and express their concerns or raise questions.

Test Blueprint: 3 F
Cognitive Code: Application

38. How can the clinical nurse educator best communicate course and assignment expectations to incoming learners?
   A. Discuss paperwork and course expectations on the first clinical day.
   B. Inform the learners that instructions are available online for them to review.
   C. Provide a handout with the expectations and policies and review this handout during the first clinical day.
   D. Remind the learners that the instructions must be followed appropriately to pass the course.

Correct Answer: C

Rationale: Learners may be overwhelmed with the clinical paperwork and course expectations. Option C allows for the clinical nurse educator to discuss the expectations and provide a handout for learners to review later. Handouts with the stated expectations allow for the learners to review when they are not as stressed (Oermann et al., 2018, p. 71). By providing verbal instructions and written materials, the clinical nurse educator provides multiple approaches to ensure that learners are properly informed. Options A, B, and D do not provide for multiple methods of communicating the expectations.

Test Blueprint: 3 F
Cognitive Code: Application

39. A learner tried to insert a Foley catheter but was not successful on the first attempt. Which is the best initial response?
   A. "I know you weren't successful, but maybe next time you should practice on a mannequin."
   B. "Did your anxiety get the best of you? You looked very nervous."
   C. "Tell me how you felt about this experience."
   D. "Go home and review the steps so that next time you are successful."

Correct Answer: C

Rationale: The learner may be embarrassed and have decreased self-confidence in the ability to complete a skill. Option C allows for the clinical nurse educator to display respect and kindness to the learner to alleviate stress and anxiety. Learners appreciate clinical nurse educators who are kind, show support, and promote confidence (Valiee, Moridi, Khaledi, & Garibi, 2016). The clinical nurse educator should strive to decrease the embarrassment and offer respect to the learner. Options A, B, and D do not support the learner in a respectful manner.

Test Blueprint: 3 F
Cognitive Code: Application

40. The clinical nurse educator is leading a postclinical conference discussion while several learners are engaging in private conversations or are using their cell phone to send text messages. How can the clinical nurse educator best address this situation?

A. Ignore the behaviors of the learners and continue to comment on the clinical evaluation tool.

B. Review the behavior expectations for postclinical conference and discuss the potential repercussions for noncompliance.

C. Encourage the learners to review the syllabus and expectations after the clinical conference.

D. After the conference send an email reminding learners about appropriate postclinical conference behaviors.

Correct Answer: B

Rationale: Uncivil behavior needs to be minimized in the clinical environment. Option B allows for the clinical nurse educator to review the expectations with learners; these expectations should be reviewed regularly (Oermann et al., 2018, p. 101). Option A does not address the uncivil behavior. Option C does not ensure that the learner reviews the expectations. Option D delays the communication; also, the clinical nurse educator would be unsure whether the learners received and read the email—thus, this may not be effective in communicating the message.

Test Blueprint: 3 F
Cognitive Code: Analysis

41. A learner approaches a clinical nurse educator and states "I forgot my stethoscope again." Which response is most appropriate?

A. "You need to be prepared for your clinical experience. This is the second time—don't let this happen again."

B. "It is important that you are ready for the clinical day. Can you borrow a stethoscope from someone?"

C. "Part of being prepared for your clinical experience includes having your stethoscope. Is there a reason you keep forgetting yours?"

D. "Because this is the second time this happened, I really could send you off the clinical unit."

Correct Answer: C

Rationale: The clinical nurse educator needs to maintain a calm, approachable manner when interacting with learners (National League for Nursing, 2018). Option C helps the learner to understand what it means to be prepared for the clinical experience. The clinical nurse educator's response also probes for a reason for the lack of preparation. Options A and D do not consider the learner needs and chastises the learner for the behavior. Option B does not address the underlying issue of the learner not being prepared for the experience.

Test Blueprint: 3 F
Cognitive Code: Application

42. Which behavior or action best reflects effective communication?
    A. The clinical nurse educator communicates to health care professionals and learners in the same manner.
    B. The clinical nurse educator uses clear, nonbiased language when communicating with all members of the health care team.
    C. When providing constructive criticism to learners, the clinical nurse educator focuses on performance errors.
    D. When providing learners with assignment feedback, the clinical nurse educator offers a list of the problems that learners had with their assignments.

Correct Answer: B

Rationale: Many factors influence communication in the health care setting. While communicating in the clinical arena, it is important for the clinical nurse educator to take into consideration several factors, such as with whom the clinical nurse educator is communicating; culture; the use of clear, explicit, fluent expressions; the use of open-communication techniques; and respect (Hou, Zhu, & Zheng, 2011). Therefore, Option B is correct. Option A states that the clinical nurse educator would communicate in the same manner to both health care professionals and learners, which would be incorrect because it does not consider learner characteristics. Option C focuses on performance errors and does not provide effective constructive feedback to assist the learner. Finally, Option D uses closed communication, which is incorrect. Additionally, in Option D, the clinical nurse educator is providing only negative feedback and offers no positive feedback for the learner.

Test Blueprint: 3 F
Cognitive Code: Analysis

43. Which statement demonstrates effective written communication on a clinical evaluation tool?
    A. "You need more practice. You did not assess the cardiovascular system."
    B. "You need to work on your assessment. While assessing the cardiovascular system, you did not assess blood pressure correctly."
    C. "You did not properly assess the cardiovascular system. While completing a blood pressure, you did not complete all the steps."
    D. "While completing a blood pressure, you did not palpate the brachial artery. Palpating the brachial artery will assist you with accuracy."

Correct Answer: D

Rationale: Written communication should be specific and precise. Feedback should identify learning that is needed for learners to improve, such as the feedback in Option D, the correct response (Oermann et al., 2018, p. 100). Options A, B, and C are vague and do not identify the exact error that occurred.

Test Blueprint: 3 F
Cognitive Code: Application

44. Which statement best demonstrates effective delivery of feedback to a learner who did not notice an intravenous (IV) infiltration during medication administration?
  A. "You need to work on your assessment skills."
  B. "I noticed that you did not assess the IV site after hanging the medication. Let me show you how to do this so you can practice."
  C. "Let's talk about how to improve your medication administration skills later today during post-conference."
  D. "You made an error. I'm busy at the moment, so please ask one of the nurses to show you the correct way to give an IV medication."

Correct Answer: B

Rationale: Option B is correct because, when evaluating psychomotor skills, the educator should provide both verbal and visual feedback to learners, explaining first where the errors were made in performance and then demonstrating the correct procedure or skill (Oermann & Gaberson, 2017). Option A does not provide the learner with precise, specific feedback or a plan for how to improve. Option C is incorrect because feedback about performance should be given to learners at the time of learning or immediately following it; the longer the period between performance and feedback from the educator, the less effective the feedback (Oermann & Gaberson, 2017). Although the statement in Option D suggests a way for the learner to gain knowledge, it is dismissive and it is not constructive feedback.

Test Blueprint: 3 F
Cognitive Code: Application

45. Several learners arrive to the clinical unit late after lunch break. Which is the best response?
  A. Monitor the situation to see if the behavior continues.
  B. Address the incident when the group meets for postclinical conference.
  C. Email the learners at the end of the clinical day.
  D. Privately discuss with the learners that they were late.

Correct Answer: D

Rationale: The clinical nurse educator needs to use clear and effective communication in the clinical learning environment (National League for Nursing, 2018). Learners should be provided with clear expectations (Oermann et al., 2018, p. 49). Option D does this by allowing the clinical nurse educator to explain that learners need to complete their lunch during the designated time. The learners should be addressed privately and not in front of the other learners, as suggested in Option B. Option A does not address the inappropriate behavior. Option C does not address the inappropriate behavior in a timely manner.

Test Blueprint: 3 F
Cognitive Code: Application

46. A learner who is working with a preceptor complains that the preceptor is mean and states, "I barely learned anything today." Which is the best initial response?

A. "This nurse just comes across that way. The nurse will teach you so much during this rotation."

B. "What do you mean by your comments? Can you further explain what happened?"

C. "Maybe you weren't making enough effort. I have never had any complaints in the past."

D. "I will reassign you to a new preceptor as soon as I can find one that is available."

Correct Answer: B

Rationale: The clinical nurse educator needs to take time to investigate learner concerns. Option B further explores the concerns and allows the clinical nurse educator to gather more information (Gardner & Suplee, 2010, p. 143). This allows the clinical nurse educator to listen to the learner in a nonthreatening manner (National League for Nursing, 2018). Options A, C, and D dismiss and disregard the learner's concerns.

Test Blueprint: 3 G
Cognitive Code: Analysis

47. Two hours after a shift has begun, a senior-level learner reports not yet completing the client assessment, collecting vital signs, or introducing oneself to staff. Which is the best response?

A. "Don't you think it's dangerous that you haven't checked on your client at all yet?"

B. "I require that you complete those assessments within an hour of starting our day. Please go do them now and report back to me right away."

C. "Our nursing assessments and client and staff interactions help us plan and prioritize care. What has prevented you from assessing the client?"

D. "That's okay—don't worry about being scared. Let's go in there together and I will show you how to perform an assessment."

Correct Answer: C

Rationale: The purpose of questioning is not to drill learners and create stress but to assess learner understanding of relevant concepts and theories that apply to client care (Oermann et al., 2018, p. 104). Option C asks the learner directly what is preventing the learner from assessing and interacting with the client without assuming intent behind the learner's behaviors. This option best helps the learner identify the cause of the delay, which may then assist in developing a corrective plan. Option A is condescending and will create a communication barrier with the learner. Although Option B is direct, it does not allow the learner to express concerns or needs. Option D assumes learner actions are motivated by fear and places the learner in a passive role.

Test Blueprint: 3 G
Cognitive Code: Application

48. On the first clinical day, a learner appears nervous and anxious about the clinical experience. How can the clinical nurse educator best decrease this learner's anxiety?
A. Discuss the learner's anxiety with the clinical group and offer support for the learner.
B. Incorporate an activity into preclinical conference for learners to identify stressors and problem-solving approaches for resolving stressors.
C. Encourage learners to express their anxiety in their postclinical experience journal assignment.
D. Email the learner after the clinical experience and ask to meet with the learner the following week to discuss stressors and clinical preparation.

Correct Answer: B

Rationale: The clinical environment can evoke a range of emotions for learners, such as anxiety. The clinical nurse educator plays a vital role in supporting learners and minimizing these feelings. Option B allows for the clinical nurse educator to work with learners to create a supportive environment through discussion. It also helps to reinforce that the clinical nurse educator wants the learner to be successful (Oermann et al., 2018, p. 68). Option A suggests discussing the learner's anxiety to the clinical group; this would be inappropriate and expose problems to others. Options C and D do not address the learner anxiety in a timely manner.

Test Blueprint: 3 G
Cognitive Code: Application

49. A clinical nurse educator is rounding on a clinical unit and finds one of the learners sitting at a computer staring at the screen. When approached by the clinical nurse educator, the learner shakes her head and says, "There is so much to do and I don't know where to start." Which is the best initial response?
A. "Are you okay?"
B. "Why are you just sitting there at the computer?"
C. "Let's go somewhere quiet to talk about what is going on."
D. "Do I need to remind you that we do not sit at the computer?"

Correct Answer: C

Rationale: The learner needs to be redirected to a quiet area. Option C allows for the clinical nurse educator to listen to the concerns of the learner in a non-threatening environment and allows the learner time to share or process. This helps to encourage and explore the emotional intelligence of the learner; the clinical nurse educator can support the learner by providing compassionate care and encourage the development of emotional intelligence and resilience (Cleary, Visentin, West, Lopez, & Kornhaber, 2018). Option A poses a yes or no response and does not help the clinical nurse educator in understanding what is happening with this learner. Option B puts the learner on the defense, needing to justify the presence at the computer. Option D is authoritarian and does not consider what is happening with the learner.

Test Blueprint: 3 G
Cognitive Code: Analysis

50. While observing a staff nurse complete a Foley catheter insertion, a learner notices that the arrangement of the sterile field is in a different manner from what was taught in the nursing skills lab. Following this procedure, the learner states to the clinical nurse educator, "This is not how I was taught this skill in lab." Which is the best response?
   A. "The way you were taught in the skills lab is correct; do not pay attention to how the nursing staff completes procedures."
   B. "Let's discuss the differences between what you were taught in lab and what you observed."
   C. "The staff nurse is correct, and we must follow the agency practices."
   D. "Which practice do you think is correct when inserting a Foley catheter?"

Correct Answer: B

Rationale: Clinical nurse educators should be cautious in labeling nursing staff as incorrect and content taught by nurse educators as correct. It would be best to identify and discuss practices that the learners observed and relate them to theories or principles (Oermann et al., 2018, p. 33). By following this approach, Option B would be the best choice. This options allows the learner and clinical nurse educator to discuss general principles such as sterile technique and determine whether those principles were followed. Options A and C disregard the multiple ways of approaching clinical problems and care. Proper evidence-based rationales should be identified instead of determining who is correct when delivering care. Option D presents a question to the learner; however, it does not necessarily require critical thinking or problem-solving. This option does not require the learner to explain the rationale for one's decision.

Test Blueprint: 3 G
Cognitive Code: Application

51. A learner approaches a clinical nurse educator and expresses concerns about caring for a client from another ethnic background because the client is "different." Which is the best initial response?
   A. "I can understand your concerns. I will immediately reassign you to a different client."
   B. "Why don't you discuss your concerns with the nurse assigned to your client?"
   C. "Can you describe your concerns for me? Let's discuss them together."
   D. "You need to put your biases aside and provide care for this client."

Correct Answer: C

Rationale: The learner needs to consider one's personal beliefs when caring for clients (Gardner & Suplee, 2010, p. 146). Option C allows the clinical nurse educator and learner to discuss the concerns together. Option A does not allow the learner to identify the concerns or address them. Although Option B may allow the learner to discuss the concerns, this should be done with the clinical nurse educator and not the nursing staff. Option D does not allow the learner to discuss the concerns first; thus, it is not the best initial response.

Test Blueprint: 3 G
Cognitive Code: Analysis

52. After a simulated learning experience, a learner looks visibly upset and states, "I performed horribly." Which is the best response?
A. "It's ok. You will do better next time."
B. "Everyone does poorly the first time in simulation."
C. "Take a break and let's discuss during debriefing."
D. "None of your peers did well either."

Correct Answer: C

Rationale: Option C acknowledges that the learner may need a break to regroup and allows for a reflective discussion during the debriefing session. Debriefing should allow for the expression of emotions and analysis of the gaps in performance (Dreifuerst, 2012; International Nursing Association for Clinical Simulation and Learning Standards Committee, 2016). Options A, B, and D attempt to pacify the learner and do not allow the learner to complete the steps in debriefing.

Test Blueprint: 3 G
Cognitive Code: Application

53. A learner approaches a clinical nurse educator regarding a short written assignment. The learner is upset and states that the assignment was graded "harder" than the peers' assignments and says it is "unfair." Which is the best response?
A. "A grading rubric was used. We can review your assignment and the rubric together."
B. "Assignments are graded fairly and I do not need to justify these grades to you."
C. "I am sorry you are upset. However, I grade assignments the same way for everyone."
D. "It is clear others spent more time on the assignment, so they received higher grades."

Correct Answer: A

Rationale: In Option A, the clinical nurse educator cites the use of a standard grading rubric, as recommended for improving evaluation reliability and validity (Oermann & Gaberson, 2017). The educator also offers to review the learner's assignment and rubric in a nonthreatening way so that the learner can understand why points were deducted. Option A allows the nurse educator to focus on the learner and provides a learning opportunity to highlight areas for improvement. Options B and D do not cite a standard evaluation approach, are defensive, and could be perceived as threatening by the learner. Although Option C acknowledges the learner's feelings, it does not mention a standard evaluation approach and could be perceived as threatening by the learner.

Test Blueprint: 3 G
Cognitive Code: Analysis

54. A nurse becomes upset when a learner has not yet administered a client's medications. Which is the best response?
   A. "I have multiple clients to administer medications to with all these learners. I have two learners that I need to give medications with and then we will give the medications."
   B. "I know that the client still needs the medications, but I am very busy. We will administer the medications as soon as we can."
   C. "Thank you for letting me know about the medications. The learner will be administering the client's medications next."
   D. "I realize we haven't given the medications. If you can't wait for us to do this then go ahead and give the medications to the client."

Correct Answer: C

Rationale: The clinical nurse educator must be calm with all communications (National League for Nursing, 2018). Option C best demonstrates effective communication in a calm manner and provides clear information to the nurse for when the medications will be given. Option A refers to "all these learners" and the response does not support the educator as a positive role model. Option B does not clearly communicate when the medications will be given. Option D does not allow the learner to administer the medications.

Test Blueprint: 3 H
Cognitive Code: Application

55. A learner who is struggling to explain medication actions becomes teary-eyed. Which is the best initial response?
   A. Ask the learner whether the learner is okay and able to continue with the medication administration.
   B. Quietly tell the learner to go to the break room until the learner stops crying.
   C. Explain to the learner that the medications need to be administered and the learner needs to "pull yourself together."
   D. Ask another learner to administer the medications and send the learner on a break.

Correct Answer: A

Rationale: Learners experience stressful situations in the clinical setting. The clinical nurse educator should display a calm and supportive demeanor when communicating with learners. Option A displays this response by the clinical nurse educator and enquires whether the learner can continue with the medication administration (National League for Nursing, 2018). Options B, C, and D do not allow the clinical nurse educator to assess learner needs and does not give the learner an opportunity to complete the medication administration.

Test Blueprint: 3 H
Cognitive Code: Analysis

56. Which response by the clinical nurse educator best demonstrates the use of empathy when providing feedback to a learner about a troubling incident that occurred?
A. "I am sorry this incident occurred."
B. "I see you are upset. Would you like to discuss the incident in more detail?"
C. "Do you want me to call the client's family for you to discuss this event with them?"
D. "Don't worry—incidents occur and you have to learn how to handle them."

Correct Answer: B

Rationale: The clinical nurse educator should use empathy during communication and is responsible for providing an educational environment that fosters empathic understanding (Williams & Stickley, 2010); therefore, Option B is correct. Option B identifies that the learner is having a difficult time with an incident that occurred and attempts to discuss the issue in further detail. Option A displays some sympathy but does not allow for further discussion about the incident. Option C does not address empathy and Option D dismisses the learner's concern and suggests that the learner has to learn to handle the situation but does not offer any strategies for how to do that.

Test Blueprint: 3 H
Cognitive Code: Analysis

57. A learner is quiet, withdrawn, and appears distracted during the clinical experience. Which initial action is most appropriate?
A. Discuss the behavior in private and inquire about potential stressors that the learner may be experiencing.
B. Do nothing, as it is normal for everyone to have some days that are better or worse than others.
C. Remind the learner that client care is a priority and point out that distracted behavior has potential to jeopardize client safety.
D. Remove the learner from the clinical environment until the learner can engage appropriately.

Correct Answer: A

Rationale: Learners experience stress and anxiety in clinical learning situations (Frank, 2012, 2016) and may exhibit these emotions and behaviors in a variety of ways. The clinical nurse educator must recognize learners' needs for supportive and collegial relationships and develop a safe learning environment in which the learner is comfortable speaking openly (Massarweh, 1999; Stokes & Kost, 2012). Discussing the behavior in private, Option A, brings the matter to the attention of the learner and allows the clinical nurse educator an opportunity to gather more information before deciding on a follow-up course of action. If personal stressors are present, this conversation also allows an opportunity for reflection, modeling of self-care, and coping skill development. Taking no action, as suggested in Option B, creates a missed opportunity for reflection, modeling of self-care, and coping skill development. Offering a harsh reminder of the learner's behavior and linking it to client safety, Option C, is not constructive and carries a punitive and accusatory tone. Removing the learner from the clinical environment, Option D, is also not constructive and is overly punitive.

Test Blueprint: 3 H
Cognitive Code: Application

58. During a clinical evaluation meeting, a learner becomes aggressive, starts to yell, and flings the evaluation paperwork across the table while stating that the evaluation was not fair. Which initial statement or action is most appropriate?
   A. "That is not acceptable behavior; you are dismissed from the clinical unit today. Please meet me in my office so we can talk after you've had a chance to think about this."
   B. Call security immediately, and do not engage in any further discussion or action regarding the behavior until security arrives.
   C. "Can we discuss this further? You need to understand why I gave you that feedback."
   D. "You are violating the learner code of conduct and I will not tolerate it! If this behavior continues, I will refer you to the dean."

Correct Answer: A

Rationale: Aggressive behavior by learners on a clinical unit mandates immediate dismissal. If the learner should resist, the clinical nurse educator should contact security to escort the learner off the clinical unit (Ehrmann, 2005). When learners violate the safety of others, it is of utmost importance to deescalate the situation; therefore, Option A is correct. Options C and D attempt to talk to the aggressive learner, which should happen later. Option B would be correct if the learner did not leave the clinical unit after the clinical nurse educator dismissed the learner.

Test Blueprint: 3 I
Cognitive Code: Application

59. A learner becomes upset and begins to speak loudly in the nursing unit hallway. Which is the best response?
   A. "I understand you're upset but your behavior is inappropriate. Can we discuss this another time?"
   B. "Why don't you take a break and calm down. We can discuss this later during lunch."
   C. "Stop yelling. I will meet with you later today to further discuss this issue."
   D. "Your behavior is violating the agency's code of conduct. I need to ask you to leave. We will meet later today to discuss the situation."

Correct Answer: D

Rationale: The clinical nurse educator may have to address incivility in the clinical setting. The learner should be confronted, and unacceptable behavior should be addressed calmly. Discussions should take place in a private location. In this situation, the learner is violating the agency's code of conduct and should be dismissed from the unit. A follow-up meeting should be scheduled after completion of the clinical day, as in Option D (Gardner & Suplee, 2010). Options A, B, and C do not involve a specific plan for addressing the problematic behavior in a specific time or appropriate location. Additionally, they allow the learner to inappropriately remain on the clinical unit.

Test Blueprint: 3 I
Cognitive Code: Analysis

60. During a clinical conference, a learner mentions that one of the nurses made demeaning comments about the learners when the clinical nurse educator was working with another learner. Which is the best response?
A. Discuss the situation in the clinical conference and suggest that the learner address the nurse.
B. Ignore the learner's comment since the clinical nurse educator was not present.
C. Ask questions about the situation and approach the nurse for clarification about concerns.
D. Plan to meet with the nurse manager to discuss how the nursing staff members are uncivil to the learners.

Correct Answer: C

Rationale: In order to be an effective team, the clinical nurse educator should ask questions and approach the nurse for clarification about concerns. Learners could feel stressed during this clinical experience; thus, the role of the clinical nurse educator is to resolve the conflict so that the learners can achieve the objectives in the clinical environment. Nursing education plays a vital role in developing conflict skills for learners—the clinical nurse educator can model a constructive conflict management style for learners (Labrague & McEnroe-Petitte, 2017). Therefore, Option C is the correct response. Option D is incorrect because the clinical nurse educator should meet with the nurse to address the concern before escalating the issue to the nurse manager. Option A expects the learner to address the nurse but the learner may not have the communication skills or knowledge to address this situation properly. Ignoring the comments is inappropriate because it role models inappropriate behavior for the learner, making Option B incorrect.

Test Blueprint: 3 J
Cognitive Code: Application

61. A clinical nurse educator overhears an upset physician speaking loudly with a learner. The physician states opposition to the learner caring for one of the clients and not trusting "beginning learners." Which is the best action?
A. After the physician leaves, discuss the experience privately with the learner to find out the learner's response to the interaction.
B. Interrupt the interaction, remove the learner from the unit, and immediately reassign care to a new client.
C. Inform the physician that the physician's behavior is inappropriate and that the client assignment will not be changed.
D. Engage in a discussion with the physician about the situation and collaboratively problem-solve alternative learner assignments for the future.

Correct Answer: D

Rationale: The clinical nurse educator should engage in discussion with the physician, Option D, to explain methods of clinical assignments and ultimately build trust with the provider. For example, the educator could discuss the multiple factors that affect selection of clinical assignments, including learning objectives of clinical activities; needs of clients; and needs, interests, and abilities of learners. Also, nursing staff members are often consulted to determine fit of clinical assignments (Oermann et al., 2018, p. 152). Allowing the physician to speak inappropriately to the learner, as in Option A, creates a hostile and abrasive learning environment. Removing the learner and reassigning client care, Option B, does not address the physician's concerns or demonstrate methods to work collaboratively to manage conflict. Confronting the physician and identifying the physician's behavior as inappropriate without discussing teaching methods and rationale for assignments, as in Option C, does not demonstrate respectful and open communication.

Test Blueprint: 3 J
Cognitive Code: Analysis

62. The clinical nurse educator hears a nurse degrading a learner. Which is the best response?
    A. Approach the learner and ask what the learner did wrong.
    B. Remind the nurse that the nurse is not role modeling appropriate behaviors for the learner.
    C. Avoid the interaction between the learner and the nurse.
    D. Suggest to the nurse that you would like to work together to understand the problem.

Correct Answer: D

Rationale: Incivility and conflict can occur in the clinical environment between learners and other health care professionals. Conflict management can be approached in a way that allows for collaboration between the disagreeing parties to find a solution for everyone (Labrague & McEnroe-Petitte, 2017). Option D shows that the clinical nurse educator is respectful of the nurse and attempts to understand the problem so that a solution can be configured; thus, this is the correct response. Option A places blame on the learner, Option B places the clinical nurse educator in an inappropriate role of evaluating the nurse, and Option C fails to address the issue.

Test Blueprint: 3 J
Cognitive Code: Analysis

63. During a clinical conference with learners, two learners get into an argument about a situation that happened on the unit. Which is the best response?
    A. Ignore the situation and continue with the planned clinical conference.
    B. Ask the learners to stay after the clinical conference to discuss the situation.
    C. Allow the learners to explain the situation and identify solutions to solve this in the future.
    D. Remind learners that this is not the time to let their emotions interfere with professional behavior.

Correct Answer: C

Rationale: Conflict resolution and management is vital in the clinical environment. Option C allows for learners to feel heard and work collaboratively to find a solution. It does not place blame and allows for exploration of the learners' behaviors. The clinical nurse educator is striving to prevent incivility and showcase respect for the learners, which can minimize misunderstandings and establish expectations about professional behaviors (Oermann et al., 2018, p. 101). Ignoring the situation does not address the issue; therefore, Option A is incorrect. Having a discussion with the learners about the situation, Option B, is important but this option does not involve the learners in resolving the issue. Option D does not sufficiently address the issue and engage the learners in resolving the problem.

Test Blueprint: 3 J
Cognitive Code: Application

64. A learner who is struggling to safely administer medications becomes upset and loudly declares, "You are constantly picking on me and not treating me fairly!" Which is the best initial response?
    A. Allow the learner to further vent frustrations.
    B. Suggest that the learner meet with the clinical nurse educator after the clinical day.
    C. Immediately dismiss the learner from the clinical unit for the day.
    D. Take the learner to a private location and explain that this behavior is inappropriate.

Correct Answer: D

Rationale: The learner is demonstrating uncivil behaviors in the clinical setting. The clinical nurse educator should discuss the issue with the learner in a private location. The clinical nurse educator should confront the learner and address the behavior as soon as possible. The learner should also be made aware that the behavior is inappropriate (Gardner & Suplee, 2010, p. 141). Options A, B, and C do not address the uncivil learning behavior immediately.

Test Blueprint: 3 J
Cognitive Code: Application

65. Which would be the best learning activity to prepare learners to address uncivil behaviors in the clinical setting?
    A. Completing a journal reflection describing a time when they experienced incivility
    B. Listening to a lecture in postclinical conference discussing uncivil behaviors in nursing
    C. Completing a simulation using cognitive behavior strategies for addressing incivility
    D. Writing a paper addressing the current state of incivility in nursing

Correct Answer: C

Rationale: The clinical nurse educator needs to prepare learners to effectively manage conflict (National League for Nursing, 2018). Cognitive behavior strategies have been an appropriate method for teaching these skills to learners (Griffin & Clark, 2014). Option A would allow learners to reflect on an experience of incivility, but Option C engages the learners in using cognitive behavior strategies. Options B and D are not the best activities because they do not actively engage the learner.

Test Blueprint: 3 J
Cognitive Code: Application

66. The clinical nurse educator is meeting with a preceptor assigned to a senior-level learner. The preceptor and learner have both expressed frustrations during the rotation. Which is the most common cause of the preceptor-learner conflict?
    A. Use of humor
    B. Unrealistic expectations
    C. Discussion of ethical issues
    D. Negative constructive feedback

Correct Answer: B

Rationale: The most common cause of learner-preceptor conflict is associated with a discrepancy in expectations. A perceived lack of competency or unclear experience outcomes can lead to conflict (Gaberson & Oermann, 2007, p. 232). Options A, C, and D are not common causes of conflict in the learner-preceptor relationship.

Test Blueprint: 3 J
Cognitive Code: Recall

67. A clinical nurse educator observes a staff nurse loudly confronting a learner for making a mistake. After speaking with the learner, the educator approaches the staff nurse. Which is the most appropriate initial response?
    A. "Do not ever shout at learners again. I am reporting you to your manager!"
    B. "I noticed you raised your voice when the learner made a mistake."
    C. "I understand that learners are frustrating, but yelling at them is not acceptable!"
    D. "You often lose your temper with learners. What is going on with you?"

Correct Answer: B

Rationale: Option B engages the staff nurse directly and focuses on the inappropriate and uncivil behavior observed, an important first step in effectively managing conflict (Luparell & Conner, 2016). The educator manages the emotions in Option B and opens the door for a collaborative solution. The educator can then outline expected behaviors and assist as needed. In Option A, the educator speaks loudly and jumps to consequences and threats, which will not be conducive to managing this conflict. In Option C, the educator makes assumptions and again speaks loudly. Option D does not focus on the inappropriate behavior observed during this scenario and may also not be well received if the educator does not have rapport with the staff nurse.

Test Blueprint: 3 J
Cognitive Code: Analysis

68. A clinical nurse educator and a learner are in the room with a client whose respiratory status is declining. The learner is attempting to place a BiPAP mask onto the client and is having difficulty. Which action by the clinical nurse educator is least appropriate?
  A. Guiding the learner to place the mask onto the client
  B. Taking the mask from the learner and stating, "You are too slow … I'll do it!"
  C. Holding the main part of the mask onto the client while the learner adjusts the straps
  D. Asking whether the learner would like help adjusting the mask

Correct Answer: B

Rationale: Clinical nurse educators must maintain an approachable, non-judgmental, and readily accessible demeanor, even in times of stress or when client status is declining (Lundeen, 2019). It is not helpful for learning and is discouraging for an educator to not only take the BiPAP mask but also tell the learner that the learner is too slow, as in Option B. Options A, C, and D are appropriate actions not only because they allow learning to occur but also because the educator remains calm, approachable, nonjudgmental, and accessible. This will help current and future learning experiences and outcomes (Lundeen, 2019).

Test Blueprint: 3 K
Cognitive Code: Analysis

69. A clinical nurse educator is reviewing a client's medications with a learner. The learner seems nervous and is struggling to respond to basic questions about the client's medications. Which response is most appropriate?
  A. "Did you review any of the client's medications today?"
  B. "These are basic questions … what exactly is confusing you?"
  C. "Take a deep breath and review the medications one step at a time."
  D. "If you cannot come prepared, perhaps you should stay home."

Correct Answer: C

Rationale: Clinical nurse educators must maintain an approachable, non-judgmental, and readily accessible demeanor (Lundeen, 2019). Option C is the most appropriate response because the educator is helping the learner calm down and tackle the task at hand. This educator is displaying an approachable, nonjudgmental, and accessible demeanor, which will help learning and outcomes. Options A, B, and D are accusatory, judgmental, and make the educator intimidating to the learner. This will not help learning; thus, these are inappropriate and incorrect responses.

Test Blueprint: 3 K
Cognitive Code: Analysis

70. A clinical nurse educator is meeting with a learner and a staff nurse preceptor to discuss the learner's progress in the course thus far. The preceptor verbalizes that the learner demonstrates proficiency in basic competencies and asks the educator for ways to challenge the learner. Which is the best response?

A. "I would stick to the course objectives, as that is the purpose of this experience."

B. "It's wonderful that you want to challenge the learner. What areas do you want to work on?"

C. "That would really be unit-specific … so I'll leave that up to you."

D. "Let's see if the objectives have been met for the course before we change directions."

Correct Answer: B

Rationale: Clinical nurse educators must maintain an approachable, non-judgmental, and readily accessible demeanor (Lundeen, 2019). Option B is appropriate because the educator recognizes the preceptor's efforts and maintains an approachable, nonjudgmental, and accessible demeanor while helping the preceptor hone in on what the preceptor is requesting; thus, this is the correct response. Options A, C, and D are dismissive and the educator seems judgmental and not approachable; these are not appropriate behaviors toward learners or other health care professionals.

Test Blueprint: 3 K
Cognitive Code: Analysis

71. A learner demonstrates significant deficits and safety concerns related to medication administration. Which approach is most appropriate?

A. Have the learner focus on other areas of client care during the clinical experience.

B. Discuss the learner's deficits and assign a medication administration review activity as a homework assignment.

C. Continue to assign the learner to multiple clients with challenging medications to allow the learner to practice this skill.

D. Develop a detailed remediation plan, including opportunities to demonstrate safe care in the skills lab prior to returning to the clinical setting.

Correct Answer: D

Rationale: The clinical nurse educator should recognize learner deficits and provide opportunities for improvement. Option D allows the learner the opportunity to correct deficiencies (Bonnel, 2016, p. 458). Options A, B, and C do not allow the learner to address the deficits. Moreover, Option C jeopardizes client safety and should not be completed until the learner has had an opportunity for remediation.

Test Blueprint: 3 L
Cognitive Code: Analysis

72. During initial rounds with senior learners working under the supervision of assigned preceptors, a learner asks the clinical nurse educator questions about complex plans of care that are unfamiliar to the educator. Which is the best action by the educator?
   A. Request that the learner submit questions in writing and independently search for the information to share with the learner.
   B. Tell the learner to go to a conference room to search online or in nursing textbooks for information.
   C. Discuss experiences from the clinical nurse educator's career that may apply to the care.
   D. Guide the learner to educational resources on the unit, including the preceptor, charge nurse, and unit educator and ask staff to help answer the inquiries.

Correct Answer: D

Rationale: Although learners value sufficient professional knowledge high among desired behaviors of clinical educators (Tang, Chou, & Chiang, 2005), the educator is admitting a lack of knowledge and helping the learner to discover the information. Option D demonstrates effective professional role modeling behaviors. Also, since the clinical nurse educator is using the preceptor model of clinical education, the preceptor can assist in helping learners discover answers to questions. This option presents important strengths of the educator, including being professional and supportive of learners and displaying scholarly attributes (Oermann et al., 2018, p. 106). Options A, B, and C do not immediately address the learner's needs or help the learner locate information and resources during clinical learning.

Test Blueprint: 3 L
Cognitive Code: Application

73. A learner is struggling with prioritizing care for multiple clients. Which is the best approach?
   A. Monitor the learner's deficits and continue to provide multiple client assignments.
   B. Email the learner after the clinical experience to share the clinical nurse educator's concerns.
   C. Immediately hold a discussion with the learner in the hallway to provide timely feedback.
   D. Privately meet at the end of the day to provide detailed feedback and develop a remediation plan.

Correct Answer: D

Rationale: The clinical nurse educator needs to communicate with the learner regarding the learner's performance (National League for Nursing, 2018). Detailed feedback and a remediation plan should be provided to communicate clear expectations (Gardner & Suplee, 2010). The learner should be aware of performance areas that need improvement. Option A does not communicate information to the learner. Option B is not the most effective means to communicate to the learner and does not include an option for remediation. Discussions about learner performance should be held in a private setting; Option C does not provide a private environment to have performance discussions.

Test Blueprint: 3 L
Cognitive Code: Application

74. The clinical nurse educator is with a learner who is administering an insulin injection to a client with diabetes. The learner administers the insulin injection and immediately recaps the needle. Which action best helps promote cognitive knowledge development regarding this skill?
    A. The learner completes a subcutaneous injection on another client to complete the skill correctly.
    B. The learner provides a rationale to support actions to show an understanding of why the needle should not have been recapped.
    C. The learner describes how the learner felt about making a mistake and how to avoid it in the future.
    D. The learner practices disposing of the syringe directly in a sharps container following all injections.

    Correct Answer: B

    Rationale: Learner development promotes independent thinking and self-reflection and is a vital part of nursing education. It facilitates achievement of personal goals (Oermann et al., 2018, p. 72). The item asks which action displays learner development of the cognitive domain; therefore, the correct response is Option B. Options A and D promote learner development of the psychomotor domain. Option C promotes learner development of the affective domain.

    Test Blueprint: 3 L
    Cognitive Code: Analysis

75. As the clinical nurse educator is reviewing laboratory findings with a learner, the learner recognizes that the primary physician needs to be notified about a low potassium level. The clinical nurse educator wants to include the situation, background, assessment, and recommendation (SBAR) approach for communication. Which is the best active learning activity using SBAR?
    A. Having the clinical nurse educator call the physician to demonstrate SBAR use
    B. Reminding the learner about the steps in SBAR to prepare for the call
    C. Encouraging the learner to read about the steps of SBAR prior to the call
    D. Discussing learner knowledge of SBAR and practicing SBAR communication prior to the call

    Correct Answer: D

    Rationale: The clinical nurse educator would review the learner's knowledge of SBAR and confidence in the learner's ability to call the physician. Option D provides support for the learner by working together to make sure that the learner is prepared prior to calling the physician. Lanz and Wood (2018) stated that clinical instruction can allow for the opportunity to practice SBAR and enhance the learner's communication. Listening to the SBAR use by the clinical nurse educator is helpful but does not allow the learner to use this skill; therefore, Option A is not the best choice. Options B and C encourage a review of SBAR content but do not allow for practice prior to calling.

Test Blueprint: 3 L
Cognitive Code: Application

76. A newly admitted client is having difficulty signing the consent form for surgery. The learner recognizes that the client does not speak much English. How can the clinical nurse educator best help the learner meet the needs of this client?
    A. Ask the unit secretary for the phone numbers for a family member who can be contacted to help translate.
    B. Refer the learner to a book of commonly used medical terminology to help communicate with the client.
    C. Offer to work with the learner to contact language services to get the client a translator.
    D. Suggest that the learner attempt to speak with the client in a slower manner and to use pictures and gestures when communicating.

Correct Answer: C

Rationale: The clinical nurse educator is a role model for learners to communicate effectively within the clinical environment. Option C allows for the learner and clinical nurse educator to work together to get the client a service to help communication with the health care team. This approach allows communication of information to clients that is understandable and seeks additional help to support the client (Oermann et al., 2018, p. 221). Options A, B, and D do not provide the most effective means of communicating with this client.

Test Blueprint: 3 M
Cognitive Code: Application

77. The clinical nurse educator reviews the importance of culture and diversity when providing care. The clinical nurse educator would anticipate which outcome following this discussion?
    A. Learners treat clients as if they are from the same culture as the learner.
    B. Learners identify all clients as unique and should be treated differently.
    C. Learners provide all activities of daily living, including shaving all clients daily.
    D. Learners allow clients to perform all personal rituals to promote their healing.

Correct Answer: B

Rationale: For learners to promote respect and appreciation for diverse clients and cultures, learners must have an overall understanding of clients from different ethnic and cultural backgrounds. By understanding the differences between and within cultures, the clinical nurse educator will begin to identify learners who act in a respectful manner to all cultures (Oermann et al., 2018, p. 44). Therefore, Option B is correct; all clients should be treated as unique individuals. Option A states the learner will treat all clients as if they are from the same culture as the learner, which is incorrect. Option C states the learner will complete all activities of daily living, which would be inappropriate to complete for all clients. Option D states the learner will allow clients to perform all personal rituals, which is incorrect because certain rituals could interfere with care; clients who perform ritualistic behavior need to discuss their plan of care with their physician.

Test Blueprint: 3 M
Cognitive Code: Analysis

78. The clinical nurse educator is working with a bilingual learner who speaks English as a second language. The learner is having difficulty understanding medical terminology in the clinical setting. Which strategy best assists the learner in overcoming this language barrier?
   A. Referring the learner to campus resources that can assist with cultural needs
   B. Suggesting additional activities and practice opportunities to reinforce content
   C. Assigning another academic adviser to work with the learner outside of class time
   D. Providing individual tutoring sessions to reteach medical terminology concepts

Correct Answer: B

Rationale: When assisting learners whose second language is English, exercises requiring the learners to communicate using the English language will strengthen their understanding of medical concepts. Practicing reading, listening, speaking, and writing will assist the learner to master the English language more effectively (Guhde, 2003). Therefore, Option B is correct. Option B provides additional activity suggestions that assist in applying the concepts learned. Option A refers the learner to campus resources, which may be appropriate, but the learner does not necessarily have specific cultural needs. Rather, the learner needs help with medical terminology and campus resources may not be best suited to assist with this need. Option C assigns the learner to another academic adviser who can provide general guidance and advice, but the learner needs practice with medical terminology. An academic adviser assignment alone may not be enough to address this need. Finally, Option D states to provide individual tutoring sessions. Individual tutoring sessions are appropriate as long as the clinical nurse educator provides additional practice activities to solidify the concept being taught. Simply reteaching the information is not sufficient.

Test Blueprint: 3 M
Cognitive Code: Application

79. When entering a client's room, a physical therapist asks the clinical nurse educator in a short-tempered tone, "are you going to be done soon? We need to begin the client's therapy and we are very busy today." Which is the best initial response?
   A. "We still have several medications to give but we can stop here and return when you are done."
   B. "I appreciate that you need to begin physical therapy, but we also need to safely administer medications. We will be done shortly."
   C. "I don't appreciate your tone. We are all working together to provide the client care."
   D. "We are very busy today too. You can provide the client care as soon as we have finished."

Correct Answer: B

Rationale: The clinical nurse educator must communicate effectively with other health care professionals in the clinical setting (National League for Nursing, 2018). Option B demonstrates effective communication with the physical therapist. Option A is not realistic for the learner or the client. Options C and D do not display effective communication.

Test Blueprint: 3 M
Cognitive Code: Application

80. Which would best prepare learners for a new clinical experience?
    A. Reviewing the nursing unit's policies and procedures manual during orientation
    B. Discussing a handout on behavioral expectations for the clinical rotation
    C. Providing learners with a list of commonly used medications on the clinical unit
    D. Completing an ice-breaker activity to allow the group members to get to know each other

Correct Answer: B

Rationale: The clinical nurse educator has a responsibility to communicate clear expectations. Although the other activities are helpful and can be used to orient learners and build group cohesiveness, learners should be provided clear expectations before the onset of the learning activities (Christensen, 2016, p. 44); therefore, Option B is correct.

Test Blueprint: 3 N
Cognitive Code: Analysis

81. During clinical conference, multiple learners report that a staff nurse coached them during the administration of an intramuscular injection for their clients. The clinical nurse educator knows that the program policy states that intramuscular injections may be given only in the presence of the clinical nurse educator. Which is the best action?
    A. Address the issue by sharing the policy with all nurses and learners on the clinical unit.
    B. Call the program administrator to discuss the policy breach and then require the learners to leave the clinical unit.
    C. Review the injection policy and procedures with all learners to ensure that they can follow the policy.
    D. Praise the learners for taking advantage of learning opportunities and encourage them to seek out more medication administration opportunities with staff nurses.

Correct Answer: A

Rationale: Clinical nurse educators have a legal duty to comply with program policies relating to teaching and learning in the health care environment. Option A is the only response that ensures that the clinical nurse educator, learners, and staff nurses maintain compliance with policy while also meeting learning objectives. It is important for educators to clarify roles and expectations with staff members, as they can serve as useful role models for nursing practice (Oermann et al., 2018, p. 78). Options B, C, and D do not ensure compliance with legal requirements or help the clinical nurse educator communicate expectations, as they are "responsible for making the learning objectives clear to all involved persons" (Oermann et al., 2018, p. 126).

Test Blueprint: 3 N
Cognitive Code: Analysis

82. A learner who has received multiple verbal warnings related to behavioral and performance issues now fails to complete a required client care assignment. Which action should the clinical nurse educator take next?
    A. Request that the nursing program chairperson meet with the learner to discuss the clinical learning deficiencies.
    B. Meet with the learner to review a formative performance evaluation and provide a written remediation plan that outlines expected performance.
    C. Ask the classroom educator who is also teaching this learner to provide information about classroom performance.
    D. Wait until the end of the clinical experience to determine final grading.

Correct Answer: B

Rationale: Principles should be followed in evaluating and grading clinical practice, such as providing evaluation and grading feedback in writing (Oermann et al., 2018, p. 355). Since verbal warnings have been ineffective, the clinical nurse educator should now move to a written remediation plan. Written remediation plans can help learners better understand plans to achieve clinical learning success while also providing educators with a formal record of conference discussions and documentation of learner performance. Option B best combines use of written learning plans and conferences to track formative feedback of a learner with performance issues. Options A, C, and D do not represent the most appropriate next action. The clinical nurse educator is the best initial person to discuss clinical learning deficiencies with the learner, not the program chairperson, as suggested in Option A. The learner's classroom performance information is not needed at this time and should not influence clinical performance evaluation, making Option C incorrect. Option D is incorrect because it does not provide an opportunity for the learner to receive feedback and modify performance.

Test Blueprint: 3 N
Cognitive Code: Application

83. Members of the health care team complain to the clinical nurse educator that learners are frequently seen on their smartphones and they believe learners are using social media and text messaging. Which is the most appropriate response?
    A. Creating and sharing guidelines regarding learners' appropriate use of mobile devices
    B. Requiring learners to leave mobile devices in the secured locker room during clinical hours
    C. Asking learners to use mobile devices only in private conference rooms or areas away from staff
    D. Informing team members that they can reprimand learners and to report any further issues

Correct Answer: A

Rationale: Although mobile devices may provide an invaluable resource for learners in the clinical setting, it is important for educators to know policies regarding mobile device use and remind learners of these policies. If this site allows mobile device use, an opportunity exists for the educator to create guidelines that will help outline appropriate device use for learners (Oermann et al., 2018, pp. 128, 231). Option A addresses concerns of the staff while also allowing learners access to helpful learning resources; Options B, C, and D do not address the issue or establish guidelines for learner conduct.

Test Blueprint: 3 N
Cognitive Code: Analysis

84. Which practice is most appropriate when implementing a preceptorship clinical education model?
    A. Since preceptors have observed the learners' performance, ask the preceptors to independently determine learners' final grades.
    B. Create a signed learning contract that includes learner, educator, and preceptor contact information as well as clinical learning objectives, activities, resources, and evaluation methods.
    C. Plan midterm and final phone call meetings with preceptors to review concerns and determine learners' midterm and final grades.
    D. Use reflective journaling for learners to write about experiences and evaluate preceptors.

Correct Answer: B

Rationale: Learning contracts are commonly used for planning and implementing clinical teaching in the preceptorship model, as they help communicate an agreement that clarifies expectations of the educator, learner, and preceptor in the learning environment (Oermann & Gaberson, 2017, p. 284). Option B demonstrates appropriate use of a learning contract and ensures that contact information is readily available for all parties, whereas Options A, C, and D focus on only one part of the learning triad. Additionally, clinical nurse educators are ultimately responsible for the final evaluation of learner performance with input from preceptors (Oermann & Gaberson, 2017, p. 284).

Test Blueprint: 3 N
Cognitive Code: Application

85. Which initial action best enhances communication when starting clinical teaching on a new unit?
    A. Giving a tour of the unit to the learners
    B. Emailing the nurse manager with the course information
    C. Meeting with the nurse manager and discussing the expectations and skills of the learners
    D. Asking the nurse manager to come to the preclinical conference to meet the learners

Correct Answer: C

Rationale: Communication among the health care team, including the nurse manager, is foundational to establish a working relationship. Option C allows for the clinical nurse educator to communicate the objectives and expectations of the clinical rotation to the nurse manager and provides an avenue to start a working relationship. When meeting with the nurse manager, the clinical nurse educator communicates the roles and responsibilities of the learners (Oermann et al., 2018, p. 220). This meeting can assist in working out the details of the unit and form an open line of communication between management, the clinical nurse educator, and learners. Option A does not enhance communication. Option B provides information to the nurse manager but does not help to establish a relationship. Also, the nurse educator may be unsure whether the nurse manager received and read the email. Option D is one method to build an effective working relationship and establish communication, but it should not be the first action.

Test Blueprint: 3 N
Cognitive Code: Analysis

86. The clinical nurse educator overhears a staff nurse complaining that the learners just sit around and "don't do anything." Which response demonstrates effective communication?
    A. Inform the nurse manager about the nursing staff demonstrating uncivil behaviors with the learners.
    B. Assertively communicate with the staff nurse the learners' responsibilities on the unit.
    C. Ignore the staff nurses' comments and remind the learners of their expectations on the clinical unit.
    D. Gather the learners in the conference room to review the clinical expectations established by the clinical nurse educator.

Correct Answer: B

Rationale: The clinical nurse educator needs to demonstrate effective communication in the clinical learning environment. Option B allows the clinical nurse educator the ability to assertively, not passively or aggressively, address the staff nurses' concerns and communicate the expectations of the learners. Speaking up is a form of effective communication used in the health care system and could minimize moral distress (Mansour & Mattukoyya, 2018). By using assertive communication, the clinical nurse educator can communicate and mitigate any potential problems in the future while showing respect for the staff nurse. Option A escalates the situation to the nurse manager, and the clinical nurse educator is not role modeling appropriate communication with the right person. Options C and D do not address the problem.

Test Blueprint: 3 N
Cognitive Code: Application

87. A learner arrives late for a clinical experience for the third time this semester. Which is the best initial response?
    A. "Do you realize you are late again? Do you arrive late for your theory classes too?"
    B. "You have been late three times. The clinical experience begins at 0645 and you are to be on the unit, prepared to receive your assignment by that time."
    C. "I need to talk to you later today. Do you realize that you have been late a few times this semester?"
    D. "Is there something going on that you can't seem to get here on time? This needs to be corrected."

Correct Answer: B

Rationale: Learner behavior issues and misconduct should be addressed by confronting the learner about the behavior. Doing so holds learners accountable for their actions and can prevent similar problems from continuing to occur. Option B provides detailed information that the learner has been late three times and includes the expectation for when the learner should arrive at the clinical site. Although Option D asks about reasons why the learner is late, it does not provide detailed information on the learner's behavior. Options A and C do not provide detailed information about the learner's behavior and could be perceived as threatening (Luparell & Conner, 2016, pp. 232–233).

Test Blueprint: 3 N
Cognitive Code: Analysis

References

Adelman-Mullally, T., Mulder, C. K., McCarter-Spalding, D. E., Hagler, D. A., Gaberson, K. B., Hanner, M. B., … Young, P. K. (2013). The clinical nurse educator as leader. *Nurse Education in Practice, 13*(1), 29–34. doi:10.1016/j.nepr.2012.07.006

Bonnel, W. (2016). Clinical performance evaluation. In D. M. Billings & J. A. Halstead (Eds.), *Teaching in nursing: A guide for faculty* (5th ed., pp. 443–462). St. Louis, MO: Elsevier.

Centre for the Advancement of Interprofessional Education. (2019). About CAIPE. Retrieved from https://www.caipe.org/about-us

Chan, Z. (2017). A qualitative study on communication between nursing students and the family members of patients. *Nurse Education Today, 59*, 33–37. doi:10.1016/j.nedt.2017.08.017

Christensen, L. S. (2016). The academic performance of students: Legal and ethical issues. In D. M. Billings & J. A. Halstead (Eds.), *Teaching in nursing: A guide for faculty* (5th ed., pp. 35–54). St. Louis, MO: Elsevier.

Cleary, M., Visentin, D., West, S., Lopez, V., & Kornhaber, R. (2018). Promoting emotional intelligence and resilience in undergraduate nursing students: An integrative review. *Nurse Education Today, 68*, 112–120. doi:10.1016/j.nedt.2018.05.018

Dreifuerst, K. T. (2012). Using debriefing for meaningful learning to foster development of clinical reasoning in simulation. *Journal of Nursing Education, 51*(6), 326–333. doi:10.3928/01484834-20120409-02

Ehrmann, G. (2005). Managing the aggressive nursing student. *Nurse Educator, 30*(3), 98–100.

Folh, K. L. (2016). A patient's rights and the nurse's responsibility to provide nonjudgmental care. *Journal of Obstetric, Gynecologic & Neonatal Nursing, 45*, S56.

Frank, B. (2012). Teaching students with disabilities. In D. M. Billings & J. A. Halstead (Eds.), *Teaching in nursing: A guide for faculty* (4th ed., pp. 55–75). St. Louis, MO: Elsevier.

Frank, B. (2016). Facilitating learning for students with disabilities. In D. M. Billings & J. A. Halstead (Eds.), *Teaching in nursing: A guide for faculty* (5th ed., pp. 55–72). St. Louis, MO: Elsevier.

Fressola, M. C., & Patterson, G. E. (2017). *Transition from clinician to nurse educator: A practical approach.* Burlington, MA: Jones & Bartlett.

Gaberson, K. B., & Oermann, M. H. (2007). *Clinical teaching strategies in nursing* (2nd ed.). New York, NY: Springer.

Gardner, M. R., & Suplee, P. D. (2010). *Handbook of clinical teaching in nursing and health sciences.* Sudbury, MA: Jones & Bartlett.

Gibbs, S. S., & Kulig, J. C. (2017). "We definitely are role models": Exploring how clinical instructors' influence nursing students' attitudes towards older adults. *Nurse Education in Practice, 26*, 64–81. doi:10.1016/j.nepr.2017.07.006

Griffin, M., & Clark, C. M. (2014). Revisiting cognitive rehearsal as an intervention against incivility and lateral violence in nursing: 10 years later. *The Journal of Continuing Education in Nursing, 45*(12), 535–542. doi:10.3928/00220124-20141122-02

Gubrud, P. (2016). Teaching in the clinical setting. In D. M. Billings & J. A Halstead (Eds.), *Teaching in nursing: A guide for faculty* (5th ed., pp. 282–303). St. Louis, MO: Elsevier.

Guhde, J. A. (2003). English-as-a-Second Language (ESL) nursing students: Strategies for building verbal and written language skills. *Journal of Cultural Diversity, 10*(4), 113–117.

Hou, X., Zhu, D., & Zheng, M. (2011). Clinical Nursing Faculty Competence Inventory—developmental and psychometric testing. *Journal of Advanced Nursing, 67*(5), 1109–1117. doi:10.1111/j.1365-2648.2010.05520.x

International Nursing Association for Clinical Simulation and Learning Standards Committee (2016). INACSL standards of best practice: Simulation^SM debriefing. *Clinical Simulation in Nursing, 12*, S21–S25. doi:10.1016/j.ecns.2016.09.008

Jeffries, P. R., Swoboda, S. M., & Akintade, B. (2016). Teaching and learning using simulations. In D. M. Billings & J. A. Halstead (Eds.), *Teaching in nursing: A guide for faculty* (5th ed., pp. 159–185). St. Louis, MO: Elsevier.

Labrague, L. J., & McEnroe-Petitte, D. M. (2017). An integrative review on conflict management styles among nursing students: Implications for nurse education. *Nurse Education Today*, *59*, 45–52. doi:10.1016/j.nedt.2017.09.001

Lanz, A. S., & Wood, F. G. (2018). Communicating patient status: Comparison of teaching strategies in prelicensure nursing education. *Nurse Educator*, *43*(3), 162–165. doi:10.1097/NNE.0000000000000440

Leh, S. K. (2011). Nursing students' preconceptions of the community health clinical experience: Implications for nursing education. *Journal of Nursing Education*, *50*, 620–627.

Lundeen, J. D. (2019). Demonstrate effective interpersonal communication and collaborative interprofessional relationships. In T. Shellenbarger (Ed.), *Clinical nurse educator competencies: Creating an evidence-based practice for academic clinical nurse educators* (pp. 39–52). Washington, DC: National League for Nursing.

Luparell, S. (2011). Incivility in nursing: The connection between academia and the workplace. *Critical Care Nurse*, *31*(2), 92–95.

Luparell, S., & Conner, J. R. (2016). Managing student incivility and misconduct in the learning environment. In D. M. Billings & J. A. Halstead (Eds.). *Teaching in nursing: A guide for faculty* (5th ed., pp. 230–244). St. Louis, MO: Elsevier.

Mansour, M., & Mattukoyya, R. (2018). A cross-sectional survey of British newly graduated nurses' experience of organization empowerment and of challenging unsafe practices. *The Journal of Continuing Education in Nursing*, *49*(10), 474–481. doi:10.3928/00220124-20180918-08

Massarweh, L. (1999). Promoting a positive clinical experience. *Nurse Educator*, *24*(3), 44–47.

National League for Nursing. (2012). *The scope of practice for academic nurse educators: 2012 revision*. New York, NY: Author.

National League for Nursing. (2018). *Certified Academic Clinical Nurse Educator (CNE®cl) 2018 candidate handbook*. Washington, DC: Author.

Niederriter, J. E., Eyth, D., & Thoman, J. (2017). Nursing students perceptions on characteristics of an effective clinical instructor. *Sage Open Nursing*. doi:10.1177/2377960816685571

Oermann, M. H., & Gaberson, K. B. (2017). *Evaluation and testing in nursing education* (5th ed.). New York, NY: Springer.

Oermann, M. H., Shellenbarger, T., & Gaberson, K. B. (2018). *Clinical teaching strategies in nursing* (5th ed.). New York, NY: Springer.

Phillips, J. M. (2016). Strategies to promote student engagement and active learning. In D. M. Billings & J. A. Halstead (Eds.), *Teaching in nursing: A guide for faculty* (5th ed., pp. 245–262). St. Louis, MO: Elsevier.

Speakman, E. (2016). Interprofessional education and collaborative practice. In D. M. Billings & J. A. Halstead (Eds.), *Teaching in nursing: A guide for faculty* (5th ed., pp. 186–196). St. Louis, MO: Elsevier.

Stokes, L. G., & Kost, G. C. (2012). Teaching in the clinical setting. In D. M. Billings & J. A. Halstead (Eds.), *Teaching in nursing: A guide for faculty* (4th ed., pp. 331–334). St. Louis, MO: Elsevier.

Tang, F., Chou, S., & Chiang, H. (2005). Students' perceptions of effective and ineffective clinical instructors. *Journal of Nursing Education*, *44*, 187–192.

Valiee, S., Moridi, G., Khaledi, S., & Garibi, F. (2016). Nursing students' perspectives on clinical instructors' effective teaching strategies: A descriptive study. *Nurse Education in Practice*, *16*, 258–262. doi:10.1016/j.nepr.2015.09.009

Vogelsang, L., & Bergen, T. (2018) Enhancing interprofessional competencies using reflective writing in clinical nursing education. *Journal of Nursing Education*, *57*(12), 768. doi:10.3928/01484834-20181119-15

Waldron, M. K., Washington, S. L., & Montague, G. P. (2016). Cooperative clinical conferences: Nursing student pediatric clinical innovation. *Journal of Nursing Education*, *55*(7), 416–419. doi:10.3928/01484834-20160615-12

Williams, J., & Stickley, T. (2010). Empathy and nurse education. *Nurse Education Today*, *30*(8), 752–755.

6

Applies Clinical Expertise in the Health Care Environment

1. Which initial action best fosters a successful role transition from an expert clinician to a new clinical nurse educator?
   A. Joining multiple university-wide and departmental committees
   B. Teaching learners in a clinical setting different from the educator's specialty area
   C. Disengaging from clinical practice in a specialty area to ensure that all professional efforts are directed toward academia
   D. Seeking out one or more mentors who can provide advice about clinical education

   Correct Answer: D

   Rationale: Mentorship is essential when transitioning to a clinical nurse educator role. A mentor can empower a novice educator with information, opportunities, and experiences that can develop and enhance teaching (Sorrell & Cangelosi, 2016). While service to the university and department is encouraged, Option A would likely be overwhelming to the novice clinical nurse educator. Option B is not an effective strategy for the novice clinical nurse educator since having knowledge of the practice area creates an environment conducive to learning (Gubrud, 2016). Option C is discouraged since maintaining clinical competence is an important aspect of the clinical nurse educator's role.

   Test Blueprint: 4 A
   Cognitive Code: Application

2. Which action would best help the clinical nurse educator maintain competence in a clinical specialty area?
   A. Participating in professional development opportunities, such as conferences and webinars
   B. Using strategies to evaluate learning in the cognitive, psychomotor, and affective domains
   C. Considering program outcomes as part of the curriculum design process
   D. Developing collaborative partnerships with other care providers in the community

   Correct Answer: A

Rationale: Option A is correct because participating in professional development opportunities in a specialty area can increase effectiveness in the educator role and is characteristic of an effective clinical nurse educator (Fisher, 2016). Maintaining and enhancing competency can be done through activities such as education, joining professional organizations, attending conferences and webinars, completing continuing nursing education modules, and becoming certified in a practice area (Strong, 2016). Options B, C, and D are important work for the clinical nurse educator but do not focus on maintaining current professional competence relevant to one's specialty area.

Test Blueprint: 4 A
Cognitive Code: Application

3. When discussing safe medication administration with learners, which statement made by the learner would most likely require clarification?
   A. "I need to check the medication with the physician's order."
   B. "I will verify the client's allergies before giving a medication."
   C. "The client must take all medication as ordered, even if they refuse."
   D. "I always check the client's name, date of birth, and allergies before giving a medication."

Correct Answer: C

Rationale: Clients have the right to refuse any medication. Therefore, Option C is incorrect and would require follow-up by the clinical nurse educator. Options A, B, and D are correct steps to ensure client safety during evidence-based medication administration (Berman, Snyder, & Frandsen, 2016).

Test Blueprint: 4 A
Cognitive Code: Application

4. Which statement by a novice clinical nurse educator best indicates commitment to maintaining clinical expertise in the health care environment?
   A. "I want to incorporate web-based assignments into the learners' clinical experiences next semester."
   B. "I am interested in becoming a member of the nursing department's curriculum committee to help prepare for the upcoming accreditation visit."
   C. "I am studying to take the Inpatient Obstetric Nursing certification exam next month."
   D. "I need to improve my skills providing timely feedback to learners about their psychomotor performance."

Correct Answer: C

Rationale: Option C is correct because obtaining formal certification in a current practice area is one way to maintain professional competence relevant to the specialty area and demonstrates a commitment to lifelong learning (Fisher, 2016; Strong, 2016). Maintaining a professional knowledge base is needed to help prepare learners for contemporary nursing practice (Fisher, 2016). Options A, B, and D are relevant to the clinical nurse educator role but do not focus on maintaining current professional competence and expertise in a specialty.

Test Blueprint: 4 A
Cognitive Code: Analysis

5. Which is considered professional service for a clinical nurse educator?
   A. Teaching theory courses in higher education
   B. Presenting a quality improvement project at a regional nursing organization meeting
   C. Participating as a board member for a nursing organization
   D. Developing a clinical course involving health care simulation

Correct Answer: C

Rationale: Service to a nursing organization is one way to impact nursing professional outcomes. Ongoing professional development and service is an expectation for nursing. Initiatives to increase the number of nurses serving on boards is a national goal for nurses, making Option C correct (Cope & Murray, 2018). Options A, B, and D involve scholarship in teaching and research.

Test Blueprint: 4 A
Cognitive Code: Application

6. Which action is most appropriate for strengthening the clinical nurse educator's competence when teaching in a new clinical learning environment?
   A. Downloading clinical applications to an electronic device to ensure access during clinical practice experiences
   B. Implementing electronic-based clinical conferences that take place online instead of in a traditional face-to-face setting
   C. Discussing clinical site selection with the program director and requesting reassignment to a more familiar medical-surgical inpatient unit
   D. Completing computer-based training that outlines unit-specific policies and procedures prior to entering the clinical setting with learners

Correct Answer: D

Rationale: Option D allows the clinical nurse educator to participate in professional development opportunities that increase one's effectiveness in the role (National League for Nursing, 2012). Having knowledge of the practice area is characteristic of an effective educator, as it creates an environment that is conducive to learning (Gubrud, 2016). While having access to digital learning technologies, as in Option A, and holding online conferences in the clinical setting, as in Option B, may be appropriate strategies for clinical learning, these actions do not directly improve the clinical nurse educator's competence on the new inpatient unit (Gubrud, 2016). Requesting reassignment, as in Option C, does not strengthen the educator's competence.

Test Blueprint: 4 A
Cognitive Code: Application

7. The clinical nurse educator is teaching learners about delegation. Which best demonstrates appropriate delegation to unlicensed assistive personnel?
   A. Obtaining a bedside glucose level of a diabetic client
   B. Reassessment of a client's blood pressure following an abnormal reading
   C. Teaching a client about dietary restrictions
   D. Ambulating a client for the first time postoperatively

Correct Answer: A

Rationale: Teaching learners how to delegate demonstrates an important clinical nurse educator skill. Allowing learners to delegate in the clinical practice setting provides practice opportunities and helps ensure learner competence with the skill (Oermann, Shellenbarger, & Gaberson, 2018, p. 23). Option A, obtaining a bedside glucose, is a psychomotor skill that can be completed by trained unlicensed assistive personnel. Options B, C, and D require further assessment by the learner or nurse and should not be delegated.

Test Blueprint: 4 A
Cognitive Code: Analysis

8. Which action best demonstrates professional competence in a clinical specialty area?
   A. Continuing membership in a national professional organization, such as the National League for Nursing (NLN)
   B. Maintaining a nursing certification in wound, ostomy, and continence
   C. Orienting to a clinical specialty area
   D. Obtaining a master's degree with a concentration in nursing education

Correct Answer: B

Rationale: Specialty certification, Option B, validates a nurse's knowledge of a specialty area of nursing and shows continued dedication and accomplishment through the recertification process (Haskins, Hnatiuk, & Yoder, 2011). Professional certification has also been shown to increase quality of care and enhance client and nurse satisfaction (Valente, 2010). The NLN does provide certification but the focus of this option is only on membership; thus, Option A is incorrect. Option C is incorrect because orienting to the clinical area will not ensure professional competence. Option D, while helping nurse educators to obtain advanced knowledge in nursing education, does not ensure clinical competence.

Test Blueprint: 4 A
Cognitive Code: Application

9. Which action best demonstrates maintenance of clinical competence by the clinical nurse educator?
   A. Working per diem as a staff nurse
   B. Completing continuing education credits for licensure
   C. Attending professional development workshops offered by the institution
   D. Maintaining membership in a professional nursing organization

Correct Answer: A

Rationale: Professional work experience supports a clinical nurse educator's credibility and assists the educator in maintaining clinical skills and clinical judgment in the practice setting (Finke, 2012, p. 1; Oermann et al., 2018, p. 61). Options B, C, and D demonstrate nurse educator competence but do not specifically enhance clinical competence.

Test Blueprint: 4 A
Cognitive Code: Application

10. Which action should receive the highest priority when preparing to teach in an unfamiliar clinical environment?
A. Reviewing learning modules provided by the clinical agency
B. Attending a face-to-face orientation in the clinical agency
C. Shadowing an experienced clinical nurse educator on the clinical unit
D. Meeting with the unit manager to discuss learner needs

Correct Answer: B

Rationale: Clinical nurse educators require formal orientation to the clinical learning environment. A formal face-to-face orientation, as in Option B, would likely include the needed information of a review of policies, procedures, and technology used at the agency (Oermann et al., 2018, pp. 58, 60). Options C and D are not the highest priority because these activities may not include all of the needed preparatory information. Online learning modules limit the ability of clinical nurse educators to demonstrate competence with client care equipment, making Option A an incorrect response.

Test Blueprint: 4 A
Cognitive Code: Analysis

11. Which professional development activity would best prepare a clinical nurse educator for practice?
A. Massive open online course (MOOC)
B. Advanced clinical skills workshop
C. Grand round discussion with an interprofessional team
D. Journal club with other nurse educators

Correct Answer: B

Rationale: Clinical competence is an essential characteristic required of clinical nurse educators (Oermann et al., 2018, p. 61). Options A, C, and D are incorrect because MOOCs, grand round discussions, and journal clubs provide only theoretical knowledge. Option B is correct because an advanced skills workshop is the only activity that includes theoretical knowledge, expert clinical skills, and clinical practice judgment (Oermann & Gaberson, 2017).

Test Blueprint: 4 A
Cognitive Code: Application

12. Which should receive the highest priority when preparing for an upcoming teaching assignment?
A. Enrollment in a formal academic class focusing on clinical teaching
B. Review of nursing program evaluation requirements
C. Orientation to clinical agency electronic health records
D. Clinical competence nursing skill updates

Correct Answer: D

Rationale: Clinical nurse educators must prepare for clinical teaching assignments. Formal academic preparation required for clinical teaching assignments, as in Option A, is determined by the college, university, and/or the state board of nursing. Familiarity with the program evaluation requirements, Option B, and orientation to the clinical agency or setting, Option C, and clinical competence, Option D, are all factors that must be considered when preparing for a clinical teaching assignment (Oermann et al., 2018, p. 60). However, clinical competence, Option D, should receive the highest priority, as it is essential that the clinical nurse educator can provide safe instruction in the clinical setting; the educator needs to be prepared for delivery of clinical care.

Test Blueprint: 4 A
Cognitive Code: Application

13. Which activity would be most effective in assisting clinical learners with translation of theory to clinical practice?
   A. Development of a research question
   B. Self-reflection paper
   C. Concept map
   D. Multiple choice quiz

Correct Answer: C

Rationale: Clinical nurse educators must assist learners to translate theory to clinical practice. Teaching plans, concept maps, and care plans allow learners to connect theory and current clinical knowledge to practice (Oermann et al., 2018, p. 242). Thus, Option C, the concept map, is correct. Development of a research question allows learners to enquire about a topic from practice but would not be the most effective in translating theory to practice; thus, Option A is incorrect. Option B would promote reflection but does not guarantee application of theory to practice. Option D would evaluate learning but not necessarily help learners translate theory into practice.

Test Blueprint: 4 B
Cognitive Code: Application

14. Which question best helps learners translate theory into clinical practice when caring for a client with congestive heart failure?
   A. "How will you administer the intravenous diuretic?"
   B. "What time is the intravenous diuretic due?"
   C. "What additional medication would you anticipate administering for this client?"
   D. "What is the client's ejection fraction?"

Correct Answer: C

Rationale: Clinical reasoning is an essential feature of nursing competence (Oermann et al., 2018, p. 21). Effective clinical reasoning requires a deep understanding of the context of a client's medical history (Oermann et al., 2018, p. 21). Option C requires a deep understanding of the pathophysiology and management considerations of congestive heart failure and forces the learner to critically think about care. Considering Bloom's taxonomy of the cognitive domain, Options A, B, and D involve knowledge and comprehension or lower levels of thinking.

Test Blueprint: 4 B
Cognitive Code: Analysis

15. Which activity best uses a client-centered approach for a graduate nursing clinical course?
   A. Shadowing a preceptor
   B. Developing a teaching plan
   C. Observing grand rounds
   D. Completing a case study

Correct Answer: B

Rationale: Option B is correct because clinical nurse educators must provide opportunities for learners to develop therapeutic client-centered relationships (Oermann et al., 2018, p. 22). A teaching plan involves building a relationship directly between a client and learner. Options A, C, and D are incorrect because, although they promote learner growth in the clinical setting, they do not directly involve the development of therapeutic client-centered relationships.

Test Blueprint: 4 B
Cognitive Code: Application

16. The learner documents a client's blood pressure as 194/76 in the electronic health record. While reviewing this documentation, the clinical nurse educator is alarmed by this finding and questions the learner. Which statement or question best assesses the learner's clinical reasoning?
   A. "Tell me about the blood pressure you documented."
   B. "Describe how you obtained the client's blood pressure."
   C. "What additional assessment data should you collect and why?"
   D. "Why didn't you report your client's blood pressure?"

Correct Answer: C

Rationale: The level of questioning used by the clinical nurse educator directs the intended learning outcomes (Oermann et al., 2018, p. 193). Option C is an analysis question that asks the learner to identify further assessment data needed and why further assessment is necessary in this situation, encouraging clinical reasoning and making this the correct response. Options A, B, and D are lower-level questions that do not help assess clinical reasoning and higher-level thinking.

Test Blueprint: 4 B
Cognitive Code: Application

17. Which question best encourages application of theory to practice?
   A. "What are the signs and symptoms of hypoxia?"
   B. "What interventions did you use to improve your client's oxygenation and were they effective?"
   C. "What further assessment data did you collect when you found out your client was anxious?"
   D. "What lab values should you check for the client on oxygen?"

Correct Answer: B

Rationale: Clinical nurse educators can help learners apply theoretical content to the clinical setting through facilitated questioning (Oermann et al.,

2018, p. 189; Stokes & Kost, 2012, p. 324). Option A explores understanding, Option B encourages application of theoretical content to practice, Option C encourages analysis, and Option D facilitates recall.

Test Blueprint: 4 B
Cognitive Code: Application

18. Which journaling prompt would best promote learner reflection?
    A. Discuss a client interaction and describe how it made you feel.
    B. Describe the clinical skills you completed on the medical-surgical unit this week.
    C. Provide a list of three goals for your outpatient oncology experience.
    D. Identify an ethical issue you observed during your clinical experience.

Correct Answer: A

Rationale: Journals help learners relate theory to clinical practice (Oermann et al., 2018, p. 244). Detailed prompts and guiding questions for journal writing facilitates learner reflection and prevents learners from simply rehashing the clinical day (Harrison & Fopma-Loy, 2010). Journal prompts should be open-ended and encourage learners to reflect on clinical experiences, clinical decisions, and/or describe feelings, as in Option A (Oermann et al., 2018, p. 245). Options B, C, and D ask learners to recall information rather than analyze their experiences, decisions, and/or feelings.

Test Blueprint: 4 B
Cognitive Code: Application

19. The clinical nurse educator is discussing implementation of client-centered care in the clinical learning environment. Which is the best example of client-centered care?
    A. Monitoring a client's vital signs every two hours following surgery
    B. Assessing a client's pain during hourly safety rounds
    C. Discussing a client's discharge needs during the interprofessional team meeting
    D. Encouraging a client to participate in the bedside shift report

Correct Answer: D

Rationale: The bedside shift report, as suggested in Option D, promotes engagement of clients and families by providing an opportunity to ask and respond to questions as well as establish client-centered goals for the shift (Agency for Healthcare Research and Quality, 2019; Sherwood & Barnsteiner, 2017, p. 76). Options A, B, and C do not promote client-centered care; rather, they focus only on the nurse providing the care and do not actively involve the client in their care.

Test Blueprint: 4 B
Cognitive Code: Application

20. A clinical nurse educator is evaluating whether a learner includes client-centered care during a community health clinical experience. Which observed learner behavior should be addressed?
   A. The learner asks the client's spouse to leave the room prior to reviewing medications.
   B. The learner helps the client develop both short- and long-term healthy lifestyle goals.
   C. The learner takes into consideration the client's culture when suggesting dietary options.
   D. The learner asks questions to assess the client's physical comfort and emotional well-being.

Correct Answer: A

Rationale: Effective clinical teaching requires clinical nurse educators to be knowledgeable about emerging clinical topics and understand theories and concepts that direct nursing practice (Gubrud, 2016, p. 288). Client-centered care has emerged as a preferred model to improve quality care (Merav & Ohad, 2017). Options B, C, and D are incorrect because they do reflect the principles of client-centered care. Excluding family, Option A, is the learner behavior that should be addressed because family members play an important contributing role in this model of care.

Test Blueprint: 4 B
Cognitive Code: Analysis

21. Which action best facilitates learner development of clinical reasoning skills when caring for a complex client with multiple comorbidities and risk factors?
   A. Change the client assignment to one with less complex care needs to decrease the learner's anxiety.
   B. Assist the learner to identify relevant subjective and objective assessment data aimed at eliminating or treating complications.
   C. Advise the learner to find a quiet place to review the client's chart while the staff nurse communicates with other health care team members.
   D. Quiz the learner during a clinical conference about the client's admitting diagnosis, medications, and recent orders.

Correct Answer: B

Rationale: Option B is correct because, to coach learners as they develop clinical reasoning skills, educators can assist learners in identifying subtle and relevant cues and start to collaborate with other health care professionals. This coaching can assist them to provide the interventions needed in anticipation of potential problems; it also helps them to consider options aimed toward eliminating or treating complications (Cappelletti, Engel, & Prentice, 2014). Option A would not provide an opportunity to develop clinical reasoning skills. Option C is incorrect because learners should be provided with opportunities to communicate with and learn from a variety of health disciplines. Option D is incorrect because exploration and questions should be encouraged without penalty; an effective clinical nurse educator promotes a learning environment that involves positive interpersonal skills, understanding, and mutual respect (Gubrud, 2016).

Test Blueprint: 4 B
Cognitive Code: Application

22. Which statement indicates the most appropriate approach for a clinical conference?
    A. "Since we do not have an available private location on the unit, we must cancel the postclinical conference to ensure client confidentiality is maintained."
    B. "The learners are typically tired at the end of the day, so I plan to review easier topics and use closed-ended questions during group discussions."
    C. "Each learner will have the opportunity to discuss an assigned client-centered clinical topic, debrief about the clinical day, and provide feedback to others."
    D. "The postclinical conference is a great time for learners to practice communication skills and learn from each other, so my role as the educator is to sit back and let the learners talk."

Correct Answer: C

Rationale: Clinical conferences provide an opportunity for learners to bridge the gap between theory and practice. Option C is correct because postclinical conferences provide a forum in which learners and educators can discuss clinical experiences, share information, analyze clinical situations, clarify relationships, identify problems, examine feelings, and develop support systems (Gubrud, 2016). Option A is incorrect because clinical conferences can take place through electronic media or online if a physical space is not available (Gubrud, 2016). Option B is incorrect because open-ended questions are preferred during clinical conferences, as they can lead to problem-solving and higher-level thinking (Oermann & Gaberson, 2017). Option D is incorrect because the clinical nurse educator should serve as conference facilitator by supporting, encouraging, and sharing information during clinical conferences (Gubrud, 2016).

Test Blueprint: 4 B
Cognitive Code: Analysis

23. A learner asks the clinical nurse educator why changes were made to the fall prevention policy at the clinical institution. The clinical nurse educator best explains that policy changes are made after completing which task?
    A. A unit-based quality improvement project
    B. A review of current literature and a client satisfaction survey
    C. A unit-based research study approved by the Institutional Review Board (IRB)
    D. A review of institution fall incidents and current literature

Correct Answer: D

Rationale: Nurses and the interdisciplinary health care team are tasked with developing and revising policies that reflect current issues within the institution as well as ensuring that the policies reflect current evidence and best practice, as in Option D. Involvement of bedside nurses and ancillary staff with this process helps to ensure compliance with policies and client safety

(Dols et al., 2017; Wonder, Martin, & Jackson, 2017, p. 336). Options A and C reflect unit-based projects, not institution-wide changes. Option B discusses client satisfaction, which is not typically reviewed for policy development.

Test Blueprint: 4 C
Cognitive Code: Analysis

24. A learner asks why nasogastric tube placement is verified using pH testing. The clinical nurse educator directs the learner to use which resource to find the answer?
    A. The nurse educator on the clinical unit
    B. Health care agency's policy on the agency's Intranet
    C. Basic Internet search
    D. Library database search

Correct Answer: D

Rationale: Clinical courses provide an opportunity to teach learners how evidence is used in day-to-day clinical practice. Learners should be challenged with finding the best possible source of evidence to answer their questions and understand practice changes based on the availability of new evidence (Dols et al., 2017; Oermann et al., 2018, p. 242). Option D provides the best source of evidence. There is no guarantee that the clinical nurse educator on the clinical unit can provide the best, current evidence-based resources. Also, this does not assist in learning how to access up-to-date information in the future. Therefore, Option A is incorrect. Options B and C may not have complete, accurate, and current evidence-based information available.

Test Blueprint: 4 C
Cognitive Code: Application

25. A learner is assigned to care for a client newly diagnosed with lupus. The clinical nurse educator assists the learner in finding evidence-based clinical guidelines to care for this client. Which resource would be the best recommendation?
    A. Centers for Disease Control and Prevention (CDC)
    B. National Database of Nursing Quality Indicators (NDNQI)
    C. Agency for Healthcare Research and Quality (AHRQ)
    D. Education Resources Information Center (ERIC)

Correct Answer: C

Rationale: Clinical nurse educators must be aware of current evidence-based resources to assist learners in providing quality evidence-based care. Most of these resources are available via the Internet and can be accessed at the institution or within the clinical agency. Option C, AHRQ, provides current clinical practice guidelines for client-related problems and diagnoses (AHRQ, 2019). Option A, the CDC, provides information on communicable disease, immunizations, and disaster preparedness. Option B, NDNQI, provides data specific to quality indicators and nurse engagement (NDNQI, 2019). Option D, ERIC, is an online library of education research and information; it provides education-focused citations, not clinical guidelines.

Test Blueprint: 4 C
Cognitive Code: Recall

26. Which database is most appropriate to recommend to a learner wanting to locate best practice guidelines for palliative care?
    A. National Guideline Clearinghouse
    B. Google Scholar
    C. PubMed/Medline
    D. Cumulative Index to Nursing and Allied Health Literature (CINAHL)

Correct Answer: A

Rationale: Clinical nurse educators assist learners to evaluate the best available evidence for clinical practice (Oermann et al., 2018, p. 242). The National Guideline Clearinghouse provides the best evidence-based recommendations for practice. Google Scholar, PubMed/Medline, and CINAHL all provide scholarly sources but do not include a synthesis of the available evidence and a recommendation for practice, making Options B, C, and D incorrect.

Test Blueprint: 4 C
Cognitive Code: Application

27. Which evidence-based practice step would the clinical nurse educator suggest to the learner to complete first?
    A. Search for evidence
    B. Critically appraise the evidence
    C. Develop a research question
    D. Cultivate a spirit of inquiry

Correct Answer: D

Rationale: Evidence-based practice (EBP) guides clinical practice and therefore must be taught and modeled by clinical nurse educators. The steps of EBP include cultivate a spirit of inquiry, ask a question, search and collect the most relevant evidence, critically appraise the evidence, integrate the best evidence with clinical expertise and client preferences, evaluate outcomes, and disseminate outcomes (Melnyk & Fineout-Overholt, 2019, p. 17). Cultivating a spirit of inquiry is the first step of the EBP process, as it prepares the organization and establishes a framework for a continued emphasis on the available evidence. Options A, B, and C would occur later in the EBP process.

Test Blueprint: 4 C
Cognitive Code: Application

28. Which statement regarding delegation is most appropriate?
    A. "Delegation is the responsibility of the primary nurse."
    B. "Your preceptor will delegate tasks to you."
    C. "Delegation is the responsibility of the charge nurse."
    D. "There are legal implications associated with delegation."

Correct Answer: D

Rationale: Clinical nurse educators should teach delegation in the clinical setting. Learners must be given the opportunity to practice delegation skills with educator guidance (Oermann et al., 2018, p. 23). Options A and

C are not accurate statements and do not allow learners to practice delegation skills. Preceptors may delegate tasks to nursing learners, as in Option B; however, the clinical nurse educator retains responsibility for education in the clinical setting. There are legal implications of delegation; thus, Option D is most appropriate, as it begins the discussion of delegation in the clinical setting with learners.

Test Blueprint: 4 D
Cognitive Code: Analysis

29. Which activity best models effective leadership skills in the clinical learning environment?
    A. Reading an evidence-based journal
    B. Serving on a unit-based evidence-based practice committee
    C. Participating in a meeting to develop a plan of care
    D. Performing a comprehensive history and physical examination

Correct Answer: B

Rationale: Clinical nurse educators should model effective leadership in the clinical setting (Oermann et al., 2018, p. 23). Options A, C, and D are incorrect because reading an evidence-based practice journal, participating in a plan of care meeting, and performing a comprehensive history and physical examination are all activities required of professional nurses. However, Option B is correct because serving on a unit-based evidence-based practice committee is an activity that is above and beyond the role of professional nurses, demonstrating leadership.

Test Blueprint: 4 D
Cognitive Code: Analysis

30. Which activity would best help a graduate learner develop leadership and management skills during a clinical practicum experience?
    A. Shadowing a unit charge nurse
    B. Attending a budget meeting
    C. Leading unit-based rounds
    D. Leading a root cause analysis meeting

Correct Answer: D

Rationale: Clinical nurse educators, at both undergraduate and graduate levels, must assist learners in developing leadership and management skills (Oermann et al., 2018, p. 23). Shadowing a unit charge nurse, Option A, and attending a budget meeting, Option B, are passive activities and do not allow learners to apply their knowledge to practice. Leading unit-based rounds, Option C, while an active skill, is a task that can be completed by unit-based nurses and does not require graduate-level knowledge. Leading a root cause analysis meeting, Option D, is the only option that requires learners to apply graduate-level knowledge to practice.

Test Blueprint: 4 D
Cognitive Code: Analysis

31. A client's spouse says to the clinical nurse educator, "it seems like all of the learners are always on their mobile devices." Which response by the clinical nurse educator is most appropriate?

A. "I agree, I was not allowed to use my mobile device when I was in nursing school."

B. "Mobile devices provide nursing learners with resources to assist with client care."

C. "The agency just changed its policy to allow nurses and learners to use mobile devices at the nurses' station."

D. "I will address the issue during our clinical post-conference today."

Correct Answer: B

Rationale: Mobile devices provide nursing learners with access to evidence-based resources to assist with client care, making Option B correct (Oermann et al., 2018, pp. 162–163). Sharing about the clinical nurse educator's experience in nursing school, Option A, does not address the spouse's comment. The clinical nurse educator should discuss the spouse's concern during post-conference, as in Option D, but this does not educate the spouse about the benefit of mobile technology in the clinical environment. Although Option C may be true, it does not address the rationale for use of the mobile devices to assist with client care.

Test Blueprint: 4 D
Cognitive Code: Analysis

32. Which best exemplifies effective leadership by the clinical nurse educator in the clinical setting?

A. Orienting learners to the clinical unit

B. Describing fall risk assessment and prevention strategies

C. Independently completing an incident report following a client fall

D. Verbalizing thought processes, decisions, and actions following a client fall

Correct Answer: D

Rationale: "Leadership in the clinical faculty role can be demonstrated by the conscious decision to be a role model for students" (Adelman-Mullally et al., 2013, p. 30). For example, a clinical nurse educator may demonstrate the appropriate way to respond to a medication error, question a physician order, advocate for a client, and delegate effectively (Adelman-Mullally et al., 2013, p. 30). While doing so, clinical nurse educators should also discuss aloud their thought processes, decisions, and actions with learners to make these transparent, as in Option D. Options A and B allow for the clinical nurse educator to share useful information but do not demonstrate role modeling, making them incorrect choices. Option C is incorrect because the clinical nurse educator assumes responsibility for the incident report completion independently and does not involve the learner in this learning opportunity.

Test Blueprint: 4 D
Cognitive Code: Application

33. The clinical nurse educator observes learners gathered together in the hallway standing in groups at the nurses' station and failing to participate in care for assigned clients. Which action should the clinical nurse educator take first?
   A. Talk to the charge nurse to brainstorm activities to keep learners remaining busy and engaged in client care.
   B. Perform an assessment of learner needs during a clinical conference to understand needs and stresses confronting the learners in the clinical environment.
   C. Evaluate learners who were not in client rooms providing care as "unsatisfactory" for the day on the clinical evaluation tool.
   D. Change future clinical assignments to use the preceptor model in which learners can be assigned care under expert nurses in the clinical setting.

Correct Answer: B

Rationale: The complex process of teaching-learning in clinical education requires an assessment of learning needs. Learner behaviors on the clinical unit may indicate issues related to stress and/or lack of prerequisite knowledge or skills needed for the clinical environment. Assessment reveals the point at which the instruction should begin (Oermann et al., 2018, p. 99). Options A, C, and D do not enable the clinical nurse educator to collect data regarding learner needs; thus, they would not be the first action the clinical nurse educator should take. Instead, the clinical nurse educator should complete an assessment of learner needs, as suggested in Option B, to identify learner problems and needs.

Test Blueprint: 4 D
Cognitive Code: Application

34. During a community health clinical experience, a clinical nurse educator assesses a learner's clinical reasoning capabilities related to a client recently diagnosed with diabetes. Which observed learner behavior should be addressed?
   A. The learner reviews the health assessment before beginning the client's discharge instructions.
   B. The learner shares with the client potential side effects of a newly prescribed diabetic medication.
   C. The learner suggests decreasing sodium when the client states having increased thirst.
   D. The learner asks the client to summarize information discussed after reviewing foot care.

Correct Answer: C

Rationale: Effective clinical teaching requires clinical nurse educators to guide and evaluate learners as they develop clinical reasoning skills (Gubrud, 2016, pp. 289–290). Clinical reasoning requires the learner to have knowledge about the clinical topic, anticipate expected outcomes, and identify subtle and relevant cues (Gubrud, 2016, pp. 289–290). Options A, B, and D are incorrect because they demonstrate appropriate clinical reasoning behaviors. Option C is the correct response since the learner failed to identify the cue of increased thirst that is associated with diabetes.

Test Blueprint: 4 E
Cognitive Code: Analysis

35. A learner approaches the clinical nurse educator and states that the client is having trouble breathing. Which action best demonstrates clinical reasoning skills?
   A. Telling the learner to notify the coassigned nurse
   B. Going with the learner to assess the client's respiratory status
   C. Calling the client's physician to report the symptoms
   D. Telling the learner to place the client on 2 L of oxygen

Correct Answer: B

Rationale: Clinical reasoning skills allow a clinical nurse educator to collect data, solve problems, and make decisions in the clinical setting to promote quality and safety of clients and learners (Stokes & Kost, 2012, p. 317). Option B allows the clinical nurse educator to assess the client with the learner and identify data indicating the severity of respiratory distress, thus demonstrating clinical reasoning skills. Option A removes the clinical nurse educator from the situation and prevents a teaching moment about clinical reasoning. Options C and D require more assessment data and should not be implemented until an assessment is complete.

Test Blueprint: 4 E
Cognitive Code: Analysis

36. The clinical nurse educator is emphasizing clinical judgment. Which learner response would most likely require follow-up?
   A. "I understand that I should have involved the client's family when I reviewed the discharge instructions."
   B. "The client voided 500 mL after administration of intravenous furosemide."
   C. "The client's blood pressure was 160/80 and I administered intravenous metoprolol."
   D. "I completed a physical assessment on my client at 10:30 a.m."

Correct Answer: D

Rationale: There are four aspects of clinical judgment, including: (a) noticing and grasping the situation; (b) interpreting and understanding the situation in order to respond; (c) responding by deciding on actions that are appropriate or that no actions are needed; and (d) reflecting, being attentive to how clients respond (Oermann et al., 2018, p. 175). Option D does not reflect clinical judgment, only completion of a psychomotor skill. Options A, B, and C require noticing, interpreting, and responding to the client care situations.

Test Blueprint: 4 E
Cognitive Code: Analysis

37. Which question would best promote clinical reasoning of learners during a clinical case study?
   A. "Is there evidence to support your treatment decision?"
   B. "What additional information would you request from the client?"
   C. "Which theoretical framework best supports the care of the client?"
   D. "Why would the client's albumin level be subtherapeutic?"

Correct Answer: D

Rationale: There are multiple strategies to promote clinical reasoning skills with case studies. Option D best achieves clinical reasoning outcomes, as it requires learners to consider multiple aspects of the client's care (Oermann et al., 2018, p. 181). Options A, B, and C do not represent the best approach for promoting clinical reasoning, as they do not require the learner to critically think prior to responding.

Test Blueprint: 4 E
Cognitive Code: Analysis

38. Which discussion prompt would best promote cognitive development during a clinical conference?
    A. "What did you learn today when observing in the emergency department?"
    B. "Which intravenous antihypertensive medication did you administer first?"
    C. "How did you coordinate the client's care with the respiratory therapist?"
    D. "What diagnostic test would be most pertinent to assist in the diagnosis of congestive heart failure?"

Correct Answer: D

Rationale: Cognitive development includes problem-solving, critical thinking, and clinical judgment skills (Oermann et al., 2018, p. 191). Clinical nurse educators can best support cognitive skill development by asking questions that encourage learners to consider alternative perspectives and viewpoints in a given situation and to provide a rationale for their thinking (Oermann et al., 2018, p. 191). Option A does not require critical thinking or clinical judgment skills. Options B and C require problem-solving and clinical judgment skills but do not require refined critical thinking skills. Option D requires the learner to use critical thinking skills.

Test Blueprint: 4 E
Cognitive Code: Analysis

39. Which activity performed by a graduate learner would best expand the learner's knowledge and skills of evidence-based practice?
    A. Participating in a root cause analysis for incorrect medication administration
    B. Examining benchmark data pertaining to congestive heart failure readmission rates
    C. Developing a question using the problem, intervention, comparison, outcomes, and time (PICOT) format
    D. Presenting key performing indicators at a staff meeting

Correct Answer: C

Rationale: An important aspect of the clinical nurse educator role is supporting evidence-based practice, client safety, and quality improvement outcomes (Oermann et al., 2018, p. 25). Options A, B, and D all refer to activities that would expand quality improvement skills. Option C is the only activity that is directly related to evidence-based practice.

Test Blueprint: 4 F
Cognitive Code: Application

40. Which activity would best help the learner expand one's clinical knowledge and skills and integrate best practices of care?
   A. Unfolding case study
   B. Grand rounds
   C. Case study
   D. Case method

Correct Answer: B

Rationale: Grand rounds, Option B, provides an opportunity to promote best practices (Oermann et al., 2018, p. 183). Learners can benefit from time spent with the clinical team and participate in the decision-making process regarding a client's care. Case studies, unfolding cases, and case methods do promote best practices; however, they are not as interactive and therefore would not be superior to participating in grand rounds.

Test Blueprint: 4 F
Cognitive Code: Application

41. Which statement by the learner regarding utilization of a continuous passive motion machine (CPM) likely requires follow-up?
   A. "The client requested the CPM."
   B. "I recently read an article demonstrating the benefits of CPMs."
   C. "The American Orthopaedic Association recommends the use of CPMs."
   D. "The provider does not use CPMs with their clients."

Correct Answer: D

Rationale: Clinical nurse educators should emphasize evidence-based practice. Client and family preferences, as in Option A, current evidence, as in Option B, and clinical expertise, as suggested in Option C, are all aspects of evidence-based practice (Oermann et al., 2018, p. 26). Option D does not represent an aspect of evidence-based practice.

Test Blueprint: 4 F
Cognitive Code: Analysis

42. Which action demonstrates best practice when making learner clinical assignments?
   A. Selecting clients who provide learners with both hands-on clinical skills and who encourage their critical thinking
   B. Picking clients recommended by the charge nurse on the clinical unit
   C. Choosing clients who consent to work with learners
   D. Selecting clients who will assist learners in meeting the learning objectives for the clinical experience

Correct Answer: D

Rationale: When planning for clinical experiences, the priority for the clinical nurse educator should be the attainment of learning objectives. This ensures that the outcomes of the clinical experience are met (Oermann et al., 2018, p. 79). Options A, B, and C are other factors that may influence the clinical nurse educator's decision, but ultimately ensuring that the client assignments meet the level and objectives for learners is best practice.

Test Blueprint: 4 F
Cognitive Code: Application

43. Effective communication between health care providers, clients, and families promotes teamwork, collaboration, and safety. To best explain this concept to learners, the clinical nurse educator reviews which during clinical orientation?
A. Basic principles of conflict resolution among team members
B. Legal and ethical considerations for communicating health information
C. Use of standardized tools for hand-off communication
D. Differences between assertive and aggressive communication approaches

Correct Answer: C

Rationale: Standardized tools decrease the risks associated with hand-offs between health care providers and promote appropriate communication (QSEN, 2019). Use of standardized tools—such as Situation, Background, Assessment, Recommendation (SBAR)—supports the Joint Commission's National Patient Safety Goal of improving communication between agency staff (Joint Commission, 2019). Options A and D provide general communication guidelines but do not necessarily promote interprofessional communication. Providing information about legal and ethical considerations is an important aspect of communication, but Option B does not focus on interprofessional communication.

Test Blueprint: 4 F
Cognitive Code: Application

44. Which action by the learner reflects clinical reasoning skills when caring for a client who begins to complain of shortness of breath?
A. Notifying the primary care provider
B. Requesting a chest x-ray
C. Obtaining vital signs and oxygen saturation
D. Calling the rapid response team

Correct Answer: C

Rationale: Clinical reasoning is the process of gathering and thinking about client information, analyzing the options, and evaluating alternatives (Gubrud, 2016). Option C demonstrates the learner's ability to detect a change in the client's condition, recognize a change in priorities, and adjust nursing care appropriately. The other options may be important interventions for this client but do not represent the best next action, thus, they are not the best reflection of clinical reasoning skills.

Test Blueprint: 4 F
Cognitive Code: Application

45. Which statement best indicates an understanding of evidence-based clinical evaluation methods?
A. "The psychomotor domain is the most important area to evaluate in the clinical setting."
B. "I will assign a letter grade to the learners' written journal reflections."
C. "Multiple evaluation methods should be used to assess learners' performance."
D. "All clinical assessment methods should be summative forms of evaluation."

Correct Answer: C

Rationale: Option C is correct because multiple strategies should be used for assessment in clinical courses owing to the breadth of competencies learners need to develop (Oermann & Gaberson, 2017). Option A is incorrect because nursing educators should be evaluating all three learning domains: affective, cognitive, and psychomotor. Option B is incorrect because grading of journals is not encouraged, as doing so would inhibit the learners' reflection and dialogue about feelings and perceptions of clinical experiences (Oermann & Gaberson, 2017). Option D is incorrect since evaluation methods can be used for either formative or summative evaluation and both are considered an essential component of most nursing courses (Oermann & Gaberson, 2017). Frequent opportunities for formative evaluation are encouraged in the clinical setting (Sorrell & Cangelosi, 2016).

Test Blueprint: 4 F
Cognitive Code: Application

46. Which initial action is most appropriate if a clinical nurse educator suspects that a learner is under the influence of alcohol while at the clinical setting?
    A. Direct the learner to a private location to allow the learner to become sober before resuming client care.
    B. Remove the learner from client care immediately and escort the the learner to a private location to address the issue.
    C. Dismiss the learner from the unit immediately and make an appointment for a follow-up meeting to discuss the implications of the learner's actions.
    D. Review the agency policy on learner intoxication before removing the learner from the client care assignment.

Correct Answer: B

Rationale: Option B is correct because educators must immediately address learner behaviors that are unsafe for client care, including substance abuse (Bonnel, 2016). O'Connor (2015) summarizes key points related to the learner who is unsafe to care for clients, noting that safety of the client is the priority in removing a learner. Also, these educators have an obligation to ensure that all learners are returned to an area of safety as well. Option A is incorrect because the learner should not be permitted to return to client care if intoxicated. Option C is incorrect in that the learner should not drive home while intoxicated; additionally, this option delays talking with the learner about the concern. Although program and agency policies must be followed in this situation, Option D is incorrect because the learner should be removed from all client care immediately.

Test Blueprint: 4 G
Cognitive Code: Application

47. A learner arrives to the clinical unit unprepared for the clinical experience. Which is the best initial response?
   A. Allow the learner to complete the preparation and reschedule the experience.
   B. Send the learner home and document the unpreparedness in the clinical evaluation.
   C. Discuss the behavior with the learner and reiterate expectations for preparation.
   D. Inform the learner that the behavior is unacceptable and implement a learning plan.

Correct Answer: C

Rationale: Immediate feedback to the learner with expectations for preparation should be reviewed first with the learner, as in Option C. This assists with learner understanding of expected behaviors, policies for clinical learning, as well as predetermined outcomes and competencies (Gaberson, Oermann, & Shellenbarger, 2015, p. 324). Other actions, such as Options A, B, and D, may follow the initial response and should be based on the existing policies and disciplinary processes within the institution.

Test Blueprint: 4 G
Cognitive Code: Application

48. The clinical nurse educator is meeting with learners individually to review their plan for the day. Which question would best ensure that learners are prepared for the clinical experience?
   A. "Why was your client transferred here from another agency?"
   B. "What nursing care will you provide first?"
   C. "Why is it important to obtain vital signs first?"
   D. "What will you do if your client falls?"

Correct Answer: B

Rationale: Preclinical conferences provide an opportunity for clinical nurse educators to assess learner preparation for the clinical experience. Questioning can be used to assess adequate knowledge to care for their assigned clients and can also be helpful in assessing a learner's understanding of important clinical care (Oermann et al., 2018, p. 66). Option B helps the clinical nurse educator assess the learner's knowledge of the plan of care and prioritization of the care to be provided. Although Options A, C, and D include relevant information, they do not assess the learner's preparedness.

Test Blueprint: 4 G
Cognitive Code: Application

49. Which initial action is most appropriate to take when a learner is not prepared to administer medications to a client?
A. Allow the learner to administer the medications and then outline the need for better preparation in the written feedback to the learner.
B. Inform the learner that due to the learner's poor preparation, the learner may not administer medications for the remainder of the term.
C. Dismiss the learner from the clinical setting immediately and arrange an appointment to discuss the implications of the actions later.
D. Instruct the learner to look up the information needed to safely administer the medications and encourage more thorough preparation practices.

Correct Answer: D

Rationale: Educators must immediately address learner behaviors that are unsafe for client care, including lack of preparation (Bonnel, 2016). Option D is correct because a learner unprepared to care for an assigned clinical client should be sent somewhere, such as the library or laboratory, to prepare (Bonnel, 2016). Option A is unsafe if the learner is not knowledgeable about the medications. Options B and C are harsh consequences and do not provide the learner with an opportunity to learn and improve on the performance.

Test Blueprint: 4 G
Cognitive Code: Application

50. Which action best helps learners meet the clinical learning outcome: *Learners will maintain safety during their clinical practice and will remain in compliance with the School of Nursing and Clinical Agency*?
A. Discussing how agency technology can help monitor client health status
B. Discussing who has the authority to make decisions for pediatric clients
C. Discussing how people from different cultures perceive and manage pain
D. Providing an example of a near miss and discussing how to manage the situation

Correct Answer: D

Rationale: Option D is a suggested activity to meet the knowledge, skills, and attitudes competencies listed in the Quality and Safety Education for Nurses (QSEN) Safety Competency (QSEN, 2019). Option A is linked to the Informatics Competency and Options B and C best correlate with the Patient-Centered Care Competency (QSEN, 2019).

Test Blueprint: 4 G
Cognitive Code: Analysis

51. Which clinical learning outcome is consistent with the Quality and Safety Education for Nurses (QSEN) Safety Competency?
A. Communicate observations or concerns related to errors to clients, families, and members of the health care team.
B. Act with integrity, consistency, and respect for differing views and opinions.
C. Assess levels of physical and emotional comfort.
D. Protect confidentiality of protected health information in electronic health records.

Correct Answer: A

Rationale: Option A is listed under the QSEN Safety Competency. Option B is consistent with Teamwork and Collaboration; Option C is noted under the Patient-Centered Care Competency; and Option D is linked to the Informatics Competency (QSEN, 2019).

Test Blueprint: 4 G
Cognitive Code: Recall

52. Which assignment would be most appropriate to balance client care and introductory learner needs during the learner's first clinical experience?
    A. Obtaining a comprehensive health history
    B. Initiating an intravenous infusion
    C. Shadowing an experienced nurse
    D. Administering oral medications

Correct Answer: A

Rationale: Clinical nurse educators should make clinical assignments based on course objectives and prerequisite knowledge, skills, and attitudes of learners (Oermann et al., 2018, p. 111). Obtaining a comprehensive health history, Option A, is the most appropriate assignment, as it introduces learners to interacting with clients and is a safe activity. Intravenous infusions, Option B, and administering oral medications, Option D, are advanced skills that may not have been developed and practiced by the first clinical experience. Option C, shadowing an experienced nurse, does not allow the nursing learner to apply knowledge to practice.

Test Blueprint: 4 G
Cognitive Code: Application

53. The clinical nurse educator removes a learner from the clinical setting because of unsafe behavior. Which activity is most appropriate for the clinical nurse educator to require next?
    A. Library assignment
    B. Skills lab remediation
    C. Self-reflection journal
    D. Attend an additional clinical day

Correct Answer: B

Rationale: Clinical nurse educators have an obligation to remove learners from the clinical setting for unsafe practice. Skills lab remediation, Option B, would be the most appropriate activity for a learner to practice psychomotor skills (Oermann et al., 2018, p. 111). An additional clinical day, Option D, would also be a consideration but it is not the most appropriate next activity because it does not focus specifically on the unsafe psychomotor activity. Library assignments, Option A, and self-reflection journals, Option C, would be appropriate for knowledge and attitude activities.

Test Blueprint: 4 G
Cognitive Code: Application

54. Which consideration should receive the highest priority when evaluating educational technologies?
A. Educator experience with technology
B. Orientation and training needs
C. Mission statement of the nursing program
D. Characteristics of the learners

Correct Answer: D

Rationale: Technology can enhance the educational experience for learners. Primary considerations when evaluating educational technologies are course objectives, cost, and characteristics of learners, as in Option D (Oermann et al., 2018, p. 159). The nursing program mission statement, as in Option C, provides a global vision for the entire academic unit and is therefore not a priority consideration. Educator experience with technology, as in Option A, and training needs, as in Option B, are considerations but not the priority consideration.

Test Blueprint: 4 H
Cognitive Code: Application

55. A clinical nurse educator would like to use social media while working with learners in diverse clinical sites. When would social media use be most appropriate?
A. Postclinical conference
B. Verification of clinical hours
C. Learner notification of clinical absence
D. Clinical orientation

Correct Answer: A

Rationale: Postclinical conferences that use social media can be an effective strategy when learners are participating in diverse clinical experiences (Oermann et al., 2018, p. 159). Clinical orientation, Option D, should be coordinated by the clinical agency and include a review of policies and procedures and electronic medical records (Oermann et al., 2018, pp. 58, 60). Clinical hours should be formally verified, as in Option B, and not visible to other learners. Option C, clinical experience absences, should be communicated directly to the clinical nurse educator and not via social media.

Test Blueprint: 4 H
Cognitive Code: Application

56. While planning for the start-of-term clinical orientation, the clinical nurse educator has created a scavenger hunt for learners to find several items in the electronic medical record that will help them understand the plan of care for their clients. This learning activity best corresponds to which Quality and Safety Education for Nurses (QSEN) competency?
A. Client-centered Care
B. Quality Improvement
C. Informatics
D. Evidence-based Practice

Correct Answer: C

Rationale: Option C is correct because this activity corresponds with the knowledge, skills, and attitudes listed in the QSEN Informatics competency (QSEN, 2019). The other options are QSEN competencies, but they would not be fully met with this learning activity.

Test Blueprint: 4 H
Cognitive Code: Recall

57. Which learning activity best facilitates learners' use of technology in the clinical learning environment?
    A. Having learners look up specific policies that are common on the clinical unit
    B. During orientation, having learners work in small groups to navigate the electronic medical record
    C. Discussing with learners how to give medications safely in the clinical area
    D. Including a care plan assignment that incorporates client-centered care for each clinical day

Correct Answer: B

Rationale: Option B is a suggested activity to meet the objectives listed in the Quality and Safety Education for Nurses (QSEN) Informatics competency. Option A links to the Evidence-based Practice competency, Option C is consistent with the Safety competency, and Option D is consistent with the Patient-centered Care competency (QSEN, 2019).

Test Blueprint: 4 H
Cognitive Code: Application

58. Which is the best method for evaluating learner competency for nasogastric tube insertion?
    A. Standardized patient
    B. Task trainer
    C. Full body mannequin
    D. Computer-based activity

Correct Answer: C

Rationale: Option C would be the method with the highest level of realism that would not involve a real person. Although Option A involves the highest level of realism or fidelity, it would be inappropriate to perform this invasive procedure on a person serving as a standardized patient. While Options B and D would be methods to consider, they would not provide learners with the highest level of fidelity mimicking a realistic client scenario (International Nursing Association for Clinical Simulation and Learning Standards Committee, 2016).

Test Blueprint: 4 H
Cognitive Code: Application

59. A learner working with a diabetic client in a community wellness center is asked questions about a new device that was prescribed to check blood sugars. The clinical nurse educator is not familiar with the device but notices a set of instructions with the device. The instructions clearly state the series of steps for the client to follow. Which would be the best action for the clinical nurse educator to take?

A. Advise the client to review the instructions for use that come with the device.

B. Refer the client to the client's primary care provider to review the product use together.

C. Review the set of instructions with the client and learner and practice using the device.

D. Recommend that the learner go home and read about the device so that the learner is prepared for client questions.

Correct Answer: C

Rationale: The clinical nurse educator acknowledges that this is an opportunity to learn about a new device. This helps to establish that the clinical nurse educator is a competent nurse. Learners desire nurse educators in the clinical environment who are competent in clinical skills and remain current in practice (Collier, 2017). Option C allows for both the clinical nurse educator and the learner to learn about a new device and provides an opportunity for the clinical nurse educator to show competency. Options A and D do not provide an opportunity to help the client or to show competence of the clinical nurse educator. Option B puts ownership of client education on the primary care provider and does not help support the client.

Test Blueprint: 4 H
Cognitive Code: Application

References

Adelman-Mullally, T., Mulder, C. K., McCarter-Spalding, D. E., Hagler, D. A., Gaberson, K. B., Hanner, M. B., ... Young, P. K. (2013). The clinical nurse educator as leader. *Nurse Education in Practice, 13*, 29–34. doi:10.1016/j.nepr.2012.07.006

Agency for Healthcare Research and Quality. (2019). Standardized shift-change process optimizes time for transfer of patient care responsibility, leads to high levels of nurse and patient satisfaction. Retrieved from https://innovations.ahrq.gov/node/4352

Berman, A., Snyder, S., & Frandsen, G. (2016). *Kozier & Erb's fundamentals of nursing: Concepts, process, and practice* (10th ed.). Boston, MA: Pearson.

Bonnel, W. (2016). Clinical performance evaluation. In D. M. Billings & J. A. Halstead (Eds.), *Teaching in nursing: A guide for faculty* (5th ed., pp. 443–462). St. Louis, MO: Elsevier.

Cappelletti, A., Engel, J. K., & Prentice, D. (2014). Systematic review of clinical judgement and reasoning in nursing. *Journal of Nursing Education, 53*(8), 453–458. doi:10.3928/01484834-20140724-01

Collier, A. D. (2017). Characteristics of an effective nursing clinical instructor: The state of the science. *Journal of Clinical Nursing, 27*(1–2), 363–374. doi:10.1111/jocn.13931

Cope, V., & Murray, M. (2018). Use of professional portfolios in nursing. *Nursing Standard, 32*(30), 55–63. doi:10.7748/ns.2018.e10985

Dols, J. D., Muñoz, L. R., Martinez, S. S., Mathers, N., Miller, P. S., Pomerleau, T. A., & White, S. (2017). Developing policies and protocols in the age of evidence-based practice. *The Journal of Continuing Education in Nursing, 48*(2), 87–92. doi:10.3928/00220124-20170119-10

Finke, L. M. (2012). Teaching in nursing: The faculty role. In D. M. Billings & J. A. Halstead (Eds.), *Teaching in nursing: A guide for faculty* (4th ed., pp. 1–14). St. Louis, MO: Elsevier.

Fisher, M. L. (2016). Teaching in nursing: The faculty role. In D. M. Billings & J. A. Halstead (Eds.), *Teaching in nursing: A guide for faculty* (5th ed., pp. 1–14). St. Louis, MO: Elsevier.

Gaberson, K. B., Oermann, M. H., & Shellenbarger, T. (2015). *Clinical teaching strategies in nursing* (4th ed). New York, NY: Springer.

Gubrud, P. (2016). Teaching in the clinical setting. In D. M. Billings & J. A. Halstead (Eds.), *Teaching in nursing: A guide for faculty* (5th ed., pp. 288–290). St. Louis, MO: Elsevier.

Harrison, P. A., & Fopma-Loy, J. L. (2010). Reflective journal prompts: A vehicle for stimulating emotional competence in nursing. *Journal of Nursing Education, 49*(11), 644–652. doi:10.3928/01484834-20100730-07

Haskins, M., Hnatiuk, C. N., & Yoder, L. H. (2011). Medical-surgical nurses' perceived value of certification study. *Medsurg Nursing, 20*(2), 71–93.

International Nursing Association for Clinical Simulation and Learning Standards Committee (2016). INACSL standards of best practice: Simulation^SM simulation design. *Clinical Simulation in Nursing, 12*, S5–S12. doi:10.1016/j.ecns.2016.09.005

Joint Commission. (2019). 2019 National patient safety goals. Retrieved from https://www.jointcommission.org/assets/1/6/2019_HAP_NPSGs_final2.pdf

Melnyk, B. M., & Fineout-Overholt, E. (2019). *Evidence-based practice in nursing and healthcare: A guide to best practice* (4th ed.). Philadelphia, PA: Wolters Kluwer.

Merav, B. N., & Ohad, H. (2017). Patient-centered care in healthcare and its implementation in nursing. *International Journal of Caring Sciences, 10*(1), 596–600.

National Database of Nursing Quality Indicators. (2019). NDNQI nursing-sensitive indicators. Retrieved from https://nursingandndnqi.weebly.com/ndnqi-indicators.html

National League for Nursing. (2012). *The scope of practice for academic nurse educators: 2012 revision.* New York, NY: Author.

O'Connor, A. B. (2015). *Clinical instruction and evaluation: A teaching resource* (3rd ed.). Burlington, MA: Jones & Bartlett.

Oermann, M. H., & Gaberson, K. B. (2017). *Evaluation and testing in nursing education* (5th ed.). New York, NY: Springer.

Oermann, M. H., Shellenbarger, T., & Gaberson, K. B. (2018). *Clinical teaching strategies in nursing* (5th ed.). New York, NY: Springer.

Quality and Safety Education for Nurses Institute. (2019). QSEN competencies. Retrieved from http://qsen.org/competencies/

Sherwood, G., & Barnsteiner, J. (2017). *Quality and safety in nursing: A competency approach to improving outcomes* (2nd ed.). Hoboken, NJ: Wiley & Sons.

Sorrell, J. M., & Cangelosi, P. R. (2016). *Expert clinician to novice nurse educator: Learning from first-hand narratives.* New York, NY: Springer.

Stokes, L. G., & Kost, G. C. (2012). Teaching in the clinical setting. In D. M. Billings & J. A. Halstead (Eds.), *Teaching in nursing: A guide for faculty* (4th ed., pp. 311–334). St. Louis, MO: Elsevier.

Strong, M. (2016). Maintaining clinical competency is your responsibility. *American Nurse Today, 11*(7), 46–47.

Valente, S. M. (2010). Improving professional practice through certification. *Journal for Nurses in Staff Development, 26*(5), 215–219. doi:10.1097/NND.0b13e31819b561c

Wonder, A. H., Martin, E. K., & Jackson, K. (2017). Supporting and empowering direct-care nurses to promote EBP: An example of evidence-based policy development, education, and practice change. *Worldviews on Evidence-Based Nursing, 14*(4), 336–338. doi:10.1111/wvn.12239

7

Facilitate Learner Development and Socialization

1. A combative client is ordered 2 mg of lorazepam intravenously (IV) prior to an invasive procedure. A learner is helping the staff nurse prepare to take the client to the procedure and notices that the staff nurse gives 1 mg of lorazepam rather than the ordered dose. In post-conference, the learner tells the clinical nurse educator and classmates what the learner observed. Which is the best response?
   A. Tell the learner that the learner should have confronted the staff nurse at the time of the incident.
   B. Ask the staff nurse about the location of the remaining dose of medication.
   C. Request a meeting with the learner and nurse manager of the unit.
   D. Remind the learner that the action of the staff nurse is a good example of nursing judgment.

   Correct Answer: C

   Rationale: Learners are held to the same professional, legal, and ethical behavior as licensed nurses (Gaberson, Oermann, & Shellenbarger, 2015, p. 98). According to the National Council of State Boards of Nursing model rules (2017), licensed nurses promote a safe environment by correcting problems or referring problems to the appropriate management level when needed (p. 4). The situation described suggests that the staff nurse may be diverting controlled substances. The learner and educator should refer the situation to the nurse manager for review, as suggested in Option C. Options A, B, and D do not appropriately address the concern.

   Test Blueprint: 5 A
   Cognitive Code: Application

2. The family member of a client angrily approaches the nurses' station and states, "The learner just told my dad that he may have lung cancer. I want to speak to the physician right now!" Which is the best initial action?
   A. Talking with the client's daughter to find out exactly what happened
   B. Meeting privately with the learner to gain more insight on the situation
   C. Asking the learner to call the physician and inform the physician of the incident
   D. Requesting the nurse manager talk with the client and his daughter

   Correct Answer: B

Rationale: Learners are held to the same legal, ethical, and professional standards as licensed nurses. According to the National Council of State Boards of Nursing model rules (2017), nurses "implement treatment and therapy" (p. 3). Physicians diagnose mental and physical conditions; licensed nurses are not permitted to make medical diagnoses (Doenges, Moorhouse, & Murr, 2016, p. 3). Thus, the learner's actions should be considered outside of the scope of the professional nurse. The best next action by the clinical nurse educator would be to talk with the learner privately about the situation, as in Option B. Options A, C, and D do not address the learner's behavior.

Test Blueprint: 5 A
Cognitive Code: Application

3. A learner in the clinical group is scheduled to administer morning medications to an assigned client at 0900. At 0915, the clinical nurse educator approaches the learner and asks whether the learner is ready to administer the medications. The learner states having administered the medications with the staff nurse at 0855. The program's policy states that all skills performed by the learner must be supervised by the clinical nurse educator. Which should be the clinical nurse educator's initial reaction?
   A. Check the medication administration record to verify that the medications were administered.
   B. While the staff nurse is on break, confront the staff nurse about the situation.
   C. Talk to the client to see whether the learner administered the medications.
   D. Send the learner to the break room to review the policy and then review it together.

Correct Answer: D

Rationale: The learner and clinical nurse educator must follow the policies of the nursing program (Oermann, Shellenbarger, & Gaberson, 2018, p. 283). In this situation, the learner failed to follow the policy of the nursing program. The clinical nurse educator should immediately remind the learner of the policy, as in Option D. Options A, B, and C do not address the learner's behavior regarding program policies.

Test Blueprint: 5 A
Cognitive Code: Application

4. A beginning learner confides in the clinical nurse educator regarding frustration that a client stated, "Get out of here, I don't want a learner today." Which is the best initial response?
   A. Instruct the learner to go back in and talk with the client to see what's bothering the client.
   B. Tell the client that the unit is short-staffed and the client would receive better care with a learner.
   C. Confirm with the client that the client does not want a learner for the day.
   D. Explain to the client that the learner will come back after breakfast.

Correct Answer: C

Rationale: Clients who encounter learners in the clinical setting may feel exploited or fearful. Clinical nurse educators must consider the rights and needs of the client as well as those of the learner (Oermann et al., 2018, p. 100). The client has the right to refuse care provided by the learner. The clinical nurse educator and learner should respect the client's autonomy; thus, Option C is correct. Options A, B, and D do not respect the client's rights.

Test Blueprint: 5 A
Cognitive Code: Application

5. The unit manager where a group of senior learners is having a clinical experience informs the clinical nurse educator that one learner sought the unit manager to inquire about a position after graduation. How should the clinical nurse educator best handle this situation?
   A. Instruct the learner to schedule a private meeting with the manager outside of designated clinical time.
   B. Express one's opinion about the learner's potential job performance to the manager.
   C. Identify the learner when discussing an example of unprofessional behavior during postclinical conference.
   D. Express one's personal opinion about working on that unit to the learner.

Correct Answer: A

Rationale: While employment after graduation is important to learners, they must be made aware that clinical experiences are for learning purposes. Learners must maintain professional behavior (Oermann et al., 2018, p. 98). The best way a learner can display professional behavior while seeking job opportunities would be to speak privately with the unit manager outside of designated clinical time. The clinical nurse educator should not give an opinion regarding the learner's clinical performance to the unit manager, as in Option B, without a written formal request. Identifying the learner as an example of unprofessional behavior during postclinical conference, as in Option C, may belittle and embarrass the learner. The clinical nurse educator should also maintain professionalism by not providing a personal opinion about the unit, as in Option D.

Test Blueprint: 5 A
Cognitive Code: Application

6. Learners are sharing their experiences of the clinical day during a postclinical conference. One learner exclaims, "I had the best day ever! One of my clients told me I was the best learner he ever had, and he gave me $50!" Which is the best action for the clinical nurse educator?
   A. Explain that it is acceptable for learners and nurses to accept tips for a job well done.
   B. Use the money to throw a pizza party for the staff on the unit.
   C. Take the money from the learner and give it back to the client.
   D. Accompany the learner to return the money to the client.

Correct Answer: D

Rationale: According to the American Nurses Association (ANA) Code of Ethics for Nurses with Interpretative Statements (2015), accepting gifts from clients is generally not appropriate. Factors to consider include the intent, value, nature, and timing of the gift (ANA, 2015, p. 7). A fifty-dollar sum of money is considerable. The learner and clinical nurse educator should return the money and explain why the learner cannot accept it.

Test Blueprint: 5 A
Cognitive Code: Application

7. In which clinical situation may a clinical nurse educator be considered liable for a negligent act?
   A. Providing senior-level nursing learners with multiclient assignments on a telemetry unit
   B. Allowing learners to pass medications after failing a medication administration quiz
   C. Requiring learners to perform clinical skills only in the presence of the clinical nurse educator
   D. Assigning entry-level learners to care for stable clients in a long-term care setting

Correct Answer: B

Rationale: Clinical nurse educators are not liable if they provide appropriate learning opportunities based on objectives and learner competence based on evaluation of the learner's knowledge, skills, abilities, and attitudes, and provide competent guidance (Oermann et al., 2018, p. 111). If a learner has not passed the medication administration quiz, the learner does not have the knowledge and skills to perform that task. Therefore, if the learner is allowed to pass medications, the clinical nurse educator can be liable for a negligent act if one occurs, as in Option B. Options A, C, and D are appropriate based on identified guidelines.

Test Blueprint: 5 A
Cognitive Code: Analysis

8. Which action by the clinical nurse educator would be a legal concern?
   A. Allowing learners to document in the electronic health record using their logins
   B. Sharing the educator's identification badge with a learner to document a glucose result
   C. Instructing learners to use their logins to document vital signs in the electronic health record
   D. Providing learners with electronic access to information for their assigned client

Correct Answer: B

Rationale: The action of giving a learner an educator's identification badge to document a glucose result, Option B, has ethical and legal ramifications. The American Nurses Association (2015) code of ethics requires that nurses safeguard clients and the public when an unethical or illegal practice occurs, which in this instance would be the use of the clinical nurse educator's badge by the learner. Also, clinical nurse educators have an obligation to role model professional nursing behaviors. Options A, C, and D align with ethical and legal expectations in the clinical environment because learners are using their own logins and functioning within their identified roles.

Test Blueprint: 5 A
Cognitive Code: Application

9. Using Bandura's Social Learning Theory, which learning activity would be most effective to enhance professionalism in the clinical environment?
   A. Researching professional nursing organizations and writing a paper regarding their influence on professional practice
   B. Creating a presentation regarding professionalism and the impact it has on nursing practice
   C. Shadowing a nurse that the clinical nurse educator has consistently observed following correct policies and procedures
   D. Interviewing a nurse on the clinical unit and writing a reflective journal

Correct Answer: C

Rationale: Social Learning Theory posits that learning occurs through role modeling. For the learning experience to be effective in enhancing professionalism, it is important that the clinical nurse educator chooses a competent individual for learners to shadow. In Option C, the response focuses on the professionalism in the nursing role through following policies and procedures. While researching professional organizations would be beneficial to learners, it does not use Bandura's Social Learning Theory, which has a central tenet of role modeling; therefore, Option A is incorrect. Interviewing a nurse does not ensure that professional attitudes and practices that enhance professionalism are discussed, making Option D incorrect. Creating a presentation, Option B, may help the learner start to understand professionalism but it does not allow learners to see the behaviors in action; it also does not require them to mirror the behaviors discussed (Bastable, 2019, p. 85).

Test Blueprint: 5 A
Cognitive Code: Application

10. A learner inserted a successful intravenous (IV) catheter and wants to photograph the accomplishment. Which is the best response?
    A. "Absolutely not, taking any type of photograph would be a direct HIPAA violation."
    B. "You can only take a photograph of the arm and IV, making sure no client identifiers are present."
    C. "I understand you are proud but remember your commitment to honor the dignity of the client."
    D. "Ask the client for verbal permission prior to taking the photograph and document the response in the client's chart."

Correct Answer: C

Rationale: Taking photographs within the clinical setting is not professional and can have legal and ethical implications. Clinical nurse educators are responsible for mentoring learners in maintaining professional boundaries and socializing to the role of the nurse. Mastering a new skill can be an exciting moment for the learner; the clinical nurse educator can acknowledge and celebrate the learner's success while also gently reminding and role modeling the fundamental commitment of nursing to the uniqueness, worth, and dignity of the client (American Nurses Association, 2015).

Test Blueprint: 5 A
Cognitive Code: Application

11. A learner approaches the clinical nurse educator and mentions having overheard a second learner in the group using inappropriate language in the presence of an unconscious client. Which is the best action?
    A. Tell the first learner "unfortunately, nothing can be done because I didn't witness the behavior."
    B. Ask other learners in the group if they have witnessed similar behaviors from the second learner.
    C. Remove the second learner from the clinical unit until a letter of apology to the client is written.
    D. Discuss the reported concerns and observed behaviors with the second learner privately.

Correct Answer: D

Rationale: The use of inappropriate language in the presence of any client, unconscious or not, is not professional. The clinical nurse educator is responsible for addressing the behavior and mentoring the learner in the development of professional nursing behaviors. Nurses establish relationships of trust and respect for the inherent dignity of clients—the clinical nurse educator is responsible for helping learners develop these skills (American Nurses Association, 2015). Options A and C ignore the concern and do not role model appropriate actions for the learner. Option D allows the nurse educator to explore the inappropriate behavior and address this issue with the learner in a respectful manner. Involving others in the situation, as in Option B, violates the privacy of the learner in question and is not appropriate. Learners have the right to expect that information about their progress in programs, academic and clinical performances, and personal concerns will be kept confidential (Christensen, 2016; Johnson, 2012). The clinical nurse educator should begin by addressing the behavior in a nonconfrontational manner to assist the learner in developing appropriate professional behaviors.

Test Blueprint: 5 A
Cognitive Code: Analysis

12. The staff nurse assigned to a learner's client is difficult to locate on the unit. Later, the learner informs the clinical nurse educator that the staff nurse smells of alcohol after returning from a break. Which is the best action?
    A. Tell the learner that because the staff nurse is impaired, the learner should prepare to accept full responsibility for the client assignment for the remainder of the shift.
    B. Bring the concern to the charge nurse on the unit and enquire about agency policy regarding this type of case.
    C. Seek the staff nurse in question to enquire about the staff nurse's whereabouts during the break and the amount of alcohol the nurse may have consumed.
    D. Ask the learner to shadow the nurse more closely and to report any further suspicious behaviors to the charge nurse.

Correct Answer: B

Rationale: Clinical nurse educators are responsible for mentoring learners in developing professional nursing behaviors, standards, and codes of ethics. Nurses have a moral obligation to uphold trust within the client relationship and, as client advocates, must support the principles of nonmaleficence (do no harm) and beneficence (do good) (American Nurses Association, 2015). Mandatory reporting of an occurrence or individual, including another nurse, is a legal requirement in some states when the public is at risk (National Council of State Boards of Nursing, 2019). Option B is correct because the clinical nurse educator should follow the chain of command and agency policy regarding this matter. Placing full responsibility for the client assignment on the learner, as in Option A, is not within the learner's scope of practice and does not address the issue of potential impairment of the staff nurse and/or mandatory reporting. The clinical nurse educator should follow the unit chain of command and agency policy regarding mandatory reporting of suspected impairment. It is not within the clinical nurse educator's scope or role to question the staff nurse about potential alcohol consumption, as in Option C. It is also not appropriate to place the learner in a position in which the learner is assessing or questioning the staff nurse about suspicious behaviors or potential alcohol consumption, as in Option D.

Test Blueprint: 5 A
Cognitive Code: Analysis

13. A learner approaches a clinical nurse educator to discuss a client assignment. The learner is concerned because the assigned client wants to follow the learner on social media. Which is the best response by the clinical nurse educator?
A. "If you feel this client is being inappropriate, I will reassign you to another client right away."
B. "Let's speak to the clinical group and see if anyone will volunteer to swap client assignments."
C. "Let's consult with the client's staff nurse to see how to handle the situation."
D. "Ignore the request for now. If it happens again, remind the client of your professional role and boundaries."

Correct Answer: D

Rationale: Clinical nurse educators are responsible for mentoring learners in maintaining professional boundaries. The work of nursing is inherently personal and the involvement of nurses in an individual's life during a stressful life event may contribute to the risk of professional boundary violations (American Nurses Association, 2015). Clinical nurse educators can mentor and equip learners in how to handle situations on their own before an intervention may be warranted. Option D helps the learner abide by professional boundaries. Reassigning the learner to another client, as in Option A, and changing the learner assignment, Option B, may immediately address the issue, but they do not allow the learner an opportunity to test out real-world solutions in a mentored environment. Option C is incorrect because the clinical nurse educator is equipped to help the learner address the issue firsthand without immediately involving the staff nurse.

Test Blueprint: 5 A
Cognitive Code: Application

14. Which active learning activity is most appropriate to emphasize the Code of Ethics for Nurses in the clinical setting?
   A. Writing a reflective summary of the daily clinical experience
   B. Attending a session on the topic of ethics in health care at an interprofessional conference
   C. Conducting an evidence-based review of the literature on the topic of professional boundaries
   D. Developing a case study with other learners about an issue identified within their clinical setting

Correct Answer: D

Rationale: A case study, as in Option D, is an in-depth analysis of a real-life situation that can help to illustrate and apply theoretical content to the real world (Phillips, 2016; Rowles, 2012). This learning activity encourages learners to apply ethical concepts to a real-world experience identified within their immediate clinical setting. Clinical nurse educators facilitate the mentoring of learners in the development of professional nursing behaviors, standards, and codes of ethics. Option A will not necessarily promote critical thinking related to the topic of ethics within the clinical environment. Option B is not an active learning strategy and, as such, does little to promote critical thinking within the clinical environment. Lecture is a teaching strategy useful for covering complex material on a topic within a specific timeframe; a disadvantage to lecture is that it decreases learner involvement (Phillips, 2016; Rowles, 2012). Option C does not focus on all aspects of the Code of Ethics for Nurses; rather, it engages only in learning about professional boundaries.

Test Blueprint: 5 A
Cognitive Code: Application

15. A learner approaches the clinical nurse educator to discuss a client assignment. The learner shares that the assignment is "hard for me because the client reminds me of my daughter." Which is the best response?
   A. "I understand this assignment may be difficult for you. How might you draw upon your experiences as a parent to establish a strong and therapeutic nurse-client relationship?"
   B. "I'll go with you during client introductions but will quietly step out once you begin your assessment."
   C. "I know this must be hard for you, and sometimes client assignments do feel personal. It is better you learn to deal with this now rather than after you graduate."
   D. "Thank you for sharing this with me. Let's identify a new client assignment together."

Correct Answer: A

Rationale: An important part of the clinical nurse educator role is to promote a learning climate of respect for all, which is accomplished through opportunities for inclusive teaching and learning within the clinical setting (Alexander, 2016). Many learners have individual responsibilities and life situations that provide a social context that affects their learning. When possible, the educator should recognize and draw on these experiences to incorporate and apply them to the learning situation, as suggested in Option A (Candela, 2012, 2016).

Accompanying a learner, Option B, can help the learner gain confidence, but does not recognize or apply the unique experience described. Option C does not support an open and trusting learning environment, nor does it recognize or apply the unique experience described. Changing clinical assignments, as in Option D, does not provide a real-world opportunity to develop resilience, nor does it recognize or apply the unique experience described.

Test Blueprint: 5 B
Cognitive Code: Application

16. A clinical nurse educator is discussing the daily client assignment with an English Language Learner (ELL). Which action would best support this learner?
    A. Assigning the learner to shadow an English-speaking staff nurse for the day
    B. Having the learner present a verbal end-of-shift report in front of the clinical group
    C. Allowing the learner to write out and organize the client care activities in the learner's native language before translating them to English
    D. Referring the learner to campus support services specific to international learners

Correct Answer: C

Rationale: Clinical nurse educators must incorporate sensitive and innovative strategies into their teaching of ELLs. Allowing ELLs time to formulate and translate their thoughts from their native language to English, as in Option C, is a helpful way to engage ELLs in organizing clinical activities (Alexander, 2016; Stokes & Flowers, 2012). Clinical nurse educators must be available and attentive to the behaviors and personal responses of ELLs that may have an impact on their feelings about English. Many ELLs express concerns about how educators, peers, clients, and staff nurses perceive them related to their English-speaking abilities (Halic, Greenburg, & Paulus, 2009). Assigning the learner to a staff nurse for the day, as in Option A, does not address these issues or concerns. The need to master the English language may impede ELL participation in group and open discussion for fear of saying the wrong thing, thus Option B is incorrect. Referring the ELL to campus support services, as in Option D, does not immediately address the clinical assignment issue. Also, the ELL may not necessarily be from another country.

Test Blueprint: 5 B
Cognitive Code: Application

17. The clinical nurse educator wants to incorporate multicultural education strategies within the clinical practice setting. Which is the best action to accomplish this goal?
    A. Creating a learning assignment that requires learners to identify an evidence-based resource for hypertension management among rural populations
    B. Assigning learners an unfolding case study that considers a multidisciplinary approach to the prevention of preterm labor in a teenage African-American client
    C. Holding a small group discussion during postclinical conference to talk about the racially diverse clients on the clinical unit
    D. Creating a database for tracking learners' client assignments and using it to ensure that learners care for diverse cultural groups

Correct Answer: D

Rationale: Inclusive teaching and learning strategies should be emphasized in the clinical practice setting as well as in the classroom. Although communities vary, clinical nurse educators must make efforts to plan and align experiences with the nature of the community and ensure that clients selected for clinical learning experiences represent diverse cultural groups (Alexander, 2016). In Option D, the use of a database to record various client demographics can assist the educator when making assignments. This database can be used to inform clinical assignments and help the educator ensure that learners care for clients from diverse cultural groups. Opportunities for inclusive teaching and learning must be provided for clinical practice so that knowledge is reinforced, skills are developed, and changes occur in learner attitudes (Alexander, 2016; Stokes & Flowers, 2012). While identifying evidence-based resources for diverse populations, Option A, is important, this activity does not promote engagement of the learner with clients from diverse cultural groups and instead may be better suited as a classroom strategy. Unfolding case studies, as in Option B, do not promote engagement of the learner with clients from diverse cultural groups and instead may be better suited as a classroom strategy. While the postclinical conference may assist learners in reflecting on their experience in the clinical setting, Option C, this activity does not promote active engagement of learners with clients from diverse cultural groups.

Test Blueprint: 5 B
Cognitive Code: Application

18. In establishing a trusting environment based on mutual respect, which action is best?
    A. Frequently reminding the learners that their success is a priority for the clinical nurse educator
    B. Providing immediate feedback to correct any errors that learners commit, regardless of severity
    C. Giving the learners ample time for breaks and socialization with each other and the staff
    D. Openly discussing learners' errors and achievements with the entire group at the end of shift

Correct Answer: A

Rationale: Before expecting learners to trust them, educators need to demonstrate their respect for learners (Oermann et al., 2018, p. 9). Option A is the only example that demonstrates respect.

Test Blueprint: 5 B
Cognitive Code: Application

19. Which statement best supports the goal of promoting professional accountability?
    A. "Before flushing the medication port, cleanse it with an alcohol swab."
    B. "Survey the client's room for any safety issues before leaving the room."
    C. "Try to let me know when you will be late for your clinical shift."
    D. "We will enter our client care error into the agency reporting system."

Correct Answer: D

Rationale: Option D involves answering to oneself and others for one's own actions—in this case, a client care error; this is the definition of professional accountability according to the American Nurses Association (ANA) code of ethics (ANA, 2015; Davis, 2017). The clinical nurse educator must encourage learners to be professionally accountable not only in the areas of safe evidence-based client care but also in the areas of self-reporting and handling errors and/or near misses appropriately (Davis, 2017). Options A and B are important safety measures but are not necessarily best for encouraging professional accountability. Option C does involve a form of professional accountability, though its nonspecific nature (that is, "try") is not best in promoting accountability (Rachel, 2012).

Test Blueprint: 5 C
Cognitive Code: Analysis

20. Upon review of preclinical preparation paperwork, the clinical nurse educator notices that two learners submitted the same typed paper. Which is the best initial response?
    A. During postclinical conference, use the paperwork as an example of what not to do for the assignment.
    B. Immediately contact the department chairperson regarding the issue.
    C. Ignore that the paperwork was the same for both learners because it was probably a mistake.
    D. Meet with each learner individually in a private location to discuss the concern.

    Correct Answer: D

    Rationale: It is imperative that clinical nurse educators enforce academic integrity policies. To effectively do this while encouraging learners to communicate with educators, the clinical nurse educator should first meet with the learners privately, as in Option D. During this meeting, the clinical nurse educator can allow each learner to "respond to the charge" (Oermann et al., 2018, p. 105). This meeting should occur prior to notification of the department chairperson as suggested in Option B, to ensure that an academic integrity violation occurred. Option A is incorrect since publicly discussing the issue in a forum such as a clinical conference may discourage other learners from communicating with the clinical nurse educator as well as have a negative impact on the learners if the concern is unfounded. Ignoring the similarities in the assignment does not address the issue; therefore, Option C is incorrect.

    Test Blueprint: 5 C
    Cognitive Code: Application

21. A staff nurse on the clinical unit is visibly upset and reports to the clinical nurse educator of having overheard a learner on the shuttle speaking negatively about the staff on the unit. When asked, the learner denies the accusation. Which is the best initial action?
    A. Tell the staff nurse that the learner denied any wrongdoing.
    B. Ask the learner to apologize to the staff nurse.
    C. Document this situation on the learner's weekly evaluation.
    D. Have a brief meeting with both the staff nurse and the learner present.

    Correct Answer: D

Rationale: Clinical nurse educators and learners must model professional behavior. Unprofessional behavior by the learner or clinical nurse educator may damage the working relationship with the clinical agency (Oermann et al., 2018, p. 98). The clinical nurse educator must make it known to the staff nurse that unprofessional behavior will not be tolerated and thus should request a brief meeting with both the staff nurse and the learner, as in Option D. Telling the staff nurse that the learner denied the accusation, Option A, does not resolve the issue. Asking the learner to apologize to the staff nurse, Option B, implies that the clinical nurse educator does not believe the learner. Noting unprofessional behavior on the learner's weekly evaluation, Option C, may be warranted; however, that should not be the initial action.

Test Blueprint: 5 C
Cognitive Code: Application

22. Which action by the learner would require the clinical nurse educator to intervene?
    A. A learner takes a photograph of a client's lab results with the learner's mobile phone in order to complete paperwork at home.
    B. A learner recognizes a neighbor who is a client on the unit while the neighbor is ambulating in the hallway and congratulates the neighbor on making progress.
    C. A learner reviews the agency procedure for urinary catheter insertion prior to performing the skill on a client.
    D. A learner gathers injection supplies and dons clean gloves prior to administering a subcutaneous injection.

Correct Answer: A

Rationale: Nursing learners are subject to the Health Insurance Portability and Accountability Act (HIPAA), which ensures clients rights to confidentiality of their health information. The action by the learner in Option A is a HIPAA violation (Westrick, 2016). Options B, C, and D are all appropriate nursing learner actions.

Test Blueprint: 5 C
Cognitive Code: Application

23. The clinical nurse educator notes multiple errors on a learner's nursing care plan. Upon further investigation, the clinical nurse educator notes that the same care plan was submitted by another learner the prior semester. Which is the best next action?
    A. Scheduling a meeting with the learner to discuss the concern
    B. Suggesting that the department chair dismiss both learners from the program
    C. Requiring that the learner resubmit a new care plan within 24 hours
    D. Asking the learner from last semester if this care plan is that learner's work

Correct Answer: A

Rationale: Dishonest acts should be taken seriously because they can have detrimental effects on learners, educators, and clients. The clinical nurse educator suspects that academic dishonesty in the form of plagiarism has occurred. However, it is important that the educator first speak with the learner privately, describe the concern, and allow the learner to respond to the situation, as suggested in Option A (Oermann et al., 2018, p. 105). Suggesting dismissal, Option B, without adequate evidence of academic dishonesty violates the learner's right to due process (Oermann et al., 2018, p. 108). Asking the learner to submit a new care plan, Option C, contributes to an environment that supports academic dishonesty. Questioning the learner from the prior semester, Option D, is not the first step in resolving the issue; the clinical nurse educator must first meet with the learner who submitted the potentially plagiarized care plan.

Test Blueprint: 5 C
Cognitive Code: Application

24. The learner tells the clinical nurse educator that vital signs were not obtained because the learner did not want to wake the client. Which is the best response?
  A. "Unfortunately, this is important assessment data that needs to be obtained. You can gently wake the client by calling their name and patting their shoulder."
  B. "You can let the client sleep for another hour and then go back to collect the vital signs."
  C. "You can shadow and watch the client care assistant collect this set of vital signs, and then you can obtain the next set in four hours when the client is awake."
  D. "Go back and try again. Many times, you can sneak in and obtain the vital signs without ever waking the client."

Correct Answer: A

Rationale: Clinical nurse educators are responsible for mentoring learners in promoting professional integrity and accountability. Equipping the learner with the tools to be successful, but without completing the task for the learner, allows the learner an active, hands-on opportunity to test out real-world solutions in a mentored environment. Option A provides guidance that will help the learner develop the needed approach for client care while respecting client dignity (American Nurses Association. 2015). Delaying the collection of important data such as vital signs, as in Option B, does not promote professional integrity and accountability. Allowing the learner to shadow a client care assistant, as in Option C, may immediately address the issue, but does not allow the learner an active, hands-on opportunity to test out real-world solutions in a mentored environment. The clinical nurse educator should role model respect for human dignity and the client's right to self-determination by not encouraging "sneaky" behavior of the learner, as suggested in Option D.

Test Blueprint: 5 C
Cognitive Code: Application

25. The clinical nurse educator has just been informed by a learner that the learner may have committed a medication administration error. The learner is visibly anxious and distraught. Which is the best response?

A. "Take a deep breath. I'll go check the client to determine how severe the side effects may be."

B. "I'm sure it's going to be okay. Let's go speak with the charge nurse together to begin the appropriate documentation process."

C. "Thank you for your accountability. Let's review the situation together in detail."

D. "Go back to the conference room and collect your thoughts. I will join you in twenty minutes to discuss the course of action."

Correct Answer: C

Rationale: An important part of the clinical nurse educator role is to facilitate and promote learners' development of professional integrity and accountability. Opportunities to discuss an error must be available to the learner immediately after an error is made and again later after the learner has had more time to process what happened (Roberts, 2005). Acknowledging the professional value of accountability, as in Option C, affirms to the learner that the right action was taken by making the clinical nurse educator aware of the situation. Option A does not involve the learner in following up about the error or involve the learner in accountability. The clinical nurse educator must obtain additional information to determine if an actual error was made before taking next steps. Option B does not verify that the error was made. Mistakes by learners—and how they are handled—are critical to professional socialization and future practice. Requiring the learner to wait twenty minutes to discuss the concern, as in Option D, is incorrect because it does not take immediate action or allow the learner to process the events.

Test Blueprint: 5 C
Cognitive Code: Application

26. A learner has been late three times in the past two weeks. When asked about this tardiness, the learner states having trouble leaving the house due to the abusive and jealous behaviors of the learner's partner. Which is the best action?

A. Letting the learner go home for the day

B. Referring the learner to the counseling office on campus

C. Giving the learner an easier assignment for the day

D. Making an appointment to discuss this with the learner during office hours

Correct Answer: B

Rationale: Aside from personal information that is disclosed, nurse educators need to consider what action would best promote learning (Gaberson et al., 2015, p. 129). Letting the learner go home for the day, Option A, or giving an easier assignment, Option C, would violate the ethical principle of justice and equal treatment for all learners. Clinical educators should avoid making special exceptions for this learner, as in Option C, that are not available to other learners (Gaberson et al., 2015, p. 129). Option D does not provide the learner with appropriate counseling resources. The clinical nurse educator should avoid assuming the counseling role. The most beneficial resource would be the counseling office on campus, Option B.

Test Blueprint: 5 D
Cognitive Code: Analysis

27. The nurse educator overhears a conversation between a learner and a client. The client is acting flirtatious and asks for the learner's phone number. The learner reciprocates the behavior and gives a personal phone number to the client. Which is the best action?
    A. Reprimand the client for this behavior.
    B. Survey the staff members to see if any have experienced similar behaviors by the client.
    C. Remind the learner about the professional nature of the nurse-client relationship.
    D. Dismiss the learner from the clinical unit for the day.

Correct Answer: C

Rationale: Learners are to abide by the same ethical, legal, and professional behavior standards as licensed nurses. The ANA Code of Ethics for Nurses with Interpretive Statements (2015) emphasizes the professional role boundaries in relationships with clients, stating that dating and sexually intimate relationships with clients are always prohibited (p. 7); therefore, it is best to remind the learner of this, as suggested in Option C. Options A, B, and D do not help ensure compliance with the code of ethics.

Test Blueprint: 5 D
Cognitive Code: Application

28. Which situation is likely an ethical concern regarding professional boundaries?
    A. Becoming friends with learners, using their personal social media accounts
    B. Sitting with learners while eating lunch in the cafeteria
    C. Asking learners about their stress levels during the semester
    D. Providing a phone contact number for learners to use if they need to call in sick

Correct Answer: A

Rationale: The clinical nurse educator must establish clear professional boundaries with learners. When these boundaries are not established, it can directly impact learner evaluation (Oermann et al., 2018, p. 102). Option A represents an ethical concern because of the use of personal social media accounts. Option B does not represent an ethical concern because the clinical nurse educator attending lunch with learners is role modeling the importance of self-care behaviors while on the clinical unit. Options C and D are correct statements regarding the development of professional boundaries with learners; it would be appropriate to enquire about learner stress levels and to provide a contact number for emergencies and illness.

Test Blueprint: 5 D
Cognitive Code: Application

29. Which action by a clinical nurse educator demonstrates the most effective communication and prudent use of social networking sites such as Facebook and Twitter?
   A. Befriending learners on their personal social media pages to use messaging functions for updates and allowing learners to openly share clinical experiences
   B. Creating an educator social media account limited to the clinical group members for information sharing within the framework of social media guidelines
   C. Inviting learners to sign up as personal friends or followers for social interactions and sharing of new nursing publications
   D. Encouraging learners to create a hashtag for the clinical group that both learners and educator can use to post and follow public announcements about clinical experiences

Correct Answer: B

Rationale: Educators can use social media for communication with learners, to build relationships, and enhance learning (Oermann et al., 2018, p. 128); however, the relationship should be collegial without being personal. As such, Option B demonstrates ethical use of a nonpersonal social media account in a closed and protected environment for effective and safe communication within the framework of agreed social media boundaries. Options A and C blur social friendship lines between learners and clinical nurse educators. Option D creates issues related to public sharing of clinical experiences and possible privacy violations of client information.

Test Blueprint: 5 D
Cognitive Code: Application

30. Which action by a clinical nurse educator would be most concerning?
   A. Encouraging learners to ask questions
   B. Following learners' personal social media accounts
   C. Offering learning resources as needed
   D. Providing learners with one's cell phone number

Correct Answer: B

Rationale: In Option B, the clinical nurse educator is not respecting and maintaining professional boundaries (Shellenbarger & Bonnel, 2019) since the clinical nurse educator is following learners' personal social media accounts; this action is not necessary to the teaching-learning process and could result in learners being concerned with issues such as favoritism and invasion of privacy. Options A and D encourage learners to contact educators as needed and are not concerning in themselves. Option C is an appropriate action by educators if they notice that learners are potentially in need of assistance resources, such as counseling sessions and/or hotlines.

Test Blueprint: 5 D
Cognitive Code: Analysis

31. Which learning activity supports learner ongoing professional development most?
   A. Attending nursing grand rounds on current issues
   B. Completing an unfolding case study assignment
   C. Interviewing a nurse regarding the nurse's client care practices
   D. Performing a urinary catheter insertion

Correct Answer: A

Rationale: Option A encourages learners to listen and cultivate understanding regarding current issues facing nursing in the formal professional development activity of attending nursing grand rounds (Shellenbarger & Bonnel, 2019). Option B may be a way to engage learners (Phillips, 2016), though it does not specifically hone ongoing professional development. Options C and D in themselves do not support ongoing professional development since they are skills based; they may be useful in promoting professional development if combined with other activities such as pre- and post-reflections.

Test Blueprint: 5 E
Cognitive Code: Analysis

32. Which learning activity encourages informal professional development best?
   A. Assigning an article for learners to read about professional role development
   B. Listening to a lecture on prioritization during clinical orientation the first week of the course
   C. Observing the insertion of a chest tube on the clinical unit
   D. Attending a continuing education session at the health care agency

Correct Answer: C

Rationale: The American Nurses Association (2018) defines formal learning as academic and professional development in practice environments and informal learning as "experiential insights gained in work, community, home, and other environments" (p. 3). While all of the options do provide professional development activities, Option C is the only one provided informally. Options A, B, and D are all provided formally in the professional practice setting.

Test Blueprint: 5 E
Cognitive Code: Application

33. Which action would best encourage formal professional development?
   A. Encouraging a senior-level learner to speak with entry-level learners about the expectations of the nursing program
   B. Having each learner provide a verbal presentation of the client and the current treatment strategies during postclinical conference
   C. Collaborating with learners to develop a poster to present at a professional nursing organization conference
   D. Requiring learners to provide client education when administering newly ordered medications during the morning medication pass

Correct Answer: C

Rationale: The American Nurses Association (2018) defines formal learning as academic and professional development in practice environments and informal learning as "experiential insights gained in work, community, home, and other environments" (p. 3). Option C is the only professional development activity that is considered formal. Educators collaborating with learners encourages learner professional development prior to entry into the profession. Options A, B, and D are considered informal venues, as they are not structured.

Test Blueprint: 5 E
Cognitive Code: Application

34. A learner asks the clinical nurse educator how to become more confident giving telephone reports. Which activity would best help the learner accomplish this goal?
   A. Asking the learner to write a reflective journal related to feelings about giving telephone reports
   B. Developing a scenario in which the learner role plays giving a telephone report to the clinical nurse educator
   C. Listening to a staff nurse give a telephone report and offering a critique of the report during post-conference
   D. Reviewing the Situation, Background, Assessment, and Recommendation (SBAR) framework for communicating client reports

Correct Answer: B

Rationale: The clinical nurse educator encourages ongoing learner professional development via formal and informal methods. Role play is an active learning approach in which the learner assumes an unscripted role and interacts with another in a spontaneous or semistructured interaction (Phillips, 2016; Rowles, 2012). As suggested in the correct response, Option B, role play has the advantage of providing the learner with immediate feedback about interpersonal and communication skills in a nonthreatening environment (Phillips, 2016; Rowles, 2012). While reflective journaling, Option A, is a strategy that activates the affective domain of learning, it does not promote an active opportunity to practice the communication skills necessary for building confidence. Critiquing the report of a staff nurse, as in Option C, does offer the learner a chance to hear a report but it does not immediately promote an active opportunity to practice the communication skills necessary for building confidence. Reviewing the SBAR framework, Option D, activates the cognitive domain of learning but does not promote an active opportunity to practice the communication skills necessary for building confidence.

Test Blueprint: 5 E
Cognitive Code: Analysis

35. The clinical nurse educator is assessing learner socialization into nursing. Which learner would be best described as an "Advanced Beginner?"
   A. The learner whose performance is inflexible and tends to be governed by context-free rules and regulations
   B. The learner who perceives situations as wholes rather than in terms of parts, and focuses on long-term goals
   C. The learner who recognizes the meaningful aspects of a real situation and makes judgments about them
   D. The learner who demonstrates organizational and planning abilities, and can differentiate important factors from less important aspects of care

Correct Answer: C

Rationale: An "Advanced Beginner" demonstrates marginally accepted performance; the learner recognizes the meaningful aspects of a real situation, as reflected in Option C. The learner has experienced enough real situations to make judgments about them (Benner, 1984). Option A describes a "Novice" in Benner's *From Novice to Expert* model; performance is limited, inflexible, and governed by context-free rules and regulations rather than experience (Benner, 1984). Option B describes a "Proficient Practitioner" in Benner's *From Novice to Expert* model. This learner has three to five years of experience; perceives situations as wholes rather than in terms of parts; uses maxims as guides for what to consider in a situation; has holistic understanding of the client, which improves decision-making; and focuses on long-term goals (Benner, 1984). Option D describes a "Competent Practitioner" in Benner's *From Novice to Expert* model. This learner has two to three years of experience, demonstrates organizational and planning abilities, differentiates important factors from less important aspects of care, and coordinates multiple complex care demands (Benner, 1984).

Test Blueprint: 5 F
Cognitive Code: Recall

36. Which best represents the purpose of a reflective journal assignment?
   A. Evaluate the learner's ability to work effectively in the clinical environment.
   B. Enable learners to identify areas that need further practice.
   C. Assist clinical nurse educators in evaluating learner's clinical performance.
   D. Provide learners with the opportunity to evaluate the clinical site.

Correct Answer: B

Rationale: Journaling is considered a formative assessment. Formative assessments provide learners with the opportunity to improve their knowledge and skills as well as identify areas of improvement, as in Option B (Oermann et al., 2018, p. 245). Journaling should be used as a diagnostic means of evaluation and should not be graded, making Options A and C incorrect since they focus on evaluation of learners' work. Reflective journaling should be focused on the learners and their skills, not the clinical agency; therefore, Option D is incorrect.

Test Blueprint: 5 F
Cognitive Code: Analysis

37. Which activity best allows learners to reflect on their clinical practice?
   A. Case study presentation
   B. Debriefing
   C. Quiz
   D. Essay examination

Correct Answer: B

Rationale: Debriefing can be used in postclinical conference for learners to discuss learning activities and analyze care provided. It requires learners to reflect on their clinical practice, making Option B correct. Furthermore, it can be used for learners to share information regarding their feelings and interactions with others during their clinical practice (Oermann et al., 2018, p. 192). Options A, C, and D are summative evaluation strategies and are focused on determining achievement of learning outcomes, whereas debriefing is a formative assessment strategy that provides learners with feedback with the intent of improving performance (Oermann et al., 2018, p. 257).

Test Blueprint: 5 F
Cognitive Code: Application

38. Which activity would best foster role socialization for senior-level baccalaureate learners?
  A. Encouraging learners to collaborate with the nursing staff responsible for their client assignment
  B. Requiring learners to report only to the clinical nurse educator about their client assignment
  C. Assigning learners to provide all aspects of care for their client assignment
  D. Focusing clinical activities primarily on knowledge learned within coursework and not the clinical environment

Correct Answer: A

Rationale: Socialization focuses on the ability to transition into a new role within a profession. To encourage socialization, clinical nurse educators should encourage learners to collaborate with the nursing staff responsible for their client assignment, as in Option A. This gives learners a sense of belonging while also allowing them to observe the practice of nursing professionals and their interactions in the health care setting (Bradshaw & Hultquist, 2017, p. 351). Option B is incorrect because if learners are allowed to report only to the clinical nurse educator, they lose an opportunity for collaboration and socialization. Option C does not allow for socialization to the role since they may be working in isolation and do not have the opportunity to experience teamwork within the health care environment, an important tenet to nursing practice. Option D is incorrect because it does not address role socialization.

Test Blueprint: 5 G
Cognitive Code: Application

39. Which activity best prepares learners for a multiple-client medication administration assignment?
  A. Simulated medication administration session prior to the first clinical day
  B. One client medication administration assignment on the clinical unit
  C. Observing a nurse with a multiple-client medication administration assignment
  D. Readings focused on medication administration prior to the first clinical day

Correct Answer: A

Rationale: Providing learners with the opportunity to learn complex skills in the simulation lab prior to entering the practice setting improves learner performance because they can perform the skill in a nonthreatening environment, as in Option A (Oermann et al., 2018, p. 67). Increased self-efficacy in performance improves learner confidence. Options B, C, and D do not provide the same level of preparation as the simulated learning environment, which allows for reflection on skill competence.

Test Blueprint: 5 G
Cognitive Code: Analysis

40. Which learning activity would be most effective to enhance interprofessional communication skills?
   A. Assigning entry-level learners to shadow the stroke team at the health care agency
   B. Providing learners with the opportunity to participate in a simulation activity focused on interprofessional collaboration
   C. Partnering an entry-level learner with a nursing assistant for delivery of basic client care
   D. Providing learners with the opportunity to practice actively listening and expressing ideas and opinions within a multidisciplinary team

Correct Answer: D

Rationale: The interprofessional competency regarding communication practices includes active participation in the health care team, which requires active listening and the provision of feedback (Oermann et al., 2018, p. 221). Providing learners with the opportunity to actively participate within a multidisciplinary team will allow them to incorporate skills from the classroom into clinical practice and enhance their ability to apply the concepts. While Options A, B, and C would provide support in role assimilation, Option D would be the most effective.

Test Blueprint: 5 G
Cognitive Code: Analysis

41. Which learning activity would help entry-level learners develop culturally sensitive communication skills best?
   A. Assigning a learner to a client who is culturally diverse from the learner
   B. Role playing in the simulation lab prior to learners reaching the clinical unit
   C. Assigning learners to research various cultures and their preferred communication methods
   D. Showing a video about culturally sensitive communication

Correct Answer: B

Rationale: Role play allows learners to practice using their communication skills prior to entering the clinical unit. They can explore situations that may be challenging for them, such as a culturally sensitive situation. The use of role play in the simulation lab provides learners with a safe environment to practice their skills. Furthermore, role playing allows learners to further examine the behaviors and feelings associated with the learning experience, making Option B correct (Bradshaw & Hultquist, 2017, p. 211). Option A may not be appropriate for an entry-level learner with no previous clinical experience; putting the learner in this situation can increase anxiety and may negatively impact care provided to the client. While Options C and D provide learners with information regarding communication, being actively engaged in the learning process has proven to be more effective in retention of content and skill acquisition.

Test Blueprint: 5 G
Cognitive Code: Analysis

42. During the first clinical experience, which assignment would be most conducive to learning and reduce learner anxiety?
A. One high-acuity client with two learners assigned
B. One low-acuity client with one learner assigned
C. Two low-acuity clients with one learner assigned
D. Two high-acuity clients with two learners assigned

Correct Answer: A

Rationale: Providing the opportunity for multiple learners to work together with one client can assist in reducing learner anxiety while also incorporating teaching strategies focused on teamwork and collaboration, as in Option A (Oermann et al., 2018, p. 126). When in this format, each learner can be assigned a specific role to enhance the learning environment. As identified by Oermann et al. (2018), this type of format allows multiple learners to effectively care for higher-acuity clients (p. 126). Options B, C, and D are potential options, but the best option to enhance learning and reduce anxiety would be Option A.

Test Blueprint: 5 G
Cognitive Code: Analysis

43. During a debriefing session following a service-learning experience, which learner comment best indicates cultural awareness?
A. "This experience allowed me to view other individuals' lived experiences."
B. "I think we may have made a difference today."
C. "The experience was different than what I was expecting."
D. "We need to make this an annual trip because it really helped my learning."

Correct Answer: A

Rationale: The learner comment in Option A conveys the ability to view the service-learning setting from the vantage point of those assisted. Cultural competence is now considered essential for providing quality care to the increasingly diverse client populations (Bauce, Kridli, & Fitzpatrick, 2014). Options B, C, and D were learner observations about the day and would not necessarily be an expression of cultural competence.

Test Blueprint: 5 G
Cognitive Code: Analysis

44. Which would best foster first-year learners' socialization to the nursing profession?
A. Asking staff nurses from various practice areas to lead discussions during post-conference each week
B. Designating one clinical day in which each learner observes the actions of the nurses on the clinical unit
C. Requiring that all learners shadow a nurse in an area of their interest in addition to designated clinical time
D. Assigning the group to read a journal article related to the role of the nurse

Correct Answer: A

Rationale: Beginning learners often have misconceptions about the role of the nurse (Ten Hoeve, Castelien, Jansen, Jansen, & Roodbol, 2017). Having nurses from various practice areas discuss their roles during post-conference each week, as in Option A, allows learners to become exposed to various nursing roles and responsibilities. Novice learners have limited clinical experience and assigning them to observe a nurse on the clinical unit may be overwhelming, as suggested in Option B. The clinical nurse educator cannot require the learners to complete additional hours for shadowing outside of designated clinical time, as in Option C. Requiring the group to read a journal article about professional nursing roles, Option D, does not allow learners to ask questions.

Test Blueprint: 5 G
Cognitive Code: Application

45. Which activity best helps learners provide constructive peer feedback?
   A. Having learners critique one another's client documentation in the electronic medical record
   B. Asking learners to observe one another in simulation and provide feedback on a peer's performance
   C. Having learners pair up to provide care for a client and use a rubric to complete a peer evaluation on one another
   D. Requiring learners to observe a classmate's medication pass

Correct Answer: C

Rationale: Peers should only evaluate competencies and assignments that they are qualified to critique (Bonnel, 2016, p. 445). Learners are still in the learning process and often have not yet refined their nursing skills. Thus, Options A, B, and D should be reserved for educator evaluation. Educator support and clear guidelines are essential for effective peer review; Option C provides learners a rubric to guide their peer review.

Test Blueprint: 5 H
Cognitive Code: Analysis

46. Which learning activity best helps senior-level learners offer constructive peer feedback regarding clinical performance?
   A. Assigning learners to act as a team leader for the day and provide each classmate basic feedback
   B. Having learners peer-review one another's quality improvement papers
   C. Assigning pairs to read one another's self-reflective journals each week and provide feedback
   D. Having learners observe one another perform a nursing skill, such as a urinary catheter insertion

Correct Answer: A

Rationale: Peers should evaluate only those competencies and assignments that they are qualified to critique (Bonnel, 2016, p. 445). Senior-level learners who are close to graduation would likely possess the ability to lead a group of their peers and provide basic feedback on individual learners. Peer feedback on a quality improvement paper, Option B, would not afford learners the experience to provide a classmate feedback on clinical performance. Journal reflections, Option C, may describe learners' personal experiences, strengths, weaknesses, and fears; opening personal thoughts and feelings to a peer may provoke feelings of anxiety, however. The opportunity for learners to perform nursing skills often varies per clinical day and not all learners may get the opportunity to perform a skill each day; therefore, Option D is not the best choice.

Test Blueprint: 5 H
Cognitive Code: Application

47. Which learning activity would develop peer feedback skills best?
   A. Completing a peer evaluation of other members of the clinical team during their first rotation
   B. Evaluating other learners' nursing notes based on provided prompts for the evaluation
   C. Working in groups to peer review and grade a written assignment
   D. Peer reviewing a nurse working on the clinical unit and providing the nurse feedback

Correct Answer: B

Rationale: Peer review is an essential skill that facilitates development of the learner. Peer review assignments can take many forms, including writing and skill critiques. Effective peer review requires learners to have the competencies and skills capable to effectively evaluate (Bonnel, 2012, p. 487). Reviewing other learners' notes and comparing that to provided prompts, Option B, would afford the learner an opportunity to develop enhanced critiquing skills. Providing prompts will facilitate feedback by focusing on the expected outcomes of the assignment. As identified by Bonnel (2012), peer feedback may be biased either negatively or positively; a structured format will assist in limiting this bias and encourage learners to reflect directly on the assignment objectives. Option A is incorrect because learners beginning their first clinical experiences have not had the opportunity to develop these skills to peer review effectively. Learners should not be grading course assignments, as suggested in Option C; this is beyond the scope of learner responsibilities. Peer review assignments should be used for formative evaluation only (Oermann et al., 2018, p. 238). Option D is incorrect because peer reviewing a staff nurse is also beyond the scope of learner responsibilities and capabilities.

Test Blueprint: 5 H
Cognitive Code: Application

48. A staff nurse informs the clinical nurse educator that a learner has done an exceptional job with client education related to a newly prescribed medication. Which initial action is most appropriate?
   A. Ask the learner to present the educational content to the clinical group during post-conference.
   B. Share the compliment with the learner, enquire about how the client education was delivered, and document the compliment in the learner's clinical evaluation.
   C. Assign the learner a reflective journal topic related to the client education experience.
   D. Do nothing, as the learner's delivery of client education was not witnessed by the clinical nurse educator.

Correct Answer: B

Rationale: One role of the clinical nurse educator is to inspire creativity and confidence in the learner. Feedback is an essential element in teaching and learning—educators should be equally equipped to point out positive aspects of learner performance, as suggested in Option B (Stokes & Kost, 2012). Options A and C are active learning strategies, but these options do not immediately inspire creativity and confidence in the learner. Feedback is an essential element in teaching and learning; educators should be equipped to point out positive aspects of learner performance as well as areas that require improvement (Stokes & Kost, 2012). Option D does not provide the learner with this needed feedback.

Test Blueprint: 5 I
Cognitive Code: Analysis

49. Which statement or question encourages learner confidence most?
   A. "I think you can handle the procedure by yourself."
   B. "What is the client's most important problem?"
   C. "Why did you ask that question in particular?"
   D. "You really have grown in your professional practice this semester."

Correct Answer: D

Rationale: Option D is an affirming statement that encourages learners and their confidence in their abilities; Option D also highlights learner growth throughout the semester, which can help learners feel confident in their hard work over the semester. Inspiring confidence is an important role of the clinical nurse educator (Shellenbarger & Bonnel, 2019). Option A may inspire confidence in the learner; however, it is not appropriate since the educator should supervise learners while they perform client care procedures. Options B and C are good questions to ask to promote critical thinking and clinical reasoning skills (Oermann, 1997; Paul & Elder, 2008), but do not necessarily encourage learner confidence.

Test Blueprint: 5 I
Cognitive Code: Application

50. Which strategy would help assist learners to effectively manage their stress best?
   A. Establish clear learner-educator boundaries indicating when learners can contact the educator with questions.
   B. Encourage learners to focus on more manageable low-priority tasks.
   C. Suggest that learners reach out to the clinical nurse educator with questions or concerns.
   D. Discuss the importance of learners staying focused on course content and eliminating extracurricular activities.

Correct Answer: C

Rationale: When clinical nurse educators are approachable and open to learners, it helps learners deal with stress. Increased contact with learners inside and outside of the clinical environment assists in establishing a positive working relationship with learners. Increased contact and encouragement improve motivation as well. Option C encourages the development of this relationship, working to effectively manage stress. Options A, B, and D can increase stress, as they do not allow learners to decompress. Furthermore, they decrease learner-educator contact (Clark, 2018).

Test Blueprint: 5 J
Cognitive Code: Application

51. Which is the best approach to alleviate anxiety or fear that learners may be experiencing during their first clinical experience?
    A. Address learner fears and concerns in a clinical conference at the end of the first day of the clinical experience.
    B. Use a preconference on the first day of the clinical experience to assess learner fears and concerns.
    C. Encourage learners to ask nurses on the clinical unit for assistance if they are unsure of clinical care activities.
    D. Tell learners to prepare questions about their experiences that can be discussed in a postclinical conference.

Correct Answer: B

Rationale: During the initial clinical experience, many learners experience fear and/or anxiety. The clinical nurse educator should work to alleviate these concerns prior to the learning experience. Providing learners with the opportunity to identify their fears and sources of anxiety during preconference, as in Option B, will encourage them to obtain guidance before beginning the clinical experience and should help learners to understand expectations. It also enhances the learners' confidence in their clinical nurse educator's desire to see them succeed; furthermore, addressing issues prior to the clinical experience will enhance the initial experience (Oermann et al., 2018, p. 68). Options A, C, and D are incorrect, as they have the potential to increase learner anxiety and fear because of the delay in identifying concerns.

Test Blueprint: 5 K
Cognitive Code: Application

52. Which clinical nurse educator is likely modeling coping and self-care skills best?
    A. After a frustrating event, the educator misses the next scheduled clinical day.
    B. An educator arrives to the clinical agency, visibly yawning several times.
    C. An educator keeps a personal reflective journal regarding a variety of topics.
    D. The educator regularly works through lunch and skip breaks.

Correct Answer: C

Rationale: Option C represents a clinical nurse educator who is engaging in the important coping and self-care activity of reflection by keeping a personal reflective journal. This educator knows that many stressors have an impact and is taking steps to make sense of these experiences and identify any insights and/or opportunities for growth (Blum, 2014). It is important to role model proper coping and self-care behaviors for learners (Shellenbarger & Bonnel, 2019). Option A represents a potentially unhealthy coping mechanism, that is, avoidance. In Option B, the educator may not be getting enough sleep and/or taking on too many responsibilities, thus not engaging in proper self-care. Similarly, in Option D, the educator is not allowing for downtime, an important aspect of proper self-care.

Test Blueprint: 5 K
Cognitive Code: Analysis

53. A group of first-semester learners are at a long-term care agency for their clinical experience. One of the learners approaches the clinical nurse educator, looking upset, and states "I just found out that the client I took care of last week passed away this morning." Which statement would best foster coping skills?
A. "I see you are upset. Let's take some time this morning and have a precon-ference with the group to discuss this situation."
B. "I'm sorry that happened to your client, but you need to get your morning care completed before the breakfast trays come."
C. "Nurses deal with death quite a bit in their career, it's good you got to experience this as a learner."
D. "You will feel more comfortable dealing with death once you learn about it in your theory class later this semester."

Correct Answer: A

Rationale: Although learners may experience a client death during their edu-cation, few feel adequately prepared for it. Clinical educators are reported to play a leading role in the training of learners in all areas regarding death and dying (Heise, Wing, & Hullinger, 2018). The clinical nurse educator should not minimize the death of a client, as in Options B, C, and D. Learners often feel a sense of inadequacy at the time of a client's death and would prefer to have the educator guide them through the experience (Heise & Gilpin, 2016). The clinical nurse educator should take time to address the learner's concern and foster an open discussion about death with the entire group.

Test Blueprint: 5 K
Cognitive Code: Application

54. The clinical nurse educator is reviewing the syllabus on the first day of a clin-ical experience. As part of the evaluation methods, learners are required to submit a self-reflective journal weekly. One of the learners groans and states, "I don't know why you make us do these!" Which is the best response?
A. "It is a course requirement and you must complete these."
B. "I don't like reading these any more than you like writing them."
C. "These allow me to see all the things you did during the day."
D. "Self-reflection is an important part of the learning process."

Correct Answer: D

Rationale: Reflection in nursing education is used to develop and engage in critical thinking. Providing opportunities for reflective learning in the clinical setting can be an effective learning strategy. Reflection helps learners con-nect classroom content to actual practice situations (Phillips, 2016, p. 258). Options A, B, and C do not convey the importance of reflection as a means to develop critical thinking and reasoning skills.

Test Blueprint: 5 K
Cognitive Code: Application

55. The clinical nurse educator is assisting a group of learners with a sterile dressing change on an unconscious client and accidentally contaminates the sterile gloves. One of the learners in the group notices and comments. Which is the best response?
   A. "Thank you for noticing my mistake—let me change my gloves and finish the dressing change and then we can talk about it."
   B. "I can't believe that. I usually never make mistakes like that. This is such a sophomoric mistake."
   C. "Evidence says most dressing changes are no longer performed using sterile technique, so sterile gloves aren't really necessary."
   D. "I don't think I contaminated my gloves so I am going to continue with the dressing change."

Correct Answer: A

Rationale: The clinical nurse educator must be able to demonstrate clinical competence. Clinical educators should be experts in clinical practice and able to explain and demonstrate nursing care in real situations. The clinical nurse educator should possess the willingness to admit limitations and mistakes honestly, as illustrated in Option A (Oermann et al., 2018, p. 84). Options B, C, and D do not allow the clinical nurse educator to admit the mistake and do not demonstrate appropriate role modeling.

Test Blueprint: 5 K
Cognitive Code: Application

56. A learner is unsuccessful at a second attempt to insert an intravenous (IV) catheter and becomes frustrated, stating, "This is awful! I hate this! I'm no good at nursing!" Which is the best response?
   A. "I can tell you're frustrated. Let's take a five-minute break and debrief this experience in the conference room."
   B. "Every nurse struggles with IVs occasionally. Getting upset with yourself isn't going to solve anything."
   C. "You just need more practice. Soon you'll be an expert at IV insertions."
   D. "Next time, watch me closely as I do the skill. Then, we can talk about where you might be getting it wrong."

Correct Answer: A

Rationale: Learners frequently report high levels of stress, anxiety, and fears related to their academic and clinical performance (Frank, 2012, 2016). The clinical nurse educator acts as a role model for self-reflection, self-care, and coping skills. A short break, as suggested in Option A, allows the learner a chance to put personal emotions in check while a private debriefing allows the learner to reflect on the experience, explore personal strengths and areas for improvement, and receive constructive feedback from the clinical nurse educator. Downplaying the emotional response of the learner, as in Options B and C, are not a constructive method for role modeling or promoting self-reflection, self-care, and coping skills. Allowing the learner to watch the skill, as in Option D, does not promote an active, hands-on opportunity to test out real-world solutions in a mentored environment.

Test Blueprint: 5 K
Cognitive Code: Application

57. The condition of a client assigned to a learner deteriorated unexpectedly and the code team was called. The code was not successful and the client passed away. The learner assigned to the client is visibly distraught and is holding back tears. Which is the best action?

A. Remind the learner that death is a natural aspect of nursing care and that supplies will need to be gathered for postmortem care.

B. Escort the learner to the restroom, allow for a few moments of privacy, and debrief the experience in a private area.

C. Assure the learner that the client's deterioration and death was not the learner's fault and use the opportunity to review theoretical concepts of end-of-life care.

D. Remove the learner from the setting to enquire about the learner's actions and nursing assessments in the moments leading up to the code.

Correct Answer: B

Rationale: Learners experience stress and anxiety in clinical learning situations (Frank, 2012, 2016; Stokes & Kost, 2012) and the death of an assigned client may trigger an emotional response from the learner. The clinical nurse educator must recognize learners' needs for supportive and collegial relationships and develop a safe learning environment in which the learner is comfortable speaking openly (Massarweh, 1999; Stokes & Kost, 2012). Offering a short, private break, as in Option B, allows the learner a chance for emotional release while debriefing allows for reflection, modeling of self-care, and coping skill development. Downplaying the emotional response of the learner, as in Option A, is not a constructive method for role modeling or promoting self-reflection, self-care, and coping skills. Instead, the clinical nurse educator must recognize the learner's need for a safe and supportive learning environment. Offering assurance, as in Option C, is not a constructive method for role modeling self-reflection regarding nursing actions that could have potentially influenced the situation. Furthermore, a visibly distraught learner may not have the emotional or mental reserves to apply critical thinking capabilities to the immediate experience. While it is appropriate to remove the learner from the setting, as in Option D, enquiring about actions and nursing assessments may feel accusatory to the emotional learner and may cause the learner to become defensive.

Test Blueprint: 5 K
Cognitive Code: Application

58. The clinical nurse educator notices that a learner is hesitant to enter an assigned client's room. The learner states, "I don't know why I'm so nervous; I've done it many times before!" Which is the best response?

A. "Do you find that your anxiety interferes with other aspects of your life, such as relationships with others?"

B. "If you are anxious, you can wait until later to begin your assessment to allow yourself some time to relax."

C. "Stress is just part of being a nurse. Unfortunately, it will never go away."

D. "What are some techniques that have been successful for you in the past whenever you are nervous?"

Correct Answer: D

Rationale: The clinical nurse educator acts as a role model for self-reflection, self-care, and coping skills. Enquiring about previously successful techniques for stress and anxiety, Option D, focuses on a self-care solution for the issue, yet also promotes educator behaviors of being supportive and understanding (Stokes & Kost, 2012). Enquiring about the effects of anxiety on the learner's personal life at this time, Option A, is assumptive, intrusive, and has the potential to negatively affect the trusting environment established by the clinical nurse educator (Stokes & Kost, 2012). In a clinical setting, it is not appropriate to delay necessary nursing care, Option B—this behavior should not be encouraged. Instead, the clinical nurse educator should redirect the conversation to methods that promote development of long-term resilience, such as techniques for self-care, coping, and stress management. While stress is commonly experienced within the clinical setting, Option C does not positively address the issue at hand.

Test Blueprint: 5 K
Cognitive Code: Analysis

59. A learner shares with the clinical nurse educator an interest in peripherally inserted central catheter (PICC) lines because the learner's father recently had one inserted after an illness. Which activity would best facilitate meeting the identified personal educational goal?
   A. Assigning the learner to shadow a staff nurse caring for several clients with PICC lines
   B. Printing the institutional policy and procedure for PICC line insertion and care for the learner to read and review
   C. Arranging an opportunity for the learner to participate on the agency's PICC line team for one clinical day
   D. Finding an educational video on PICC lines for the learner to view outside of clinical time

Correct Answer: C

Rationale: One aspect of the clinical nurse educator role is to empower learners to be successful in meeting professional and educational goals. Active learning involves the learner through participation and an investment in exploring content knowledge in all phases of the learning process (Scheckel, 2012). Arranging for the learner to spend one clinical day participating on a specialty team, Option C, allows exposure to expert-level knowledge in the area of PICC lines. Simply shadowing a staff nurse caring for clients with a PICC line, as in Option A, is not the best option for promoting active learning. Reading and reviewing policies and procedures, Option B, and watching an educational video, Option D, do not constitute active learning activities.

Test Blueprint: 5 L
Cognitive Code: Application

60. The clinical nurse educator notes that a learner consistently struggles to set up and maintain sterile fields. In a private discussion, the learner responds, "I agree. I cannot seem to master this skill for some reason because there are too many things to remember." Which activity would best facilitate performance of this skill?

A. Reviewing the principles of surgical asepsis, then having the learner set up a sterile field

B. Having the learner read and review the textbook chapter related to surgical asepsis

C. Assigning the learner to return to the clinical practice laboratory to practice the skill repeatedly

D. Showing an educational video on surgical asepsis to the clinical group during post-conference

Correct Answer: A

Rationale: The clinical nurse educator empowers learners to be successful in meeting professional and educational goals. Reviewing the principles of the concept, as in Option A, triggers recall from the cognitive domain; then, immediately putting these principles into practice stimulates the psychomotor domain (Scheckel, 2012). The educator would also have the learner reflect on the learning experience. Reading and reviewing, Option B, activates only the cognitive domain and does not constitute the best example of active learning. Repeated practice of the skill, Option C, activates only the psychomotor domain and does not constitute the best example of active learning. Watching a video, as in Option D, activates only the cognitive domain and does not constitute the best example of active learning.

Test Blueprint: 5 L
Cognitive Code: Application

61. A learner informs the clinical nurse educator of being caught up on all client assignment tasks and readily volunteers to assist others. Which initial action is most appropriate?

A. Assign the learner to shadow a staff nurse caring for multiple clients.

B. Enquire about personal clinical objectives that the learner would like to explore for that day.

C. Allow the learner to take a long break as a reward for strong time management skills.

D. Ask the learner to develop a case study and present it during post-conference.

Correct Answer: B

Rationale: The clinical nurse educator empowers learners to be successful in meeting professional and educational goals. This learner demonstrates strong clinical practice and time management skills and should be offered more challenging learning opportunities. The clinical nurse educator should enquire about personal clinical objectives, Option B, that the learner may have and then assist the learner in identifying opportunities to meet them (Scheckel, 2012). Option A, simply shadowing a nurse caring for multiple clients, is not the best option for promoting active learning. Allowing the learner to take a long break, Option C, does not challenge and stimulate learning. While developing a case study, Option D, could constitute an active learning strategy, this option does not consider the personal educational goals or clinical outcomes that the learner may have.

Test Blueprint: 5 L
Cognitive Code: Application

62. Midway through the semester, a senior learner confides to the clinical nurse educator about not feeling prepared to assume a four-client assignment, which is an identified course competency. Which is the best action?
   A. Remind the learner that learners must care for four clients before the semester ends or potentially fail the course.
   B. Assign the learner to shadow a classmate who has been caring for four clients without difficulty.
   C. Work with the learner to develop goals that will enable the learner to fulfill this requirement by the end of the semester.
   D. Review the learner's final clinical evaluation from the prior semester to gain further insight into the situation.

Correct Answer: C

Rationale: Learners differ in their learning styles. The clinical nurse educator must make a concerted effort to balance learning needs and styles when selecting clinical assignments (Gubrud, 2016, p. 286). The clinical nurse educator should assist the learner in developing goals and using strategies to help achieve the course competency of caring for four clients. The learner is already aware of needing to fulfill this competency; thus, a reminder, Option A, would not be beneficial. Shadowing a classmate, Option B, removes the clinical nurse educator as the facilitator of learning. While it is common for clinical nurse educators to communicate information about learner performance, Option D, evaluative statements about learner performance, should not be shared with other educators (Oermann et al., 2018, p. 102).

Test Blueprint: 5 L
Cognitive Code: Application

63. On the first day of the clinical experience, a learner approaches the clinical nurse educator about a hearing disability. The learner is fearful that without a special stethoscope, the learner will not be able to adequately assess clients. Which is the best action?
   A. Enquire as to how the learner ascertained the disability and if it is temporary or permanent.
   B. Pair the learner up with another learner without a hearing problem for the duration of the clinical experience.
   C. Instruct the learner to contact the office of disability services on campus.
   D. Assign the learner to perform only activities of daily living (ADLs) needs for clients so that a stethoscope will not be needed.

Correct Answer: C

Rationale: Learners with disabilities are responsible for informing the institution of the disability and requesting reasonable accommodations (Oermann et al., 2018, p. 107). The clinical nurse educator should not attempt to determine the nature of the disability, whether accommodations are needed, or provide accommodations, but rather should refer the learner to the appropriate campus resource that can assist in obtaining appropriate accommodations.

Test Blueprint: 5 L
Cognitive Code: Application

64. A group of first-semester learners is having a clinical conference in which they are discussing personal and professional goals. One learner states the desire to become a nurse anesthetist someday. Which statement or question by the clinical nurse educator is most supportive of this learner?
    A. "I wouldn't worry about that yet—you have to finish nursing school first."
    B. "Nurse anesthetists make big salaries; you will do well in this area."
    C. "What are some strategies that you can use now to help you achieve this goal?"
    D. "Nurse anesthesia sounds like a good career, but I would never want to do that."

Correct Answer: C

Rationale: The clinical nurse educator's interpersonal skills may affect learner outcomes. Showing respect for learners, being supportive, and not belittling or making assumptions about learner intent or motivation is important (Gubrud, 2016, p. 291). Assisting the learner in professional goal setting is an important role of the clinical nurse educator, as in Option C. Options A, B, and D belittle the learner's aspirations.

Test Blueprint: 5 L
Cognitive Code: Application

65. A clinical nurse educator must identify appropriate preceptors for senior-level learners to complete their final clinical practicum experience. Which action best supports learners in meeting their educational goals for the preceptorship?
    A. Asking nurses with whom the educator has a personal relationship to be preceptors
    B. Telling learners to find their own preceptors and then making plans to contact them
    C. Seeking input from learners regarding their interest in a specific clinical specialty
    D. Finding the closest agency to the learner's address so that the commute is manageable

Correct Answer: C

Rationale: The selection of preceptors and settings should consider the learners' interest in specific clinical specialties as well as their need to develop particular skill sets (Oermann et al., 2018, p. 204), as in Option C. Asking personal contacts or seeking the closest clinical agency, as in Options A and D, will not necessarily assist learners in meeting their goals. Learners can provide input into their potential preceptor, but the initial contact should come from the clinical nurse educator, making Option B incorrect.

Test Blueprint: 5 L
Cognitive Code: Application

66. The clinical nurse educator is making visits to senior learners enrolled in a preceptorship experience and notices that one learner does not have a client assignment. When asked, the learner tells the educator that the preceptor called off for the day and the nurse manager asked the learner to fill in as the nursing assistant because the unit is short-staffed. Which is the best response?
   A. Talk with the nurse manager and remind the manager of the goals of the preceptorship experience.
   B. Reprimand the learner for not notifying the clinical nurse educator of the situation immediately.
   C. Take over the nursing assistant role and tell the learner to precept with another nurse.
   D. Tell the learner to go home for the day and give the learner a make-up assignment.

Correct Answer: A

Rationale: The clinical nurse educator must be able to assist learners in achieving their educational goals (Gubrud, 2016, p. 289). Talking with the nurse manager about the goals of the preceptorship experience, as in Option A, ideally will trigger the nurse manager to find a suitable replacement preceptor and prevent the situation from recurring. While the learner should have notified the educator of the situation, the learner should not be reprimanded, as in Option B. The nurse manager, who is in a position of power, asked the learner to perform a function and the learner followed the instructions. It is not the duty of the clinical nurse educator to fill in due to short-staffing, as in Option C. Option D, sending the learner home and giving the learner a make-up assignment, would not assist the learner in meeting the goals of the preceptorship.

Test Blueprint: 5 L
Cognitive Code: Application

67. Which best promotes learner empowerment?
   A. The clinical nurse educator instructs the learner to call the pharmacy regarding a question about medications and a client allergy.
   B. A learner assists a staff nurse on the clinical unit with a client transfer after the nurse requests help.
   C. The staff nurse instructs the learner to review the steps of a procedure before providing the care to the client.
   D. The clinical nurse educator and the learner use the computer system to look up a new medication assigned to a client.

Correct Answer: A

Rationale: Empowerment is impacted directly by confidence and knowledge. Learners who do not feel like an integral part of their client's care may feel as though they have no power and that their input is not valued. It is important for the clinical nurse educator to provide experiences in which the learner can advocate for the client and perform tasks directed at this advocation; this will enhance learners' sense of empowerment (Bradshaw & Hultquist, 2017, p. 314). Encouraging the learner to contact resources within the agency will enhance learner empowerment; thus, Option A is correct. Options B, C, and

D assist learning in the clinical setting but do not necessarily promote empowerment.

Test Blueprint: 5 L
Cognitive Code: Analysis

68. Which is the best learning activity to assist learners in understanding quality improvement practices?
    A. Analyzing fall precaution practices at their clinical agency and using evidence-based practice guidelines to identify strategies for improvement
    B. Watching videos discussing quality improvement practices in the clinical setting and identifying how this relates to their clinical agency
    C. Writing a paper discussing current quality improvement practices in health care agencies
    D. Listening to a presentation discussing quality improvement practices in health care agencies and methods for improvement

Correct Answer: A

Rationale: While all of these strategies will help learners to understand quality improvement practices, the most effective in helping them understand is to engage them actively in the process. As identified by the Quality and Safety Education for Nurses (QSEN) Institute (2019), quality improvement requires both monitoring outcomes and identifying improvement methods to continuously improve the quality and safety of health care. Actively participating in the quality improvement process enhances learners' engagement and requires them to use critical thinking, further assisting in the understanding and application of these processes (Keating, 2011, p. 83), making Option A the correct response. Options B, C, and D do not actively engage learners or are missing key components of the QSEN recommendations.

Test Blueprint: 5 M
Cognitive Code: Application

69. A clinical nurse educator is reinforcing the concept of quality improvement and evidence-based practice. Which is the most appropriate assignment?
    A. Asking learners to identify a quality improvement issue on the clinical unit and using a research journal article on that topic to identify a potential solution
    B. Requiring learners to complete a guided journal reflection on a quality improvement topic observed on the clinical unit
    C. Assigning learners to write a three-page research paper on a quality improvement topic of their choice
    D. Arranging for each learner to spend a clinical day with the charge nurse to observe delegation skills

Correct Answer: A

Rationale: The clinical nurse educator is reinforcing prior learned content; asking learners to identify a quality improvement (QI) issue on the clinical unit and to use a research article to identify a potential solution, Option A, allows learners to apply the principles of QI and evidence-based practice (Oermann et al., 2018, p. 242). Option B, asking learners to write a journal reflection related to a QI topic on the clinical unit, is a more appropriate assignment for the introduction of QI concepts. Having learners write a QI paper on a topic of their choice, Option C, does not provide the opportunity for application of QI and evidence-based practice. While charge nurses may sometimes be involved in QI measures, QI is often monitored and assessed by the nurse manager or a designated QI nurse; Option D also states that the purpose of the observation is to observe delegation, which is not the identified goal.

Test Blueprint: 5 M
Cognitive Code: Analysis

70. The clinical nurse educator observed a learner enter a client's room without putting on the required personal protective equipment. Which is the most appropriate initial action?
    A. Addressing the learner privately when the learner exits the room
    B. Waiting until post-conference and discussing isolation precautions with all learners
    C. Providing each learner with a copy of the agency infection control policy
    D. Following the learner into the room after putting on the required personal protective equipment

Correct Answer: D

Rationale: Option D is correct because following the learner in the room with the appropriate personal protective equipment will allow the learner to identify the appropriate behavior and prompt a behavior change. Learners tend to imitate behaviors they observe on the clinical unit. The clinical nurse educator should role model appropriate behaviors for learners to encourage proper nursing practice (Oermann et al., 2018, p. 27). Options A, B, and C do not address the lack of use of appropriate precautions immediately and could put the learner at risk.

Test Blueprint: 5 M
Cognitive Code: Analysis

71. An interprofessional team conference is scheduled about an end-of-life decision regarding a learner's client. Which strategy most actively engages the learner in applying best practices for this client?
    A. Ask the learner to develop a poster on end-of-life care issues to present on the clinical unit.
    B. Review concepts of palliative and end-of-life care with the learner during preconference so that the learner knows what to expect.
    C. Direct the learner to the online End-of-Life Nursing Education Consortium (ELNEC) website for additional resources and training modules.
    D. Arrange for the learner to participate in the team conference to provide input on client assessments and nursing care.

Correct Answer: D

Rationale: One role of the clinical nurse educator is to actively engage learners in applying best practices. The best strategy for this objective is one in which the learner is actively participating in the team conference and practicing communication and teamwork skills by providing assessment and nursing care input, as suggested in Option D. Preparing and presenting a poster on the topic, Option A, can certainly strengthen the cognitive domain, but does not provide an opportunity for the learner to engage actively in best practices. Reviewing concepts during preconference, Option B, may help prepare the learner for the day but does not provide an opportunity for the learner to engage actively in best practices. Option C, directing the learner to the ELNEC website (Relias Learning, 2019) is a strategy to strengthen the cognitive domain but does not provide opportunities for the learner to engage actively in best practices.

Test Blueprint: 5 M
Cognitive Code: Analysis

References

Alexander, G. R. (2016). Multicultural education in nursing. In D. M. Billings & J. A. Halstead (Eds.), *Teaching in nursing: A guide for faculty* (5th ed., pp. 263–281). St. Louis, MO: Elsevier.

American Nurses Association. (2015). Code of ethics for nurses with interpretive statements. Retrieved from https://www.nursingworld.org/coe-view-only

American Nurses Association. (2018). Competency model. Retrieved from https://www.nursingworld.org/~4a0a2e/globalassets/docs/ce/177626-ana-leadership-booklet-new-final.pdf

Bastable, S. B. (2019). *Nurse as educator: Principles of teaching and learning for nursing practice* (5th ed.). Burlington, MA: Jones & Bartlett Learning.

Bauce, K., Kridli, S. A., & Fitzpatrick, J. J. (2014). Cultural competence and psychological empowerment among acute care nurses. *Online Journal of Cultural Competence in Nursing and Healthcare, 4*(2), 27–38. doi:10.9730/ojccnh.org/v4n2a3

Benner, P. (1984). *From novice to expert: Excellence and power in clinical nursing practice.* Menlo Park, CA: Addison-Wesley.

Bonnel, W. (2012). Clinical performance evaluation. In D. M. Billings & J. A. Halstead (Eds.), *Teaching in nursing: A guide for faculty* (4th ed., pp. 485–502). St. Louis, MO: Elsevier.

Bonnel, W. (2016). Clinical performance evaluation. In D. M. Billings & J. A. Halstead (Eds.), *Teaching in nursing: A guide for faculty* (5th ed., pp. 443–462). St. Louis, MO: Elsevier.

Blum, C. A. (2014). Practicing self-care for nurses: A nursing program initiative. *The Online Journal of Issues In Nursing, 19*(3), 3. doi:10.3912/OJIN.Vol-19No03Man03

Bradshaw, M. J., & Hultquist, B. L. (2017). *Innovative teaching strategies in nursing and related health professions* (7th ed.). Burlington, MA: Jones & Bartlett Learning.

Candela, L. (2012). From teaching to learning: Theoretical foundations. In D. M. Billings & J. A. Halstead (Eds.), *Teaching in nursing: A guide for faculty* (4th ed., pp. 202–243). St. Louis, MO: Elsevier.

Candela, L. (2016). Theoretical foundations of teaching and learning. In D. M. Billings & J. A. Halstead (Eds.), *Teaching in nursing: A guide for faculty* (5th ed., pp. 211–229). St. Louis, MO: Elsevier.

Christensen, L. S. (2016). The academic performance of students: Legal and ethical issues. In D. M. Billings & J. A. Halstead (Eds.), *Teaching in nursing: A guide for faculty* (5th ed., pp. 35–54). St. Louis, MO: Elsevier.

Clark, C. (2018). How nurse faculty can help students de-stress. *Reflections on Nursing Leadership.* Retrieved from https://www.reflectionsonnursingleadership.org/features/more-features/how-nurse-faculty-can-help-students-de-stress

Davis, C. (2017). The importance of professional accountability. *Nursing Made Incredibly Easy, 15*(6), 4. doi:10.1097/01.NME.0000525557.44656.04

Doenges, M. E., Moorhouse, M. F., & Murr, A. C. (2016). *Nursing diagnosis manual: Planning, individualizing, and documenting patient care* (5th ed.). Philadelphia, PA: F. A. Davis.

Frank, B. (2012). Teaching students with disabilities. In D. M. Billings & J. A. Halstead (Eds.), *Teaching in nursing: A guide for faculty* (4th ed., pp. 55–75). St. Louis, MO: Elsevier.

Frank, B. (2016). Facilitating learning for students with disabilities. In D. M. Billings & J. A. Halstead (Eds.), *Teaching in nursing: A guide for faculty* (5th ed., pp. 55–72). St. Louis, MO: Elsevier.

Gaberson, K. B., Oermann, M. H., & Shellenbarger, T. (2015). *Clinical teaching strategies in nursing* (4th ed.). New York, NY: Springer.

Gubrud, P. (2016). Teaching in the clinical setting. In D. M. Billings & J. A. Halstead (Eds.), *Teaching in nursing: A guide for faculty* (5th ed., pp. 282–303). St. Louis, MO: Elsevier.

Halic, O., Greenburg, K., & Paulus, T. (2009). Language and academic identity: A study of the experiences of non-native English speaking international students. *International Education, 38*(2), 73–94.

Heise, B. A., & Gilpin, L. C. (2016). Nursing students' clinical experience with death: A pilot study. *Nursing Education Perspectives, 37*(2), 104–106. doi:10.5480/13-1283

Heise, B. A., Wing, D. K., & Hullinger, A. H. R. (2018). My patient died: A national study of nursing students' perceptions after experiencing a patient death. *Nursing Education Perspectives, 39*(6), 355–359. doi:10.1097/01.NEP.0000000000000335

Johnson, E. G. (2012). The academic performance of students: Legal and ethical issues. In D. M. Billings & J. A. Halstead (Eds.), *Teaching in nursing: A guide for faculty* (4th ed., pp. 34–54). St. Louis, MO: Elsevier.

Keating, S. B. (2011). *Curriculum development and evaluation in nursing* (2nd ed.). New York, NY: Springer.

Massarweh, L. (1999). Promoting a positive clinical experience. *Nurse Educator, 24*(3), 44–47.

National Council of State Boards of Nursing. (2017). Model rules. Retrieved from https://www.ncsbn.org/17_Model_Rules_0917.pdf

National Council of State Boards of Nursing. (2019). Nursing regulation: Filing a complaint. Retrieved from https://www.ncsbn.org/7127.htm

Oermann, M. H. (1997). Evaluating critical thinking in clinical practice. *Nurse Educator, 22*(5), 25–28.

Oermann, M. H., Shellenbarger, T., & Gaberson, K. B. (2018). *Clinical teaching strategies in nursing* (5th ed.). New York, NY: Springer.

Paul, R., & Elder, L. (2008). Critical thinking: The art of Socratic questioning, part III. *Journal of Developmental Education, 31*(3), 34–35.

Phillips, J. M. (2016). Strategies to promote student engagement and active learning. In D. M. Billings & J. A. Halstead (Eds.), *Teaching in nursing: A guide for faculty* (5th ed., pp. 245–262). St. Louis, MO: Elsevier.

Quality and Safety Education for Nurses Institute. (2019). QSEN competencies. Retrieved from http://qsen.org/competencies/pre-licensure-ksas/

Rachel, M. M. (2012). Accountability: A concept worth revisiting. *American Nurse Today, 7*(3). Retrieved from https://www.americannursetoday.com/accountability-a-concept-worth-revisiting/

Relias Learning. (2019). End-of-Life Nursing Education Consortium (ELNEC). Retrieved from https://elnec.academy.reliaslearning.com/

Roberts, F. B. (2005). Socialization into nursing: Forming a professional attitude. In L. Caputi & L. Engelmann (Eds.), *Teaching nursing: The art and science, Vol. 2* (pp. 1082–1100). Glen Ellyn, IL: College of DuPage Press.

Rowles, C. J. (2012). Strategies to promote critical thinking and active learning. In D. M. Billings & J. A. Halstead (Eds.), *Teaching in nursing: A guide for faculty* (4th ed., pp. 258–284). St. Louis, MO: Elsevier.

Scheckel, M. (2012). Selecting learning experiences to achieve curriculum outcomes. In D. M. Billings & J. A. Halstead (Eds.), *Teaching in nursing: A guide for faculty* (4th ed., pp. 170–187). St. Louis, MO: Elsevier.

Shellenbarger, T., & Bonnel, W. (2019). Facilitate learner development and socialization. In T. Shellenbarger (Ed.), *Clinical nurse educator competencies: Creating an evidence-based practice for academic clinical nurse educators* (pp. 63–72). Washington, DC: National League for Nursing.

Stokes, L. G., & Flowers, N. (2012). Multicultural education in nursing. In D. M. Billings & J. A. Halstead (Eds.), *Teaching in nursing: A guide for faculty* (4th ed., pp. 291–310). St. Louis, MO: Elsevier.

Stokes, L. G., & Kost, G. C. (2012). Teaching in the clinical setting. In D. M. Billings & J. A. Halstead (Eds.), *Teaching in nursing: A guide for faculty* (4th ed., pp. 331–334). St. Louis, MO: Elsevier.

Ten Hoeve, Y., Castelein, S., Jansen, W. S., Jansen, G. J., & Roodbol, P. F. (2017). Nursing students' changing orientation and attitudes towards nursing during education: A two year longitudinal study. *Nurse Education Today, 48*, 19–24. doi:10.1016/j.nedt.2016.09.009

Westrick, S. J. (2016). Nursing students' use of electronic and social media: Law, ethics, and e-professionalism, *Nursing Education Perspectives, 37*, 16–22.

8

Implement Effective Clinical Assessment and Evaluation Strategies

1. Which evaluation method is used when providing learners with feedback after performing a skill?
   A. Formative evaluation
   B. Emergent evaluation
   C. Summative evaluation
   D. Comprehensive evaluation

   Correct Answer: A

   Rationale: Formative evaluation is "conducted while the teaching-learning process is unfolding" (Scheckel, 2016, p. 169). This type of evaluation method occurs throughout learning. Option C is incorrect because this method measures learner outcome achievement and course and program effectiveness (Scheckel, 2016, p. 170). Options B and D are incorrect because they are not forms of evaluation.

   Test Blueprint: 6 A
   Cognitive Code: Recall

2. Which learning outcome best represents the affective domain?
   A. Conduct an initial physical assessment of a client.
   B. Develop basic plans of care using the nursing process.
   C. Respond to aspects of sociocultural influences that impact the health of families.
   D. Apply relevant principles of pathophysiology to current client health status.

   Correct Answer: C

   Rationale: The affective domain reflects learners' growth in feelings or emotional awareness; learners demonstrate belief in the value of individuals and respond appropriately (Oermann, Shellenbarger, & Gaberson, 2018b). Thus, Option C represents the affective domain and is the correct response. Options B and D represent the cognitive domain and Option A involves the psychomotor domain.

   Test Blueprint: 6 A
   Cognitive Code: Recall

3. Which evaluation method is based on outcomes or competencies associated with a course?
   A. Objective Structured Clinical Examination (OSCE)
   B. Summative evaluation
   C. Criterion-referenced
   D. Norm-referenced

   Correct Answer: C

   Rationale: Criterion-referenced evaluation measures learner performance with predetermined criteria or standards for the course, as in Option C. In contrast, norm-referenced evaluation, Option D, measures learners against the performance of other learners within the same group or course. Summative evaluation, Option B, is given at the end of a specific time, such as the end of the course, and could theoretically be either norm- or criterion-referenced (Oermann & Gaberson, 2017, pp. 217–219). Finally, an OSCE, Option A, is an incorrect choice because it is generally for assessing the performance of a single skill rather than an entire set of course outcomes (Patrick, 2019, p. 76).

   Test Blueprint: 6 A
   Cognitive Code: Recall

4. A clinical nurse educator has decided to implement concept maps as a clinical learning assignment. Which is true about concept maps?
   A. Concept maps improve learners' writing and research skills.
   B. Concept maps are easy to interpret and understand.
   C. Concept maps help learners explore their values, attitudes, and beliefs.
   D. Concept maps help learners see how concepts are connected.

   Correct Answer: D

   Rationale: As suggested in Option D, concept maps help learners see how concepts are connected as opposed to concentrating on content (Oermann et al., 2018b, p. 239). Concept maps are not designed to improve writing and research skills; therefore, Option A is incorrect. It is often hard to understand learners' intent with concept maps as keywords and phrases are used, and written concept maps are complex and sometimes lack clarity (Kirkpatrick & DeWitt, 2016); thus, Option B is incorrect. Concept maps are not designed to help learners explore their values, attitudes, and beliefs, as suggested in Option C.

   Test Blueprint: 6 A
   Cognitive Code: Recall

5. The clinical nurse educator wants to create an assignment to help learners examine their beliefs and values that might affect care. Which learning activity would be most helpful to meet this goal?
   A. Weekly journal
   B. Electronic concept map
   C. Written care plan
   D. Evidence-based practice paper

   Correct Answer: A

   Rationale: Option A is correct because the use of journals helps learners reflect on and examine their beliefs and values (Oermann et al., 2018b, p. 237). Options

B, C, and D are useful teaching and learning activities that enhance cognitive learning but do not typically help learners examine values and beliefs.

Test Blueprint: 6 A
Cognitive Code: Analysis

6. A clinical nurse educator is evaluating a learner on the ability to perform a head-to-toe assessment of an adult client. Which evaluation method is least appropriate?
   A. A checklist that outlines step-by-step what needs to be completed for a head-to-toe assessment of an adult client
   B. A journal entry in which the learner is asked to describe the perceived value of a head-to-toe assessment
   C. A self-evaluation activity that requires the learner to list strengths and weaknesses when performing a head-to-toe assessment
   D. A written care plan that involves a head-to-toe assessment and identifies care priorities

Correct Answer: B

Rationale: Although journals can be functional in the clinical environment, writing about the perceived value of this experience would not provide ample evidence to support evaluation by a clinical nurse educator, as suggested in Option B (Bonnel, 2016, p. 454). Criterion-referenced tools, Option A, self-evaluation activities, Option C, and care plans, Option D, all give more information regarding the determination of achievement of learning outcomes.

Test Blueprint: 6 A
Cognitive Code: Application

7. Which written assignment prompt best encourages development of higher-level thinking skills?
   A. Summarize and explain the purpose of a research article.
   B. Compare client assessment findings with the physiological processes of heart failure.
   C. Write a paper about the pathophysiology of a health problem impacting the client.
   D. List data collection and assessments for an assigned client.

Correct Answer: B

Rationale: Written assignment prompts, such as comparing physiological conditions, encourage the analysis and evaluation of client problems and help learners develop ideas and connections, as in Option B. Summarizing an article and listing data, such as the assignment in Option A, may assist in understanding and comprehension; however, it does not promote higher-level thinking skills. Writing a paper, as suggested by Option C, helps the learner understand and explain ideas but does not necessarily encourage higher-level thinking abilities. Listing data collection and assessment, as suggested in Option D, involves remembering information only, a lower-level cognitive process (Gaberson, Oermann, & Shellenbarger, 2015, pp. 296–298).

Test Blueprint: 6 A
Cognitive Code: Analysis

8. Which is an example of formative evaluation?
  A. Providing feedback to a learner following administration of medications
  B. Summarizing competencies that a learner has achieved at midterm
  C. Documenting learner achievement of course clinical outcomes
  D. Assigning a grade to a clinical learning activity

Correct Answer: A

Rationale: Formative clinical evaluation provides feedback to learners about their ongoing progress in meeting skills, outcomes, and competencies and further identifies learner needs regarding skill development. Providing feedback regarding medication administration, Option A, is specific to a skill that the learner would work on to improve performance (Gaberson et al., 2015, p. 323). Options B, C, and D are all examples of summative evaluation methods.

Test Blueprint: 6 B
Cognitive Code: Recall

9. Which feedback statement is most appropriate when completing formative evaluation?
  A. "You need to improve on your assessment skills. I recommend you go to the lab for assistance."
  B. "You failed to notice an abnormal assessment finding; you will receive a learning contract in order to further develop."
  C. "You require improvement with cardiac assessment and auscultation of key landmarks. Review the appropriate procedure to enhance knowledge and skills in this area."
  D. "You did a nice job on the assessment; however, you missed a few key areas. I would recommend that you attend open lab to continue to work on your skills."

Correct Answer: C

Rationale: Formative feedback should be precise and specific for learners to correct their behaviors. Option C provides specific information and direction for improvement. Options A, B, and D provide general statements and are negative; feedback with negative reinforcement should be avoided in formative evaluation, as they do not assist with performance improvement (Gaberson et al., 2015, p. 326).

Test Blueprint: 6 B
Cognitive Code: Analysis

10. A clinical nurse educator wants to follow best practices when providing feedback to learners in the clinical environment. Which action best represents providing appropriate feedback?
  A. Informing learners of progress at the beginning of each clinical day
  B. Engaging learners at predetermined times throughout the semester
  C. Discussing performance measures at midterm and at the end of the semester
  D. Providing feedback on an ongoing basis, at midterm, and at the end of the semester

Correct Answer: D

Rationale: Any protocol for clinical evaluation should include extensive formative evaluation and periodic summative evaluation (Oermann & Gaberson, 2017, p. 218). Option D presents feedback on an ongoing basis and at midterm and the end of the semester, which includes both formative and summative evaluation. Option A, informing learners of progress at the beginning of each clinical day, omits summative assessment. Engaging the learner only at predetermined times throughout the semester, Option B, as well as at only the midterm and end of the term, Option C, do not promote formative assessment.

Test Blueprint: 6 B
Cognitive Code: Application

11. A clinical nurse educator has a group consisting of eight learners on a large medical-surgical unit. Typically, the learners are assigned clients through-out the unit and are not in close proximity. Considering these factors, which method would best evaluate learners' prioritization skills?
    A. Having learners complete a reflective learning activity at the end of the shift
    B. Interviewing learners periodically throughout the shift
    C. Spending 15-minute segments of direct observation with each learner during the shift
    D. Having learners complete nursing care plans by the end of the shift

Correct Answer: D

Rationale: Nursing care plans allow clinical nurse educators to evalu-ate learners' ability to determine and prioritize care (Bonnel, 2016, p. 450). Option D provides a means to evaluate prioritization while still managing the volume of learners in this scenario. A reflective activity, such as Option A, may offer discussion about prioritization but this learning activity is largely dictated by the learner; there is no guarantee that prioritization skills will be discussed. Option B, interviewing learners throughout the shift, can assist with critical thinking processes and prioritization but may be difficult to achieve in a timely fashion with the volume of learners and distance between each learner. With direct observation on a rotational basis, Option C, there is a chance that the clinical nurse educator would not be able to visualize learner prioritization.

Test Blueprint: 6 B
Cognitive Code: Application

12. A learner does not understand why some evaluations count as a grade and others do not. Which response is most appropriate?
    A. "Daily evaluations are used as part of your grade for the clinical course."
    B. "Some evaluations do not align with competencies so they cannot be used for a grade."
    C. "The course coordinator decides which feedback will count for a grade and which will not."
    D. "Some feedback supports improvement while some is used for final evalu-ation and grading."

Correct Answer: D

Rationale: Formative evaluation does not count for a grade whereas summative evaluation is used for grading purposes (Oermann & Gaberson, 2017, p. 217). Option D describes how formative evaluation or feedback is used for improvement while summative feedback is used for grading. A daily evaluation, Option A, refers to formative assessment and does not inform the learner of the summative evaluation component. All evaluations must align with competencies or desired learning outcomes, making Option B incorrect. Although the course coordinator does likely determine which feedback will ultimately count for a grade, more transparency is needed to fully answer the question.

Test Blueprint: 6 B
Cognitive Code: Analysis

13. Which statement best describes formative and summative evaluation methods?
    A. Formative evaluation is based on observation whereas summative evaluation is obtained from an exam score.
    B. Formative evaluation occurs throughout learning whereas summative evaluation occurs at the end of learning.
    C. Formative evaluation is formal and graded whereas summative evaluation is informal and is not graded.
    D. Formative evaluation is used to help determine a final course grade whereas summative evaluation provides an assignment grade.

Correct Answer: B

Rationale: Formative evaluation occurs throughout the learning process, as found in Option B. Learners can benefit from formative evaluation by using it to identify strengths and weaknesses and meet the objectives and outcomes efficiently. Option A is incorrect because this statement is not always true; there are multiple ways to evaluate learners formatively and summatively, depending on many factors (Oermann & Gaberson, 2017). Summative evaluation provides a grade at the end of a specific time, such as at the end of a semester, and provides an assessment of performance, making Option C incorrect. Summative evaluation can be used for the course grade; thus, Option D is incorrect. Formative evaluation supports summative decisions (Bonnel, 2016, pp. 445–446; DeYoung, 2015, pp. 214–215; Oermann & Gaberson, 2017, pp. 217–218).

Test Blueprint: 6 B
Cognitive Code: Recall

14. Which best describes the purpose of keeping detailed anecdotal notes about learner performance and feedback given?
    A. Notes will help the clinical nurse educator remember learner performance.
    B. Notes will document learner progress made or lack of progress.
    C. Notes will provide evidence to support the summative evaluation.
    D. Notes will identify trends and learner performance gaps.

Correct Answer: C

Rationale: Clinical nurse educators should keep anecdotal notes about learners' progress to provide evidence for their summative evaluation. If a learner contests the grade, the clinical nurse educator is protected against charges of violating due process; anecdotal notes should provide evidence to show that the learner was clearly observed and kept aware of strengths and weaknesses. Keeping such notes supports summative decisions; thus, Option C is correct (Bonnel, 2016, pp. 448, 458; DeYoung, 2015, pp. 214–215; Kan & Stabler-Haas, 2018, p. 94). Options A, B, and D help the clinical nurse educator when determining a summative grade, but they do not adequately describe the purpose of keeping anecdotal notes.

Test Blueprint: 6 B
Cognitive Code: Analysis

15. Which evaluation method would be considered summative?
    A. Weekly logs documenting learner progress
    B. Criterion-referenced clinical evaluation tool
    C. Summarizing learner performance of a skill
    D. Feedback during medication administration

Correct Answer: B

Rationale: Summative evaluation is designed for assigning clinical grades and summarizing the performance of a learner in a certain time, as in Option B (Oermann et al., 2018b, p. 257). Options A, C, and D are incorrect because they describe formative evaluations.

Test Blueprint: 6 B
Cognitive Code: Recall

16. Which evaluation activity would best provide the learner with formative evaluation information?
    A. Completing a checklist to grade performance of a procedure
    B. Completing a final clinical evaluation tool
    C. Providing just-in-time feedback regarding sterile technique
    D. Reviewing the grading rubric for a final written assignment

Correct Answer: C

Rationale: Option C provides the learner with timely feedback about progress in meeting a clinical competency (Oermann & Gaberson, 2017), in this case, regarding sterile technique. Formative feedback is diagnostic and should not be graded, and should help the learner to improve subsequent performances (Oermann & Gaberson, 2017). Options A and B represent examples of summative evaluations in that they are final, graded evaluations that summarize competency (Oermann & Gaberson, 2017). Option D may provide formative feedback since it could help performance; however, it does not provide specific feedback and is regarding a final assignment; thus, it is not the best example of formative evaluation.

Test Blueprint: 6 B
Cognitive Code: Analysis

17. A learner is having difficulty connecting high-level concepts in the clinical setting. Interventions by the clinical nurse educator have proven ineffective. Which is the best next action?

A. Discuss the curriculum concerns with the course coordinator.

B. Encourage the learner to withdraw from the course.

C. Continue to try new techniques to help the learner progress.

D. Anticipate that the learner will need to repeat this clinical experience.

Correct Answer: A

Rationale: The curriculum should guide clinical practice (Gubrud, 2016, p. 285). Engaging the course coordinator, as suggested in Option A, allows for a better understanding of learner progress in connection to the curriculum. It also provides an opportunity to discuss the potential theory-practice disconnect. Withdrawing from a course, Option B, does not fix the problem. As interventions by the clinical nurse educator have proven ineffective, attempting new techniques, Option C, will likely not be successful. Although a repeat of the clinical experience may be necessary, as in Option D, reasonable steps should be taken to support the learner before this occurs.

Test Blueprint: 6 C
Cognitive Code: Application

18. A clinical nurse educator has just been reassigned to a new clinical group starting next week. Which action best limits personal influence on learner performance evaluations?

A. Reflecting on personal values before beginning the new clinical experience

B. Focusing on making fair evaluations throughout the clinical experience

C. Treating this clinical group the same as all previous clinical groups

D. Considering changing personal values to help remove bias toward certain learners

Correct Answer: A

Rationale: Developing awareness of values helps avoid influencing clinical evaluations to the point of unfairness to the learner (Oermann & Gaberson, 2017, p. 216). Option A engages the clinical nurse educator in understanding one's own values. Fair evaluation throughout the clinical experience, Option B, does not include an understanding of personal values. Option C, treating the clinical group the same as previous groups, does not account for changes with the new clinical group nor does it promote self-awareness. Changing values is likely not achievable, making Option D incorrect.

Test Blueprint: 6 D
Cognitive Code: Analysis

19. Which action is best when a learner accuses the clinical nurse educator of not being fair in evaluation?

A. Reassure the learner that bias is eliminated with proper evaluation.

B. Tell the learner to speak with the course coordinator regarding fair evaluation practices.

C. Request for the learner to be reallocated to another clinical group.

D. Provide evidence on how fairness in evaluation is reinforced.

Correct Answer: D

Rationale: There are a variety of ways to improve evaluation fairness, including identifying one's own values, focusing clinical evaluation on predetermined outcomes or competencies, and developing a supportive learning environment (Oermann & Gaberson, 2017, p. 218). Option D supports helping the learner understand specific actions that are taken to improve evaluation fairness. Option A, providing reassurance, is helpful but some degree of bias is typically present. Asking the learner to approach the course coordinator, Option B, does not promote a learner-educator relationship nor does it answer the learner's question. A discussion should occur first to understand the concerns, making Option C incorrect.

Test Blueprint: 6 D
Cognitive Code: Application

20. A learner arrives to the clinical setting 30 minutes late. The program's policy states that learners arriving more than 10 minutes late should be sent home and receive an incomplete for the day. Which is the best action?
    A. Send the learner home and then notify the course coordinator.
    B. Give the learner a warning that the next late arrival will result in being sent home.
    C. Send the learner to the unit and then call the course coordinator for instructions.
    D. Ask the learner to wait in the conference room and then call the program chairperson for advice.

Correct Answer: A

Rationale: The clinical nurse educator should follow the program's policy; thus, the learner should be sent home, as in Option A. The incident should be written in the learner's file and the course coordinator should be notified as soon as possible (O'Connor, 2015). Options B, C, and D do not adhere to the program's policy.

Test Blueprint: 6 D
Cognitive Code: Application

21. Which best describes how to maintain integrity during the learner evaluation process?
    A. Being aware of personal values that could bias judgments
    B. Considering evaluation an objective measure
    C. Maintaining a complete set of anecdotal notes for a learner performing unsatisfactorily
    D. Assigning a course grade as soon as enough data is collected to support the grade

Correct Answer: A

Rationale: Clinical evaluation is a subjective process requiring the clinical nurse educator to pass judgment about learners and their performance. To maintain integrity in the evaluation process, educators must examine their values, beliefs, and attitudes to fairly evaluate each learner. The clinical nurse educator must not let learner differences (e.g., speed, outgoing personality, or other factors not related to clinical performance) influence the evaluation process (Bonnel, 2016, p. 444; Oermann & Gaberson, 2017, pp. 216–217), making Option A correct. Clinical evaluation is a subjective process, making Option B incorrect. Option C will assist in making grading decisions but will not necessarily help maintain integrity of the evaluation process. Option D is incorrect, as a learner may continue to improve or show evidence of decline after this grading decision.

Test Blueprint: 6 D
Cognitive Code: Application

22. Which is the best approach to reading written assignments?
    A. Random order
    B. Alphabetical order by last name
    C. Submission order
    D. From shortest to longest in length

Correct Answer: A

Rationale: To ensure grading consistency, the clinical nurse educator should read written assignments in a random order, as suggested in Option A (Oermann et al., 2018b, p. 251). Options B, C, and D may introduce bias in the evaluation.

Test Blueprint: 6 D
Cognitive Code: Application

23. Which action best prevents incorrect evaluations?
    A. Discussing observations of learners with other educators
    B. Obtaining learners' perceptions of their behavior
    C. Relying on staff to evaluate learner performance
    D. Trusting first impressions

Correct Answer: B

Rationale: To prevent incorrect judgments and misconceptions, it is helpful to discuss observations with learners and obtain learners' perceptions of their behavior, as suggested in Option B (Oermann et al., 2018b, p. 262). It would be inappropriate to discuss observations of learners with other educators, Option A, especially if they do not have a legitimate educational interest. Clinical nurse educators should not defer evaluation to staff, as in Option C, or trust first impressions, as in Option D, as they might not be correct (Oermann et al., 2018b, p. 272).

Test Blueprint: 6 D
Cognitive Code: Application

24. A learner has difficulty meeting safe practice competencies on the clinical unit. Which action is most appropriate?
    A. Allowing the learner additional time to meet the competencies
    B. Documenting the pattern of marginal or unsafe behavior
    C. Working with the course coordinator to transfer the learner to another clinical area
    D. Assigning additional paperwork to support knowledge development

Correct Answer: B

Rationale: Objective documentation of the unsafe behavior is necessary to support decision-making related to learner progression and to develop a plan for remediation, as in Option B (Bonnel, 2012, p. 498). Allowing additional time to meet competencies, Option A, transferring the learner, Option C, and assigning additional paperwork, Option D, would be inappropriate as they potentially cause legal issues since the same opportunities are not offered to all learners.

Test Blueprint: 6 D
Cognitive Code: Application

25. Which setting would be most appropriate to review midterm evaluations with learners?
A. On the nursing unit at the end of the clinical day
B. In a shared office space and conference area
C. In a private room with a scheduled appointment time
D. In the clinical learning laboratory

Correct Answer: C

Rationale: The setting and environment in which an evaluation conference takes place should be comfortable and privacy must be maintained at all times. Appointment times away from the clinical site, as suggested in Option C, are encouraged; this promotes a comfortable and private setting for learners to listen and receive constructive commentary (Bonnel, 2012, p. 498). Options A, B, and D are not private and thus are not appropriate for learner evaluation conferences.

Test Blueprint: 6 D
Cognitive Code: Application

26. A learner has been having difficulty meeting deadlines for required paperwork and often arrives late to the clinical learning experience. The learner states having "personal and financial" issues that have been hindering the learner's performance. Which initial action is most appropriate?
A. Extending paperwork deadlines for the learner to allow for more flexibility
B. Documenting the learner's statements in the formative evaluation
C. Asking the learner to elaborate on issues affecting performance
D. Making a referral to the counseling or learner support services department

Correct Answer: D

Rationale: Learners at risk for failing to meet clinical learning outcomes may have personal problems that affect their performance. Clinical nurse educators should refer these learners to counseling or support services, as suggested by Option D. The clinical nurse educator should not attempt to counsel the learner, as in Option C, as this may lead to bias with evaluation of clinical performance (Gaberson et al., 2015, p. 358). Extending paperwork deadlines, Option A, is not initially appropriate. Documentation of the learner's statements related to personal problems, as in Option B, should not occur in formative evaluation.

Test Blueprint: 6 D
Cognitive Code: Analysis

27. When preparing to evaluate a learner in the clinical setting, which is the most important to consider?
   A. The difference between formative and summative feedback
   B. One's own values and beliefs that may influence evaluation
   C. Agency policy and procedure
   D. The learner's age and life experience

Correct Answer: B

Rationale: Due to the subjective nature of clinical evaluation, it is important for the clinical nurse educator to identify one's own values and beliefs that influence how one evaluates, as in Option B. A clinical nurse educator's values often lead to judgments about the quality of learner performance (Gaberson et al., 2015, p. 322). Understanding the difference between formative and summative feedback is important, as in Option A, but does not play a role in preparation. Learners should not be evaluated according to agency policy, as in Option C. Learners' age and life experience, as in Option D, should not factor into performance evaluation and may lead to bias.

Test Blueprint: 6 D
Cognitive Code: Analysis

28. During a Foley catheter insertion skill evaluation, the clinical nurse educator notes that the learner incorrectly performed the procedure. During debriefing, the learner responds by stating, "this is how I was taught during open lab." Which is the most appropriate initial action?
   A. Inform the learner that the learner was unsuccessful and will need to repeat the competency.
   B. Communicate with the lab educator prior to assigning a grade.
   C. Assign a passing grade and follow up with the lab educator to review the procedure.
   D. Report concerns regarding inconsistent practices to the program dean and/or director.

Correct Answer: B

Rationale: Prior to assigning a failing grade, the clinical nurse educator should verify that the data collected and the tools used for evaluation are consistent. If the learner, in fact, was instructed differently and failed, this could lead to a legal concern. Verification of skill performance can assist with reliability when assigning the grade (Bonnel, 2012, p. 488). Informing the learner that the learner was unsuccessful, Option A, and assigning a passing grade, Option C, are not appropriate, as more clarity is required at this time. Reporting concerns to the dean or director, as in Option D, may occur after working with the educator who taught the skill.

Test Blueprint: 6 D
Cognitive Code: Analysis

29. After providing feedback, the clinical nurse educator asks the learner to sign the written clinical evaluation form. The learner verbalizes concerns about signing the form. Which is the best response?
A. "Your signature indicates that you agree with the commentary provided on the form."
B. "The signature indicates that you understand the end-of-course competencies."
C. "Your signature means that you have read and received the evaluation."
D. "The signature means that you understand the areas that you need to improve on."

Correct Answer: C

Rationale: The signature on a clinical evaluation form is verification that the learner has met with the clinical nurse educator, read, and received the clinical evaluation, as in Option C. The signature does not indicate understanding or agreement with the commentary, making Options A, B, and D incorrect (Gaberson et al., 2015, p. 356).

Test Blueprint: 6 D
Cognitive Code: Application

30. The clinical nurse educator is observing a learner administer an intravenous medication. When is the best time to provide feedback?
A. At the end of the scheduled clinical experience
B. During the medication administration process
C. During the weekly scheduled meeting with the learner
D. Immediately after completion of the medication administration

Correct Answer: D

Rationale: Feedback related to psychomotor skills and procedures should occur promptly following the task, as in Option D. Providing prompt feedback is essential for skill performance improvement. As time passes, the learner or clinical nurse educator may not remember specific areas of clinical skill practice that require improvement (Gaberson et al., 2015, p. 326). At the conclusion of the clinical experience, Option A, and during a weekly review, Option C, involve too great of a time lapse between the skill and feedback. Although providing feedback during a skill, as in Option B, may be needed at times for safety reasons, it is not the best time to deliver feedback. It is not clear that a safety concern exists in this scenario, making it incorrect. Delivering feedback during a skill for reasons other than ensuring safety can be distracting and compromise confidence. Delivering feedback should most often be delayed until after a skill is completed.

Test Blueprint: 6 E
Cognitive Code: Application

31. Which feedback statement would be most beneficial for learners?
A. "You need to go to the skills lab for more practice."
B. "You need to work on calculation of IV drip rates."
C. "You need to reread the chapter on neurology."
D. "You need to practice your physical assessment skills."

Correct Answer: B

Rationale: Option B provides specific feedback that can guide performance and represents an important component of effective feedback (Oermann et al., 2018b, p. 259). Options A, C, and D are general statements that do not provide specific information.

Test Blueprint: 6 E
Cognitive Code: Analysis

32. When would feedback be most effective?
    A. Immediately after skill performance
    B. At the end of the clinical day
    C. At the end of the experience
    D. At the midpoint of the semester

    Correct Answer: A

    Rationale: Option A represents the best time to give feedback, that is, in that moment or shortly after (Oermann et al., 2018b, p. 259). The more time that passes between the performance and the feedback, the less useful it will be (Oermann et al., 2018b, p. 259). Options B, C, and D offer delayed feedback and do not best assist in development.

    Test Blueprint: 6 E
    Cognitive Code: Application

33. The clinical nurse educator identifies performance issues and deficiencies that may influence a learner passing the course. Which initial step is best?
    A. Discuss the issue with other educators teaching in the course.
    B. Hold a conference with the learner and create a remediation plan.
    C. Note the issue on the learner's evaluation form.
    D. Place a note in the learner's academic file.

    Correct Answer: B

    Rationale: Since there are areas of concern that may influence passing the course, the clinical nurse educator should hold a conference to discuss issues and develop a remediation plan, as in Option B (Oermann et al., 2018b, p. 282). It is not appropriate to discuss performance issues with others, especially if they do not have a legitimate educational interest, as in Option A. Though noting performance issues on the evaluation form, Option C, or in the learner's academic record, Option D, may be appropriate, they are not the best initial actions.

    Test Blueprint: 6 E
    Cognitive Code: Application

34. The clinical nurse educator is reviewing a draft of a written assignment. Which statement represents the most appropriate feedback?
    A. "Your writing is a little vague—dig deeper and provide more supportive details."
    B. "In this assignment, you did not describe the client's presenting problem."
    C. "Explain the problem of increased falls and use supporting data when revising your paper."
    D. "You have grammatical errors throughout your paper. Please visit the writing center for help."

    Correct Answer: C

Rationale: Option C offers the best feedback because it identifies the problem areas and makes specific suggestions about changes that are needed (Oermann et al., 2018b, p. 248). General statements such as those in Options A, B, and D do not help learners understand the problems with their work or what needs to be altered (Oermann et al., 2018b, p. 248).

Test Blueprint: 6 E
Cognitive Code: Application

35. Which represents the best time to provide performance feedback?
    A. During post-conference so that the entire clinical group can benefit
    B. After the learner has had sufficient time to independently reflect on the activity
    C. Immediately after the activity has been observed
    D. After the clinical nurse educator has had time to write an anecdotal note

Correct Answer: C

Rationale: One of the principles that makes feedback the most beneficial is to provide it immediately after a learning activity, as in Option C. Prompt feedback helps maintain effectiveness. If immediate feedback cannot be given, the clinical nurse educator should write a note to remember the details (Gubrud, 2016, p. 289; Oermann & Gaberson, 2017, p. 221). Option A does not provide privacy. Option B is incorrect because the learner may forget details about performance if there is a delay in feedback. Option D is incorrect because a note should be written after the feedback to include learner response and plans for improvement.

Test Blueprint: 6 E
Cognitive Code: Analysis

36. Which statement likely represents a clinical nurse educator who strives to maintain objectivity when providing feedback?
    A. "Your head-to-toe assessment was not thorough. You forgot a few systems."
    B. "You need to auscultate all four quadrants of the abdomen, not two, when doing assessments."
    C. "You are showing improvement and building confidence when auscultating lung sounds."
    D. "You did a good job performing a bedside assessment on your client."

Correct Answer: B

Rationale: Though clinical evaluation is subjective (Oermann & Gaberson, 2017, p. 216), providing objective feedback is critical for learners to understand how they can improve their performance; it is not enough to say that the learner did a good or bad job. The clinical nurse educator should instead use precise, specific feedback. Specific, direct feedback providing insight for observed performance and ways to improve are more valuable to the learner, as in Option B (Gubrud, 2016, p. 289; Oermann & Gaberson, 2017, p. 221; Robb & Shellenbarger, 2018). Options A, C, and D are incorrect because they do not provide specific feedback, nor do they offer suggestions for improvement.

Test Blueprint: 6 E
Cognitive Code: Application

37. Which question or statement would best encourage learner self-reflection?
A. "Why don't you feel comfortable giving injections? You practiced in the lab."
B. "I noticed you were hesitant about giving the medication. Can you tell me about that?"
C. "You don't have sufficient knowledge of the actions of beta-blockers; look that up."
D. "I am concerned about the timeliness of your medication administration."

Correct Answer: B

Rationale: Approaching feedback with a sense of curiosity will help the clinical nurse educator better understand the learner's concerns and will encourage self-reflection. Posing the observed behavior or concern in a question rather than a statement can open a dialogue and create an opportunity for learning; talking about it can help identify the steps to take to progress, as in Option B (Robb & Shellenbarger, 2018, p. 13). Options A, C, and D are accusatory and do not pose a question or statement that would open dialogue with the learner.

Test Blueprint: 6 E
Cognitive Code: Analysis

38. A clinical nurse educator is observing a learner perform a dressing change at the bedside. The learner correctly performs the dressing change but does not communicate with the client during the dressing change. Which action best reflects delivering effective feedback?
A. Emailing general feedback at the end of the clinical day
B. Discussing the lack of communication immediately after the dressing change
C. Providing face-to-face, private feedback mixing both positive and negative feedback
D. Telling the learner to communicate more effectively during the dressing change

Correct Answer: C

Rationale: Important considerations are needed when giving learners feedback, including specificity, timing, consistency, continuity, and approach (Gubrud, 2016, p. 289). Positive aspects should be pointed out as well as areas that need improvement, as in Option C. Clinical nurse educators need to recognize which feedback should be given immediately and which can be slightly delayed. In this case, feedback can be slightly delayed, rather than providing feedback directly after the encounter. Option A is incorrect because it suggests providing feedback later via email instead of face-to-face immediately. Option B allows for immediate feedback but it does not highlight positive aspects of performance. Feedback is provided in front of the client in Option D, which is not appropriate.

Test Blueprint: 6 E
Cognitive Code: Application

39. Which practice best supports the goal of evaluating learners fairly?
A. Developing a supportive learning climate
B. Providing negative feedback
C. Setting clear and high expectations
D. Tailoring evaluation strategies to each learner

Correct Answer: A

Rationale: Option A is an important aspect of a fair clinical evaluation system (Oermann & Gaberson, 2017). Learners who are comfortable and feel supported by their educators will value feedback as tools to help them improve (Oermann & Gaberson, 2017). Option B is not the best way to ensure that learners are evaluated fairly; mixing feedback types is important (Patrick, 2019). Option C is not the best response because, although it is important to set clear expectations for performance, setting expectations too high may intimidate learners and not create the supportive learning climate needed for fair evaluation (Oermann & Gaberson, 2017). Option D is not appropriate because educators should use the same evaluation methods for all learners. Notably, using a mix of evaluation methods per clinical competency and/or course outcome is important but should be implemented for all learners (Oermann & Gaberson, 2017).

Test Blueprint: 6 E
Cognitive Code: Analysis

40. Which statement or question provides the most helpful feedback?
   A. "It seems you are having a difficult time organizing your day. What suggestions do you have for improving your time management?"
   B. "We have been here for two hours and the client assessment has not been completed. I am concerned that you are not organizing your time well."
   C. "You need to work on your time management. It looks like you are not ready to give your nine o'clock medications."
   D. "You do realize that we have been on the unit for two hours and you have not completed your client assessment yet?"

Correct Answer: B

Rationale: It is helpful for the learner to receive specific examples of behaviors that do not meet the learning outcomes. Options A and C do not provide a specific example of why the clinical nurse educator is concerned. Option D identifies a specific behavior but does not connect the behavior with a learning outcome and the tone might be considered nonsupportive (DeYoung, 2015, p. 218). Option B provides the most helpful feedback by identifying a specific behavior that is concerning.

Test Blueprint: 6 E
Cognitive Code: Analysis

41. Which feedback approach is most appropriate regarding psychomotor skill performance?
   A. Immediately explain where the error was made, demonstrate the correct skill, and allow the learner to practice.
   B. Avoid discussing the error in front of the client and plan to outline areas for improvement in the learner's weekly written feedback.
   C. Discuss the error with the other learners during postclinical conference to prevent them from making the same error.
   D. Prohibit the learner from performing all psychomotor nursing skills for the remainder of the clinical day.

Correct Answer: A

Rationale: When evaluating psychomotor skills, the clinical nurse educator should provide both verbal and visual feedback to learners, explaining first where errors were made in performance and then demonstrating the correct procedure or skill (Oermann & Gaberson, 2017). Options B and C are incorrect because clinical evaluation feedback should be given promptly in a private setting at the time of performance or immediately following (Oermann & Gaberson, 2017). Option D is an inappropriate and unnecessary action that punishes the learner and does not facilitate learning.

Test Blueprint: 6 E
Cognitive Code: Application

42. A new clinical nurse educator is discussing clinical evaluations with a more experienced clinical nurse educator. Which statement by the newer educator likely requires follow-up?
    A. "I will include input from the unit nurse to provide additional evaluation information."
    B. "I will provide general information about each learner's behavior and clinical performance."
    C. "I need to identify beliefs and biases that may influence how I complete my learner evaluations."
    D. "I will complete the learner evaluations using predetermined outcomes and competencies."

Correct Answer: B

Rationale: Feedback should be precise and specific. General information, such as "you need more practice," does not indicate which behaviors need improvement or how to develop them (Oermann & Gaberson, 2009, p. 256). Options A, C, and D are correct statements regarding the completion of clinical evaluations that do not require follow-up.

Test Blueprint: 6 E
Cognitive Code: Application

43. A learner struggled to administer medications to a client. Which response best demonstrates thoughtful and constructive feedback?
    A. "You did okay administering the medications but there are some opportunities for improvement."
    B. "How do you feel you did administering the medications?"
    C. "You didn't check the client's identification by asking name and date of birth."
    D. "You had issues related to safety when administering the medications."

Correct Answer: C

Rationale: The clinical nurse educator should provide timely and constructive feedback to learners. Option C provides the most specific feedback by explaining exactly what the learner did incorrectly (Oermann et al., 2018b). Options A and D do not provide specific information that would guide learner development; only general information is provided. Option B does not provide feedback and asks only for the learner to self-reflect on performance.

Test Blueprint: 6 E
Cognitive Code: Analysis

44. Which feedback example would be most effective for a learner to gauge performance?
   A. "You are doing a great job! Keep up the good work. It is great to have you in this clinical group!"
   B. "Good job turning in your assignment on time. Keep doing what you are doing."
   C. "I was impressed with how you spent time answering the client's questions and offered them educational materials on their new medications."
   D. "I think that you are doing just fine in the clinical environment, especially with your documentation."

Correct Answer: C

Rationale: Feedback allows for a learner to reflect on performance and strive to make changes moving forward. Option C offers clear, concise feedback on the performance of the learner. The clinical nurse educator should present specific details when offering feedback to the learner (Horner, 2018). Options A, B, and D do not provide specific information to guide the learner.

Test Blueprint: 6 E
Cognitive Code: Application

45. Which feedback method is most appropriate?
   A. Implementation of standard evaluation phrases such as "lacks depth of content"
   B. Documentation and communication of feedback through written evaluation methods
   C. Provision of feedback with others present who can serve as witnesses in case issues arise later
   D. Provision of specific feedback that occurs at the time of the experience or shortly thereafter

Correct Answer: D

Rationale: Prompt feedback helps the educator summarize the extent of learning achieved in the course and targets specific outcomes or objectives that are met or unmet (Oermann & Gaberson, 2017, pp. 285–286). Option D ensures that feedback is given as close to real time as possible so that the time between performance and feedback is lessened; prompt feedback helps learners recall specifics of their performance that need to be modified (Oermann & Gaberson, 2017, p. 286). Option A does not provide specific, detailed feedback that can assist learning and improvement. While written documentation can be helpful, Option B does not provide details about the nature or quality of the feedback. Feedback should be delivered in a private setting, making Option C incorrect.

Test Blueprint: 6 E
Cognitive Code: Application

46. A clinical nurse educator is conducting skill validations in a lab environment. Upon receiving an unsatisfactory score, a learner pleads with the clinical nurse educator to allow one further attempt at the skill. The learner begins to cry and angrily packs up personal belongings. Which is the best response?

A. "Take a deep breath. Tell me what's going on outside the classroom that may be affecting your clinical performance."

B. "It's going to be okay. One unsatisfactory score on a validation isn't going to end your nursing career."

C. "I can't allow you another attempt at the skill right now. That would be unfair to the rest of the class."

D. "I understand you may be upset; however, this is inappropriate behavior. Let's set up an appointment to discuss your skill validation after you have had some time to regroup."

Correct Answer: D

Rationale: One aspect of the clinical nurse educator role is to assist learners in giving and receiving constructive feedback in a safe and professional learning environment. Opportunities to dialogue about mistakes must be available to the learner immediately after a mistake is made, and again later after the learner has had more time to process what happened, as suggested in Option D (Roberts, 2005). However, the learner will not be receptive to feedback during a heightened emotional state; therefore, the clinical nurse educator must call attention to the inappropriate behavior and work to diffuse the situation. Making an assumption about the learner's personal matters, as in Option A, may come across as invasive, too personal, and can disrupt the trusting environment. Learners are often unaware of how their behaviors are perceived; in a trusting environment in which learners' professional development is a priority, clinical nurse educators have a responsibility to provide concrete and specific feedback regarding behaviors that may impede progress (Luparell & Conner, 2016; Whitney & Luparell, 2012). Downplaying the validation score, Option B, offers false assurance and does not promote an opportunity to develop professional resilience associated with receiving constructive feedback. Allowing a repeat attempt at the skill validation, Option C, is unfair to the other learners who don't get a repeat attempt and it doesn't address the learner's emotional response.

Test Blueprint: 6 E
Cognitive Code: Analysis

47. A clinical nurse educator observes a learner administering medications inefficiently. Which is the best approach to provide feedback to this learner?

A. Offer guidance and suggestions while in the client's room to accelerate medication administration and reinforce positive change throughout the shift.

B. Speak to the learner at postclinical conference about the learner's proficiency with medication administration.

C. Immediately after leaving the client's room, discuss with the learner in a private location specific ways to improve medication administration.

D. Talk with the learner after completing medication administration about being more prepared for routine tasks.

Correct Answer: C

Rationale: Feedback should be specific, timely, and consistent (Gubrud, 2016, p. 289). Option C, engaging the learner outside of the client's room in a private location and discussing ways to improve, is timely, specific, and appropriate. Having this discussion outside the client's room allows the clinical nurse educator to ensure feedback is given one-on-one and in a private setting, thereby being sensitive to the learner. Accelerating medication administration through assistance, Option A, is not appropriate, as it can interfere with learner development. Option B is incorrect because speaking with the learner at postclinical conference is not timely. Providing general recommendations for improvement, as suggested in Option D, does not provide specific feedback that will help the learner improve.

Test Blueprint: 6 E
Cognitive Code: Analysis

48. The clinical nurse educator is providing feedback to a learner. Which statement is most appropriate?
A. "You did a great job completing wound care. I look forward to evaluating your abilities each time I have the opportunity to do so."
B. "You were able to dress the wound appropriately. In the future, consider the client's pain level before starting wound care."
C. "I am not sure I would have completed wound care in that fashion, but good job completing the task."
D. "It is clear to me that you did not adequately prepare for this skill. I suggest you go back to simulation to practice."

Correct Answer: B

Rationale: There are five principles to providing feedback as part of clinical evaluation; feedback should be precise and specific, be both verbal and visual, be timely, have a varying amount of feedback and positive reinforcement, and be diagnostic (Oermann & Gaberson, 2017, p. 221). Option B is positive, specific, and diagnostic. Without offering recommendations for improvement, the clinical nurse educator omits a valuable aspect of feedback, as found in Option A. Remarks that are indifferent, such as Option C, do not guide the learner. Option D, which contains negative feedback with nonspecific guidance, is also not appropriate.

Test Blueprint: 6 E
Cognitive Code: Application

49. After observing a registered nurse (RN) loudly berating a nursing assistant (NA) when discussing expected performance, the learner approaches the clinical nurse educator to discuss this situation. Which is the best response?
A. "Lateral violence unfortunately occurs between staff members. Tell me how you feel about what you just witnessed."
B. "This happens all the time. I am sure the staff is used to this by now."
C. "Understand that lateral violence behaviors, such as raising your voice to a colleague, are not okay but are a reality in today's workplace."
D. "It is unacceptable to raise your voice to a colleague in the workplace. Management is aware and is taking action to correct the problem."

Correct Answer: A

Rationale: Lateral or horizontal violence behaviors, such as raising one's voice, are often observed and witnessed by learners. When observed or witnessed, the clinical nurse educator has the opportunity to help learners understand what is occurring and soften, but not deny, the existence of violence in the nursing workplace (Gubrud, 2016, p. 284). Confirming the reality of lateral violence while probing for more information from the learner to support understanding, as in Option A, is appropriate. Statements such as Options B, C, and D that do not provide an understanding of lateral violence, that do not seek to gain input from the learner's perspective on lateral violence, or that do not offer a viable response to the problem are not appropriate.

Test Blueprint: 6 F
Cognitive Code: Analysis

50. Upon reviewing a learner's midpoint self-evaluation, the clinical nurse educator discovers that the learner lacks confidence with clinical skills. Which is the best action to take?
A. Wait for the learner to mature and gain confidence, as this is a normal part of the clinical learning experience.
B. Continue to monitor the learner and intervene if the learner starts to not achieve learning outcomes.
C. Request an appointment with the learner to discuss strategies to overcome barriers to confidence with clinical skills.
D. Reevaluate learner confidence through another self-evaluation at the conclusion of an additional clinical shift.

Correct Answer: C

Rationale: The ability to critically reflect influences the individual performance of the learner (Bonnel, 2016, p. 454). Option C involves building a learner-educator relationship and supporting reflective abilities, which is indicated in this scenario. Option A, not intervening, neglects an opportunity for the clinical nurse educator to better support the learner. Similarly, Option B, continuing to monitor, is passive when action is indicated at this point in time. Reevaluating through another self-reflection, Option D, does not help correct the apparent problem in a timely manner.

Test Blueprint: 6 F
Cognitive Code: Application

51. A learner is having difficulty preparing for a sterile dressing change and states, "I just can't do this anymore." Which response is most appropriate?
A. "I understand your frustration, but you have completed this skill before."
B. "Let me finish the procedure and we can talk after we leave the room."
C. "I will help you get started by walking you through the first steps."
D. "Come back in the room in 15 minutes after you review the procedure."

Correct Answer: C

Rationale: Developing a supportive learning environment facilitates learning (Oermann & Gaberson, 2017, p. 219). Option C is supportive and fosters learner development. Option A, acknowledging feelings without offering additional support, is insufficient in this scenario. Taking control of the situation, as suggested in Option B, does not promote learning. Having the learner leave the room and revisit the skill independently, Option D, is isolative and not supportive.

Test Blueprint: 6 F
Cognitive Code: Analysis

52. At the beginning of a clinical experience, learners exhibit signs of being fearful of negative comments. Which action helps create a supportive learning environment best?
    A. Limiting feedback to summative evaluations
    B. Approaching each learner in a neutral tone
    C. Exhibiting leniency with evaluations
    D. Establishing trust at the initial meeting

Correct Answer: D

Rationale: Establishing trust is integral to developing a supportive learning environment (Oermann & Gaberson, 2017, p. 219), as suggested in Option D. Feedback should not be limited to summative evaluations, Option A. Approaching learners with a neutral tone may be off-putting to some learners, making Option B incorrect; a positive tone is often indicated. Leniency in evaluations undermines learner achievement of clinical outcomes, making Option C incorrect.

Test Blueprint: 6 F
Cognitive Code: Application

53. Which time period would best help a clinical nurse educator assess learner progress and determine future teaching-learning needs?
    A. During calculations of learners' theory grades
    B. During classroom discussions about client care problems
    C. During a feedback session after a skill performance in the learning lab
    D. During postclinical conference where learners debrief about their day

Correct Answer: D

Rationale: Postclinical conferences are a time when learners can debrief about their clinical day and discuss their client-care experiences, as in Option D. This allows learners to discuss concerns or uncertainties about their performance, enabling the clinical nurse educator to ask further questions and to plan and design future learning experiences (Gubrud, 2016, pp. 295, 444; Kan & Stabler-Haas, 2018, p. 118). Options A and B do not directly relate to learner needs for teaching-learning strategies in the clinical setting. Option C allows for sharing of feedback but does not provide insight from the learners' perspective about their needs.

Test Blueprint: 6 F
Cognitive Code: Analysis

54. After evaluating a learner in the simulation laboratory, a clinical nurse educator notes that the learner has difficulty performing a focused head-to-toe assessment. When developing a learning plan, which it essential to include?
A. Learning and remedial activities involving client assessment
B. A referral to the academic counselor for study skills
C. A copy of the policy for standards of safe practice
D. Preparation guidelines for the simulation laboratory

Correct Answer: A

Rationale: When developing a learning plan, it is essential to include specific learning and remedial activities that may assist a learner in the achievement of the clinical outcome—in this case, assessment skills—as in Option A (Gaberson et al., 2015, p. 357). Option B, a referral to the academic counselor for study skills, would not be indicated for psychomotor skills. Options C and D are not necessarily important to include in a performance improvement plan in which a learner is having difficulty with assessment skills.

Test Blueprint: 6 F
Cognitive Code: Application

55. Which activity is most appropriate to evaluate skill competence?
A. Case study
B. Gaming
C. High-fidelity simulation
D. Return demonstration

Correct Answer: D

Rationale: Observation of a return demonstration is the most effective way to evaluate skill sets and provide structured feedback, as in Option D. While high-fidelity simulation often includes skills, as in Option C, this activity is best used for analysis of clinical scenarios and clinical judgment (Gaberson et al., 2015, pp. 329–344). Case studies and gaming, suggested in Options A and B, are not effective for evaluating skill acquisition and may be more appropriate for evaluating cognitive knowledge.

Test Blueprint: 6 G
Cognitive Code: Application

56. During an Objective Structured Clinical Examination (OSCE), the learner continues to ask the clinical nurse educator questions related to the scenario. Which is the best response?
A. Tell the learner that questions may be asked after the examination is complete.
B. Allow the learner to take a break to ask questions during the examination and then resume.
C. Review the expectations and learning outcomes with the learner.
D. Inform the learner that continuing to ask questions will result in a failing grade.

Correct Answer: C

Rationale: During an OSCE, learners may be asked to demonstrate skill performance in a simulated environment for a grade or competency. It is essential that learners understand the purpose of the activity and outcomes

(Gaberson et al., 2015, p. 347). Learners may often exhibit anxiety during high-stress evaluation situations. It is important to redirect the learners' focus to the expectations and outcomes of the scenarios. Options A, B, and D are inappropriate in an OSCE situation.

Test Blueprint: 6 G
Cognitive Code: Analysis

57. During a summative evaluation, the clinical nurse educator assigned a failing grade to a learner because of consistent unsafe performance. The learner responds by stating, "This is unfair, you treated the other learners as your favorites and did not help me." Which initial action is most appropriate?
   A. Allow the learner to state the case and reconsider the grade.
   B. Reiterate specific findings that led to failure to meet learning outcomes.
   C. Provide the learner with a copy of the grievance policy.
   D. Refer the learner to the program dean or director.

Correct Answer: B

Rationale: The failing learner may react in a variety of ways; it is important for the clinical nurse educator to redirect the learner's attention and promote understanding of specific instances of poor performance in relation to learning outcomes (Bonnel, 2012, p. 499), thus supporting Option B as the correct response. Allowing the learner to bargain about the evaluation, as suggested in Option A, should not occur, as the grading decision has already been made. Options C and D should occur after discussing findings with the learner and thus do not represent the most appropriate initial actions.

Test Blueprint: 6 G
Cognitive Code: Application

58. Which is a major difference between undergraduate prelicensure and advanced practice graduate-level Objective Structured Clinical Examinations (OSCEs)?
   A. OSCEs are used for evaluation of communication skills in prelicensure education, whereas they are used in advanced practice for holistic skill evaluation.
   B. OSCEs are used to evaluate psychomotor skills in prelicensure programs and affective skills in advanced practice.
   C. OSCEs assess knowledge in prelicensure programs and application in advanced-practice programs
   D. OSCEs are a formative evaluation measure in prelicensure programs and are a summative evaluation measure in advanced practice.

Correct Answer: D

Rationale: In OSCEs, learners respond to client scenarios to demonstrate cognitive and psychomotor skills. OSCEs are primarily formative for prelicensure learners and summative for advanced-practice learners (Bonnel, 2016, p. 453; DeYoung, 2015, pp. 216–217). OSCEs can be used for a variety of skills in any level of education, making Options A and B incorrect. OSCEs can be used to assess knowledge and application at any level of education, making Option C incorrect.

Test Blueprint: 6 G
Cognitive Code: Analysis

59. Which is most important to consider when determining clinical assignments?
   A. The assignment is a repetitive measure of outcomes already met.
   B. The purpose of the assignment is clear to learners.
   C. The assignment allows for summative evaluation.
   D. The assignment helps learners meet course outcomes.

Correct Answer: D

Rationale: Assessment and evaluation in the clinical setting should be done with carefully selected assignments; assignments should always be designed to meet course objectives or outcomes, as in Option D. Though timing and other logistical concerns are important when planning assignments, the most important factor is choosing assignments that help learners attain the course outcomes (Bonnel, 2016, p. 456; Oermann & Gaberson, 2017, p. 229). Options A, B, and C are components to consider but they are not the most important considerations.

Test Blueprint: 6 G
Cognitive Code: Analysis

60. Which statement made by an inexperienced clinical nurse educator warrants clarification?
   A. "I will make sure to define the knowledge and skills learners are expected to demonstrate at the beginning of the clinical experience."
   B. "I will point out both strengths and areas for improvement when providing feedback to learners."
   C. "I will focus primarily on the learner's ability to perform skills safely and effectively in my evaluation."
   D. "I will document learner behavior over time to determine if patterns are present."

Correct Answer: C

Rationale: Multidimensional evaluation is most appropriate in the clinical environment (Bonnel, 2016, p. 444). Although providing safe and effective care is integral to clinical experiences, Option C does not support using a variety of strategies to determine achievement of learning outcomes and thus warrants clarification. Option A, providing clear expectations, is appropriate to guide learners. Pointing out strengths and areas for improvement in feedback is appropriate, as suggested in Option B. Option D, documenting over time, is appropriate for identification of patterns.

Test Blueprint: 6 G
Cognitive Code: Analysis

61. A clinical nurse educator has been asked to evaluate learners using a criterion-referenced approach. Which statement shows that the educator is using this approach?
   A. "I will provide feedback to learners throughout the term via weekly documented notes."
   B. "I will use a check sheet with competencies to indicate learner performance."
   C. "I will compare learner performance to other learners in the group for evaluation purposes."
   D. "After the experience, I will create a tool that I can use to rate learner performance."

Correct Answer: B

Rationale: Criterion-referenced clinical evaluation involves comparing clinical performance with predetermined criteria (Oermann & Gaberson, 2017, p. 217). A check sheet with competencies, as provided in Option B, could be a tool used in criterion-referenced evaluation. Providing feedback through documented notes, Option A, describes formative feedback that may not be criterion-referenced. Option C, comparing learner performance to other learners, is norm-referenced. Criterion-referenced tools are created in advance; they are not created after the performance, as suggested in Option D.

Test Blueprint: 6 G
Cognitive Code: Recall

62. How should the clinical nurse educator best ensure fair evaluation of learner performance?
    A. Using learning outcomes as a guideline for evaluation of clinical performance
    B. Avoiding giving a critique about a learner's clinical performance until after several clinical days
    C. Meeting with the course educator to review the past performance of each learner
    D. Seeking feedback from the unit nurse before confronting the learner about performance issues

Correct Answer: A

Rationale: Focusing on learning outcomes when evaluating learner performance may decrease the influence of personal values and biases when evaluating performance (Oermann et al., 2018b, p. 257), as in Option A. Learners should be given feedback as often as possible so that they will not be surprised about their performance and have adequate time to adjust the behaviors, making Option B incorrect. Obtaining information about a learner's past performance, as in Option C, may create an unfair bias. Although the nurse's input may be helpful, obtaining this type of feedback is not always required, making Option D incorrect.

Test Blueprint: 6 G
Cognitive Code: Application

63. Which statement made by a clinical nurse educator colleague would likely warrant correction and/or further clarification?
    A. "I am going to speak to a learner next week about the clinical performance."
    B. "I had midterm meetings with each learner to discuss their performance."
    C. "I spoke to a learner privately about cellphone use during the clinical day."
    D. "I use the same clinical evaluation tool to appraise learner performance."

Correct Answer: A

Rationale: Option A needs correction and/or further clarification because the nurse educator is not providing timely feedback to the learner (Patrick, 2019); in other words, why is the educator waiting until next week to speak to the learner? It is important to provide feedback as close to an event as possible and to allow time for improvement (Oermann & Gaberson, 2017). Options B and D are appropriate because the educator appears to be acting fairly and with integrity. Option C is an appropriate way to provide feedback, that is, privately.

Test Blueprint: 6 G
Cognitive Code: Analysis

64. Which evaluation strategy is likely concerning?
    A. Completing checklists during skill performances
    B. Documenting anecdotal notes
    C. Providing graded feedback only
    D. Using a variety of evaluation methods

Correct Answer: C

Rationale: Option C is concerning because nurse educators should provide formative nongraded feedback as well as summative graded evaluations (Oermann & Gaberson, 2017; Patrick, 2019). Options A, B, and D are all appropriate evaluation strategies and do not raise any direct concerns (Oermann & Gaberson, 2017; Patrick, 2019).

Test Blueprint: 6 G
Cognitive Code: Analysis

65. Which is the best way to strengthen the validity of a simulation scenario?
    A. Use subject matter clinical experts to review the scenario and provide feedback.
    B. Ask the learners what actions would be best in the scenario.
    C. Consult with another simulation clinical nurse educator who can help write the scenario.
    D. Design a scenario that mimics a clinical experience that resulted in a poor client outcome.

Correct Answer: A

Rationale: Option A is correct because subject matter clinical experts will provide the best clinical experiential knowledge for simulation validity (Gaberson et al., 2015; International Nursing Association for Clinical Simulation and Learning Standards Committee, 2016). Options B and D do not use the best clinical knowledge and, even though Option C involves consultation with others, it is unclear whether the simulation educator is an expert in scenario design.

Test Blueprint: 6 G
Cognitive Code: Application

66. A clinical nurse educator is concerned that there may be other issues affecting the performance of a learner who is in danger of course failure. Which is the best action?
    A. Refer the learner to counseling and other support services.
    B. Practice visualization with the learner.
    C. Advise the learner to take a leave of absence.
    D. Discuss coping skills that can be used to deal with personal problems.

Correct Answer: A

Rationale: The clinical nurse educator should refer learners to counseling and other support services if they feel there are other issues affecting performance, as suggested in Option A (Oermann et al., 2018b, p. 282). Clinical nurse educators should not advise the learner to take a leave of absence without investigating circumstances further, as in Option C, as this is a major decision that involves multiple factors. The learner should be referred to an academic adviser for assistance with such decisions. The clinical nurse educator should not assume the role of counselor and offer interventions, as suggested in Options B and D.

Test Blueprint: 6 G
Cognitive Code: Application

67. Which is the best strategy when observing clinical performance?
    A. Make a minimum number of observations for all learners.
    B. Observe and document performance of only the learners at risk for failure.
    C. Focus on observing specific skills for each clinical day.
    D. Observe invasive procedures only for learners who have already demonstrated safe care.

Correct Answer: A

Rationale: The clinical nurse educator should complete a minimum number of observations and document findings for all learners regardless of level of performance, as suggested in Option A (Oermann et al., 2018b, p. 283). The clinical nurse educator should not evaluate and document performance on only the poor or at-risk learners, as suggested in Option B, as this treats learners differently (Oermann et al., 2018b, p. 283). The clinical nurse educator should not pick specific skills to observe, as suggested in Options C and D, but rather should use the course objectives and program policies to guide observations.

Test Blueprint: 6 G
Cognitive Code: Application

68. Which question would best help evaluate basic understanding of concepts?
    A. "What information would you use to prioritize client care?"
    B. "What data did you use to evaluate the client's condition?"
    C. "What is the most important client finding?"
    D. "How would you define hyperglycemia?"

Correct Answer: D

Rationale: Option D represents a low-level thinking question that can be used in the clinical setting to help build learners' confidence (Oermann, De Gagne, & Phillips, 2018a, p. 194). Asking lower-level questions will help evaluate whether learners have a basic understanding of concepts. Options A, B, and C are incorrect because they are higher-level thinking questions; though these options should also be used in clinical settings, they are not best to evaluate basic understanding of concepts.

Test Blueprint: 6 H
Cognitive Code: Application

69. Which clinical outcome is written most effectively?
   A. Collaborates appropriately with the interprofessional health care team.
   B. Communicates effectively with family members and includes them in client care.
   C. Uses the nursing process in the care of clients with mental illness.
   D. Provides an organized shift change report and makes care recommendations.

Correct Answer: D

Rationale: Option D provides the most specific clinical outcome (Oermann et al., 2018b, p. 260). Vague outcomes such as "collaborates appropriately," as in Option A, "communicates effectively," as in Option B, and "uses the nursing process," as in Option C, are open to interpretation and are not clear.

Test Blueprint: 6 H
Cognitive Code: Analysis

70. Which question helps develop higher-level thinking skills best?
   A. "What would you suggest we do next for the client?"
   B. "How would you identify whether your client was hypoglycemic?"
   C. "What do you remember about myocardial infarctions?"
   D. "What happens when you administer furosemide (Lasix)?"

Correct Answer: A

Rationale: Higher-level questions, such as Option A, require the learner to consider the client situation and make judgments about care, stimulating a deeper understanding of the information (Oermann et al., 2018a, p. 194). Asking higher-level questions will help the clinical nurse educator evaluate whether the learner is able to critically think about the concepts. Options B, C, and D are all lower-level thinking questions because they involve knowledge and comprehension.

Test Blueprint: 6 H
Cognitive Code: Application

71. The clinical nurse educator is choosing a written assignment for a clinical course. Which is the most appropriate initial consideration?
   A. The expected course outcomes and competencies
   B. The writing experience and other abilities of learners
   C. The time needed to grade the assignment
   D. The writing support available on campus

Correct Answer: A

Rationale: As suggested in Option A, clinical nurse educators should consider outcomes and competencies that learners need to achieve in a course before choosing a written assignment (Oermann et al., 2018b, p. 235). Although other factors such as writing experience and other abilities, Option B, time for grading, Option C, and available supports, Option D, might influence the decision, the first consideration should be related to outcomes and competencies.

Test Blueprint: 6 H
Cognitive Code: Application

72. Which learner action best indicates clinical reasoning abilities?
   A. Making a detailed list of every medication the client has taken for the last two weeks
   B. Correctly performing the steps to insert an indwelling urinary catheter
   C. Communicating with the client and family about upcoming surgery and postoperative care
   D. Anticipating the need to administer antibiotics if a urinary tract infection develops

Correct Answer: D

Rationale: Clinical reasoning is the process of gathering and thinking about client information, analyzing the options, and evaluating alternatives (Gubrud, 2016). Options A, B, and C are important nursing actions, but only Option D demonstrates the learner's ability to identify the details of a clinical situation and what is salient (Benner, Sutphen, Leonard, & Day, 2010).

Test Blueprint: 6 H
Cognitive Code: Analysis

73. A clinical nurse educator is evaluating learners' ability to perform initial physical assessments on clients at midterm. One learner appears very nervous and makes numerous errors with assessment techniques. Which initial action is most appropriate?
   A. Inform the learner of concerns about lack of skills and give a failing grade.
   B. Assess the learner's needs and assign the learner practice time in the lab prior to reevaluation.
   C. Realize that physical assessment is difficult, and give positive feedback and a passing evaluation.
   D. Call the course coordinator and discuss the need to potentially fail the learner.

Correct Answer: B

Rationale: Clinical nurse educators should allow plentiful learning time with ample opportunity for feedback before summatively evaluating learner performance (Oermann et al., 2018b, p. 8). Offering the learner more time to practice helps learning; therefore, Option B is the correct response. The other options do not contribute to learning and do not assist the learner in enhancing performance before the end of the course.

Test Blueprint: 6 H
Cognitive Code: Application

74. Which type of clinical evaluation compares a learner's clinical performance with the performance of a group of learners, indicating that the learner has more or less clinical competence than other learners?
   A. Criterion-referenced
   B. Norm-referenced
   C. Comparative-referenced
   D. Self-referenced

Correct Answer: B

Rationale: Norm-referenced scores are based on a comparison of learner performance to a group of learners, as in Option B (Oermann & Gaberson, 2017). Option A refers to criterion-referenced and Option D compares learner performance to oneself. Option C does not indicate what is being compared and is incorrect.

Test Blueprint: 6 H
Cognitive Code: Recall

75. Which type of evaluation judges learners' progress in meeting the learning outcomes and developing competencies for practice?
    A. Summative
    B. Feedback
    C. Formative
    D. Course

Correct Answer: C

Rationale: With formative evaluation, Option C, the clinical nurse educator judges learners' progress in meeting learning outcomes (Oermann & Gaberson, 2017). Summative evaluation, Option A, summarizes learner competencies and performance. Feedback, Option B, provides information that can be used to correct performance. Option D is used to assess the course, not the learner.

Test Blueprint: 6 H
Cognitive Code: Recall

76. Which type of evaluation is the end-of-instruction evaluation designed to determine what the learner has accomplished?
    A. Summative
    B. Feedback
    C. Formative
    D. Course

Correct Answer: A

Rationale: Option A summarizes learner competencies and performance and represents summative evaluation (Oermann & Gaberson, 2017). Option B represents formative evaluation. Option C offers information that can be used to correct performance. Option D is used to assess the course, not the learner.

Test Blueprint: 6 H
Cognitive Code: Recall

77. Which is the best example of appropriate use of an assessment tool?
    A. Rubric used to assess safety procedures used in medication administration
    B. Observation used to assess learner's knowledge of nursing care plan development
    C. Multiple-choice exam that assesses ethical decision-making in the clinical setting
    D. Objective Structured Clinical Examination (OSCE) assessing internalization of professionalism

Correct Answer: A

Rationale: During evaluation, it is imperative that the objectives or outcomes can be assessed in a way that allows the nature of the task to be evaluated. Though multiple measures of the same outcome are best, the measurement tool used must accurately measure what it is supposed to be measuring (Bonnel, 2016, p. 444; Oermann & Gaberson, 2017, pp. 227–229; Patrick, 2019, p. 75). Safety during medication administration could be evaluated by a rubric in which the clinical nurse educator can select a level of competency for each step of safe administration. The educator cannot observe learner knowledge, as in Option B, during care plan development. Option C does not allow the educator to easily confirm the display of ethical decision-making on an exam. Option D is incorrect because the clinical nurse educator cannot assess the internalization of professionalism through an OSCE because OSCEs are meant to assess cognitive and psychomotor skills rather than the affective domain.

Test Blueprint: 6 H
Cognitive Code: Analysis

78. Which learning activity would best evaluate the outcome *identifies and prioritizes problems based on relevant data*?
   A. Development of a nursing care plan
   B. Administration of scheduled medications
   C. Participation in client care rounds
   D. Providing client discharge instructions

Correct Answer: A

Rationale: Evaluation of the learner's ability to develop a nursing care plan best assists in the achievement of a clinical outcome that asks the learner to prioritize and reason (Gaberson et al., 2015, p. 297). Options B, C, and D incorporate client problems but are not the best methods to evaluate the learner's ability to prioritize.

Test Blueprint: 6 H
Cognitive Code: Analysis

79. After reviewing a learner's summative evaluation data, the clinical nurse educator has decided to fail the learner because of a consistent pattern of unsatisfactory performance. Prior to meeting with the learner, which action is essential?
   A. Referring to the program's policy and procedure regarding unsafe clinical performance
   B. Asking the learner to complete a self-evaluation of clinical performance
   C. Developing a new learning plan and remediation strategies for improvement
   D. Consulting with the course educator to verify the learner's theory course grade

Correct Answer: A

Rationale: As soon as the decision is made to fail a learner, the clinical nurse educator should refer to program policies regarding safe clinical practice, clinical failure, and progression, as in Option A (Bonnel, 2012, p. 499; Gaberson et al., 2015, p. 359). Policy and procedure will help to guide the clinical nurse educator in decision-making and delivering the information to the learner in a proactive manner. Asking the learner to complete a self-evaluation, Option B, and the development of a new remediation plan, Option C, will not change the outcome of the unsafe practice at the final summative evaluation period. Consultation with the course educator about the theory course grade, as in Option D, is not necessary to determine satisfactory clinical progression.

Test Blueprint: 6 H
Cognitive Code: Application

80. Which describes criterion-referenced evaluation?
    A. A learner's clinical performance is compared to that of another learner.
    B. The learner is evaluated based on predetermined competencies and behaviors.
    C. A learner's clinical performance is rated in relation to the clinical group.
    D. The learner is evaluated only at the end of the clinical experience.

Correct Answer: B

Rationale: Criterion-referenced evaluation involves evaluating a learner compared to predetermined criteria or performance behaviors (Gaberson et al., 2015, p. 323), as in Option B. A comparison of learners to one another or a group is considered norm-referenced evaluation, making Options A and C incorrect. Evaluation at the end of the clinical experience, as in Option D, is considered summative evaluation.

Test Blueprint: 6 I
Cognitive Code: Recall

81. Which is the most important consideration when writing performance standards?
    A. Performance standards must match with the National Council Licensure Examination (NCLEX).
    B. Performance standards must align with previous and subsequent levels in the program.
    C. Performance standards must be measurable.
    D. Performance standards must be clearly explained.

Correct Answer: C

Rationale: Performance standards must be written in a measurable way, as in Option C. Learners should be aware of how they are being evaluated and they must be able to exhibit a performance that can meet the standard. Vague, unmeasurable objectives are useless (DeYoung, 2015, p. 218). Options A, B, and D, though valuable for writing performance standards, are not the most important consideration to ensure that the standards can be used for evaluation.

Test Blueprint: 6 I
Cognitive Code: Application

82. A learner is performing below passing based on a criterion rating scale at midterm. Which action would best address this concern?
  A. Requiring the learner remediate in the skills laboratory
  B. Contacting the course coordinator to request copies of didactic examinations
  C. Discussing concerns with the learner to better understand deficiencies
  D. Requesting that the learner meet with the course coordinator to develop an improvement plan

Correct Answer: C

Rationale: Understanding learners can help align learner needs, interests, and abilities with expected competencies and outcomes (Gubrud, 2016, p. 286). Option C involves engaging in discussion with the learner so that the clinical nurse educator can better understand how to support the learner. Though remediation, Option A, may be helpful, determining the cause of poor progression is most appropriate. Reviewing examination content, Option B, may be helpful but could also not be the primary area of concern for the learner's progression. Meeting with the course coordinator, Option D, defers an intervention by the clinical nurse educator; this step may be necessary in the future, but other options are available that are more appropriate.

Test Blueprint: 6 I
Cognitive Code: Application

83. A clinical nurse educator uses an evaluation tool in the clinical environment but is concerned that the tool does not adequately describe competency. Which initial action is most appropriate?
  A. Use the tool and inform the learner of the score regardless of feelings about the tool.
  B. Score with the tool according to how the clinical nurse educator has always scored the tool but adjust grades as needed.
  C. Use the tool as a baseline for performance but speak with the learner to discern additional strengths and areas for improvement.
  D. Do not use the tool to evaluate since it is not accurate.

Correct Answer: C

Rationale: Deviation in rating scale interpretation can occur after the initial development and agreement on the competencies to be rated and how the scale will be used (Oermann & Gaberson, 2017, p. 238). However, the tools can still be used to gain greater insight into the abilities of the learner. Option C allows for gaining understanding of strengths and areas for improvement of the learner in the midst of this limitation. Limiting evaluation to the tool itself, Option A, does not address the concern. Using the tool the same way it has always been used, Option B, and adjusting scores is not appropriate. A tool should be used with observation of learner performance in the clinical setting, making Option D incorrect.

Test Blueprint: 6 I
Cognitive Code: Analysis

84. Which approach to documenting performance is most appropriate for a clinical nurse educator working with eight learners on a medical-surgical unit?
A. Taking mental notes and writing these notes as time permits
B. Documenting detailed information on an electronic device while observing learners in real time
C. Documenting performance during regularly scheduled breaks during the day
D. Writing notes about significant events concerning performance on notecards throughout the day

Correct Answer: D

Rationale: An efficient method of making brief written or electronic notes should be used by the clinical nurse educator to support feedback (Gubrud, 2016, p. 289). Option D is efficient, as only significant or major notes are recorded; this approach allows for quick notation for reference when evaluating learners. Mental notes, as in Option A, are quick but may not be accurate, as they are not immediately recorded. Given the number of learners in the clinical group, the clinical nurse educator may not have time to record extensive detailed notes, as suggested in Option B; extensive documentation is inefficient and takes time away from working with learners in this clinical group. Also, mandating built-in breaks during the clinical day for documentation purposes, as in Option C, artificially imposes constraints on the educator and hinders the ability to adapt to the ever-changing pace of the clinical environment.

Test Blueprint: 6 J
Cognitive Code: Application

85. A clinical nurse educator is offering feedback to a learner who just completed tracheostomy care. Which statement is most appropriate?
A. "You did a great job explaining the tracheostomy care to the client and you completed the procedure effectively."
B. "It would have been best to start by introducing yourself when entering the room as opposed to right before you began the tracheostomy care."
C. "You can make improvements with tracheostomy care by reviewing this skill in the laboratory environment."
D. "It was great to see that you were able to complete the tracheostomy care effectively, but you can still work to decrease the time spent on the skill."

Correct Answer: D

Rationale: One method for providing feedback includes offering both positive aspects of performance and areas that require improvement (Gubrud, 2016, p. 290), as in Option D. Options A, B, and C either lack positive remarks or lack areas of improvement.

Test Blueprint: 6 J
Cognitive Code: Application

86. A clinical nurse educator is concerned that a learner may not pass the clinical course and holds a conference to discuss performance with the learner. Which best represents the primary goal of this conference?
   A. To discuss perceptions of the learner's intelligence and ability
   B. To develop remedial learning activities to address specific performance problems
   C. To provide instruction about clinical performance deficiencies
   D. To review other factors that could be influencing learner performance

Correct Answer: B

Rationale: A conference should be conducted to discuss learner performance issues and develop a remediation plan for learners who are not meeting performance standards, as suggested in Option B (Oermann et al., 2018b, p. 282). It is inappropriate for the clinical nurse educator to share one's perceptions of the learner's intelligence and ability, as suggested in Option A (Oermann et al., 2018b, p. 282). The conference is not the appropriate time to provide instruction, as suggested in Option C; instead, the conference provides time to focus on the specific issues that need to be addressed (Oermann et al., 2018b, p. 282). The clinical nurse educator can discuss other factors that could be influencing performance, as suggested in Option D, but this is not the primary goal of the conference.

Test Blueprint: 6 J
Cognitive Code: Application

87. A learner completes an inaccurate self-evaluation. Which action would best prepare a clinical nurse educator for a discussion regarding this inaccuracy?
   A. Outlining clear expectations at the beginning of the experience so that the learner is not surprised
   B. Keeping anecdotal notes of the learner's performance, feedback given, and progression
   C. Reviewing the course and clinical objectives with the learner
   D. Comparing the learner's performance with that of other learners in the clinical course

Correct Answer: B

Rationale: Maintaining anecdotal notes on clinical performance, feedback given, and comments on progression is essential because it provides objective evidence as to how the clinical nurse educator evaluated the learner during the clinical experience. Learners need specific, concrete examples of how they have performed. Relying on documentation, rather than memory, will enable the educator to provide specific examples to help the learner understand and to support the grading decisions, as in Option B (Bonnel, 2016, pp. 444, 458; Kan & Stabler-Haas, 2018). Options A and C both help prepare the clinical nurse educator because they deal with the course expectations and objectives, but they do not relate to the learner's performance.

Option D is incorrect because clinical evaluation is typically based on meeting objectives, not comparisons with other learners.

Test Blueprint: 6 J
Cognitive Code: Application

88. A novice clinical nurse educator is completing formative evaluations of learners in the assigned clinical group. Which statement would warrant correction from a mentor?
    A. "I will share my formative evaluation comments with the learners individually."
    B. "I will have the learners sign the evaluation forms following the review."
    C. "I am going to develop a plan for improvement for a learner who is not meeting outcomes."
    D. "I am only going to document about those learners who are not performing well."

Correct Answer: D

Rationale: There should be a minimum number of observations and documentation of all assigned learners, not just those who are not meeting outcomes, as in Option D. Therefore, this statement warrants correction by a mentor. Formative documentation is imperative for all learners to provide feedback and guide learning (Gaberson et al., 2015, p. 358). Options A, B, and C are all appropriate statements and thus do not warrant correction.

Test Blueprint: 6 J
Cognitive Code: Application

89. The clinical nurse educator is completing documentation about a learner who is unsafe during medication administration. Which statement is best to include in the formative evaluation?
    A. "The learner is unsafe with medication administration."
    B. "The learner required significant direction with each step of medication administration."
    C. "The learner was not able to identify the rationale and had difficulty preparing the injection."
    D. "The learner struggles with medication administration and should continue to practice this skill."

Correct Answer: C

Rationale: Formative feedback should be precise and specific for the learner to understand and correct the behavior. Option C provides specific information regarding the unsafe issue that was observed; this is essential not only when documenting poor performance and in establishing a pattern of performance but also for learners to improve based on feedback (Gaberson et al., 2015, p. 359). Options A, B, and D do not provide specific and precise feedback.

Test Blueprint: 6 J
Cognitive Code: Analysis

90. The clinical nurse educator is evaluating a unit as a potential clinical education site. Which finding would likely be a barrier to the achievement of learning outcomes?
   A. The clients on the unit were diagnosed with common clinical problems taught in the course.
   B. The nurse manager and staff nurses are accepting of learners.
   C. The nursing staff rarely engages in evidence-based practice and quality improvement.
   D. The nursing staff is composed of novice nurses with only two to three years of experience.

Correct Answer: C

Rationale: To meet clinical learning outcomes, positive learning environments should be used that are supportive and current with evidence-based practice (Bonnel, 2012, p. 497). Clinical learning environments that do not demonstrate evidence-based practice and promote quality improvement, as in Option C, could lead to unsafe environments and provide a barrier to achievement of learning outcomes. While a nursing staff that is mostly novice, as suggested by Option D, is not ideal, the clinical nurse educator is present to provide direction for learning. Client diagnoses that align with content, Option A, and an accepting nurse manager and staff, Option B, are favorable for learning.

Test Blueprint: 6 K
Cognitive Code: Application

91. When completing an end of the semester site evaluation, which observation would limit the quality of the learning experience most?
   A. High staff turnover rate on the clinical unit
   B. More independent client population with fewer care needs
   C. Many of the same client diagnoses seen throughout the semester
   D. Lack of professionalism in nursing staff on the clinical unit

Correct Answer: D

Rationale: Learners, when properly instructed by the clinical nurse educator, should be able to make any situation into a positive learning experience. The clinical nurse educator should be able to work through and make the most out of the learning experiences offered by Options A, B, and C. Option D, however, might impact the development of professionalism and should be a concern. Although client safety is not an immediate risk, this should be addressed with the coordinator of the course (Kan & Stabler-Haas, 2018, pp. 41–42).

Test Blueprint: 6 K
Cognitive Code: Analysis

92. Two hours into a clinical day, a unit manager approaches the clinical nurse educator and requests that the learners not care for clients due to the presence of an accrediting site visitor on the unit. Which is the best approach in response to this request?

A. Complete case studies off the unit while periodically checking in with the unit manager to see whether the accrediting site visitor is no longer on the unit.

B. Leave the unit and contact the clinical educator department to dispute the request.

C. Cancel the experience for the day to accommodate the request of the unit manager and have learners finish care plans outside of the clinical setting.

D. Refuse to leave the unit, as the agency agreed to have learners on this particular unit and approval had been granted for this day.

Correct Answer: A

Rationale: Clinical nurse educators have the primary responsibility to teach and guide learners in the clinical environment. When barriers arise, the clinical nurse educator must reason effectively and sustain relationships to facilitate learning (Gubrud, 2016, p. 285). Completing work that relates to the clinical experience but occurs off the unit fulfills the unit manager's request and supports the objectives of the clinical experience. Options B and D, contacting the clinical educator department to dispute the request and refusing to leave the unit, do not support relationships between the clinical nurse educator and the clinical site. Canceling the clinical experience, Option C, and completing care plans does support some of the goals of the clinical experience but is not the ideal use of allocated clinical time.

Test Blueprint: 6 K
Cognitive Code: Analysis

93. A clinical nurse educator is evaluating the clinical environment for an assigned rotation. Which finding is most concerning?

A. The unit manager does not respond within 24 hours to email communication on a consistent basis.

B. The clinical staff have not worked with beginning-level learners before.

C. The charge nurse on the unit refuses to allow learners to perform basic nursing skills due to a poor experience with learners from another program.

D. The clinical unit often has low acuity and limited variation in types of clients.

Correct Answer: C

Rationale: Effective communication and relationship building are essential when establishing a supportive and effective learning environment for learners (Gubrud, 2016, p. 285). Overcoming the preconceived ideas of the charge nurse, Option C, needs to be achieved. It is understandable that unit managers are not able to respond within 24 hours via email communication, Option A, based on workload in the clinical environment. The clinical nurse educator can clarify learner expectations with staff, as in Option B; thus, this should not be a concerning finding. Although low acuity and limited varia-tions in clients may not be ideal, as in Option D, these circumstances give learners an opportunity to focus on fundamental skills. Advanced concepts can be introduced through other modalities when low acuity is present.

Test Blueprint: 6 K
Cognitive Code: Application

94. The clinical nurse educator is determining the appropriateness of a health care agency for a clinical learning experience. Which factor is the least impor-tant consideration?
    A. The orientation process for new clinical nurse educators
    B. The culture of the immediate unit's clinical environment
    C. The client population for needed experiences
    D. The health care agency's accreditation status

Correct Answer: A

Rationale: Clinical nurse educators, not the health care agency, have the pri-mary responsibility for teaching and guiding learners in the clinical environ-ment. Clinical nurse educators are responsible for orienting themselves to the practice setting and for building relationships with personnel within the health care agency environment, supporting Option A as the correct response (Stokes & Kost, 2012). The culture of the immediate clinical environment, Option B, affects teaching and learning; for example, staffing levels, work-load, and acuity of clients can influence the time that staff members have to devote to learners (Stokes & Kost, 2012). Assessing the client population for needed experiences, Option C, will ensure that expected course outcomes are met (Stokes & Kost, 2012). Assessing the health care agency's accreditation status, Option D, will ensure that the nursing program's own accreditation standards are met (Stokes & Kost, 2012).

Test Blueprint: 6 K
Cognitive Code: Analysis

95. Which method would help evaluate the quality of the clinical learning expe-rience most?
    A. Clinical evaluation tool
    B. Learner observation
    C. Learner survey
    D. Simulation

Correct Answer: C

Rationale: Option C allows the learner to provide feedback on the clinical learning experience (Patrick, 2019), which can be helpful data for educators evaluating the quality of clinical learning experiences. Options A, B, and D can be useful evaluation methods to assess learner competency and/or course outcomes (Oermann & Gaberson, 2017), but do not usually capture evaluation data regarding the clinical learning experience itself.

Test Blueprint: 6 K
Cognitive Code: Analysis

References

Benner, P., Sutphen, M., Leonard, V., & Day, L. (2010). *Educating nurses: A call for radical transformation.* San Francisco, CA: Jossey-Bass.

Bonnel, W. (2012). Clinical performance evaluation. In D. M. Billings & J. A. Halstead (Eds.), *Teaching in nursing: A guide for faculty* (4th ed., pp. 485–502). St. Louis, MO: Elsevier.

Bonnel, W. (2016). Clinical performance evaluation. In D. M. Billings & J. A. Halstead (Eds.), *Teaching in nursing: A guide for faculty* (5th ed., pp. 443–462). St. Louis, MO: Elsevier.

DeYoung, S. (2015). *Teaching strategies for nurse educators* (3rd ed.). Boston, MA: Pearson.

Gaberson, K. B., Oermann, M. H., & Shellenbarger, T. (2015). *Clinical teaching strategies in nursing* (4th ed.). New York, NY: Springer.

Gubrud, P. (2016). Teaching in the clinical setting. In D. M. Billings & J. A. Halstead (Eds.), *Teaching in nursing: A guide for faculty* (5th ed., pp. 282–323). St. Louis, MO: Elsevier.

Horner, M. D. (2018). Maximizing learning opportunities in interprofessional clinical environments through precepting. *Journal of Continuing Education in Nursing, 49*(12), 545–546. doi:10.3928/00220124-20181116-04

International Nursing Association for Clinical Simulation and Learning Standards Committee (2016). INACSL standards of best practice: Simulation[SM] simulation design. *Clinical Simulation in Nursing, 12,* S5–S12. doi:10.1016/j.ecns.2016.09.005

Kan, E. A., & Stabler-Haas, S. (2018). *Fast facts for the clinical nursing instructor* (3rd ed.). New York, NY: Springer.

Kirkpatrick, J. M., & DeWitt, D. A. (2016). Strategies for evaluating learning outcomes. In D. M. Billings & J. A. Halstead (Eds.), *Teaching in nursing: A guide for faculty* (5th ed., pp. 398–422). St. Louis, MO: Elsevier.

Luparell, S., & Conner, J. R. (2016). Managing student incivility and misconduct in the learning environment. In D. M. Billings & J. A. Halstead (Eds.), *Teaching in nursing: A guide for faculty* (5th ed., pp. 230–244). St. Louis, MO: Elsevier.

O'Connor, A. (2015). *Clinical instruction and evaluation: A teaching resource* (3rd ed.). Boston, MA: Jones & Bartlett.

Oermann, M. H., De Gagne, J. C., & Phillips, B. C. (2018a). *Teaching in nursing and role of the educator: The complete guide to best practice in teaching, evaluation, and curriculum development* (2nd ed.). New York, NY: Springer.

Oermann, M. H., & Gaberson, K. B. (2009). *Evaluation and testing in nursing education* (3rd ed). New York, NY: Springer.

Oermann, M. H., & Gaberson, K. B. (2017). *Evaluation and testing in nursing education* (5th ed.). New York, NY: Springer.

Oermann, M., H., Shellenbarger, T., & Gaberson, K. B. (2018b). *Clinical teaching strategies in nursing* (5th ed.). New York, NY: Springer.

Patrick, A. M. (2019). Implementing effective clinical assessment and evaluation strategies. In T. Shellenbarger (Ed.), *Clinical nurse educator competencies: Creating an evidence-based practice for academic clinical nurse educators* (pp. 73–83). Washington, DC: National League for Nursing.

Robb, M., & Shellenbarger, T. (2018). Constructive feedback: How to have the difficult conversation. *American Nurse Today, 13*(6), 12–13. Retrieved from https://www.americannursetoday.com/constructive-feedback-difficult-conversation/

Roberts, F. B. (2005). Socialization into nursing: Forming a professional attitude. In L. Caputi & L. Engelmann (Eds.), *Teaching nursing: The art and science, Vol. 2* (pp. 1082–1100). Glen Ellyn, IL: College of DuPage Press.

Scheckel, M. (2016). Designing courses and learning experiences. In D. M. Billings & J. A. Halstead (Eds.), *Teaching in nursing: A guide for faculty* (5th ed., pp. 159–185). St. Louis, MO: Elsevier.

Stokes, L. G., & Kost, G. C. (2012). Teaching in the clinical setting. In D. M. Billings & J. A. Halstead (Eds.), *Teaching in nursing: A guide for faculty* (4th ed., pp. 331–334). St. Louis, MO: Elsevier.

Whitney, K. M., & Luparell, S. (2012). Managing student incivility and misconduct in the learning environment. In D. M. Billings & J. A. Halstead (Eds.), *Teaching in nursing: A guide for faculty* (4th ed., pp. 244–257). St. Louis, MO: Elsevier.

Certified Academic Clinical Nurse Educator (CNE®cl) Examination Test Blueprint

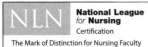 National League for Nursing Certification — The Mark of Distinction for Nursing Faculty	Certified Academic Clinical Nurse Educator (CNE®cl) Examination Test Blueprint	
Category	**Major Content Areas**	**Percent of Examination**
1	Function within the Education and Health Care Environments	18%
2	Facilitate Learning in the Health Care Environment	19%
3	Demonstrate Effective Interpersonal Communication and Collaborative Interprofessional Relationships	15%
4	Applies Clinical Expertise in the Health Care Environment	15%
5	Facilitate Learner Development and Socialization	15%
6	Implement Effective Clinical Assessment and Evaluation Strategies	17%

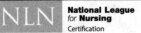

Certified Academic Clinical Nurse Educator® (CNE®cl) Examination

Detailed Test Blueprint

National League
for **Nursing**
Certification

The Mark of Distinction for Nursing Faculty

1. Function within the Education and Health Care Environments	18%

A. Function in the Clinical Educator Role
   1. Bridge the gap between theory and practice by helping learners to apply classroom learning to the clinical setting
   2. Foster professional growth of learners (e.g., coaching, reflection, and debriefing)
   3. Use technologies to enhance clinical teaching and learning
   4. Value the contributions of others in the achievement of learner outcomes (e.g., health team, families, social networks)
   5. Act as a role model of professional nursing within the clinical learning environment
   6. Demonstrate inclusive excellence (e.g., student-centered learning, diversity)

B. Operationalize the Curriculum
   1. Assess congruence of the clinical agency to curriculum, course goals, and learner needs when evaluating clinical sites
   2. Plan meaningful and relevant clinical learning assignments and activities
   3. Identify learners' goals and outcomes
   4. Prepare learners for clinical experiences (e.g., facility, clinical expectations, equipment, and technology-based resources)
   5. Structure learner experiences within the learning environment to promote optimal learning
   6. Implement clinical learning activities to help learners develop interprofessional collaboration and teamwork skills
   7. Provide opportunities for learners to develop problem-solving and clinical reasoning skills related to course objectives (e.g., learning outcomes).
   8. Implement assigned models for clinical teaching (e.g., traditional, preceptor, simulation, dedicated education units)
   9. Engage in theory-based instruction (e.g., constructivism, social cognitive theory)
  10. Provide input to the nursing program for course development and review

C. Abide by Legal Requirements, Ethical Guidelines, Agency Policies, and Guiding Framework
   1. Apply ethical and legal principles to create a safe clinical learning environment
   2. Assess learner abilities and needs prior to clinical learning experiences
   3. Facilitate learning activities that support the mission, goals, and values of the academic institution and the clinical agency
   4. Inform others of program and clinical agency policies, procedures, and practices
   5. Adhere to program and clinical agency policies, procedures, and practices when implementing clinical experiences
   6. Promote learner compliance with regulations and standards of practice
   7. Demonstrate ethical behaviors

2. Facilitate Learning in the Health Care Environment	19%

A. Implement a variety of clinical teaching strategies appropriate to learner needs, desired learner outcomes, content, and context
B. Ground teaching strategies in educational theory and evidence-based teaching practices
C. Use technology (e.g., simulation, learning management systems, electronic health records) skillfully to support the teaching-learning process
D. Create opportunities for learners to develop critical thinking and clinical reasoning skills
E. Promote a culture of safety and quality in the health care environment
F. Create a positive and caring learning environment
G. Develop collegial working relationships with learners, faculty colleagues, and clinical agency personnel
H. Demonstrate enthusiasm for teaching, learning, and nursing to help inspire and motivate learners

3. Demonstrate Effective Interpersonal Communication and Collaborative Interprofessional Relationships	**15%**

A. Value collaboration and coordination of care
B. Foster a shared learning community and cooperate with other members of the health care team
C. Create multiple opportunities to collaborate and cooperate with other members of the health care team
D. Support an environment of frequent, respectful, civil, and open communication with all members of the health care team
E. Act as a role model showing respect for all members of the health care team, professional colleagues, clients, family members, as well as learners
F. Use clear and effective communication in all interactions (e.g., written, electronic, verbal, non-verbal)
G. Listen to learner concerns, needs, or questions in a non-threatening way
H. Display a calm, empathetic, and supportive demeanor in all communications
I. Manage emotions effectively when communicating in challenging situations
J. Effectively manage conflict
K. Maintain an approachable, non-judgmental, and readily accessible demeanor
L. Recognize limitations (self and learners) and provide opportunities for development
M. Demonstrate effective communication in clinical learning environments with diverse colleagues, clients, cultures, health care professionals, and learners
N. Communicate performance expectations to learners and agency staff

4. Applies Clinical Expertise in the Health Care Environment	15%
A. Maintain current professional competence relevant to the specialty area, practice setting, and clinical learning environment B. Translate theory into clinical practice by applying experiential knowledge, clinical reasoning, and using a patient-centered approach to clinical instruction C. Use best evidence to address client-related problems D. Demonstrate effective leadership within the clinical learning environment E. Demonstrate sound clinical reasoning F. Expand knowledge and skills by integrating best practices G. Balance client care needs and student learning needs within a culture of safety H. Demonstrate competence with a range of technologies available in the clinical learning environment	

5. Facilitate Learner Development and Socialization	15%
A. Mentor learners in the development of professional nursing behaviors, standards, and codes of ethics B. Promote a learning climate of respect for all C. Promote professional integrity and accountability D. Maintain professional boundaries E. Encourage ongoing learner professional development via formal and informal venues F. Assist learners in effective use of self-assessment and professional goal setting for ongoing self-improvement G. Create learning environments that are focused on socialization to the role of the nurse H. Assist learners to develop the ability to engage in constructive peer feedback I. Inspire creativity and confidence J. Encourage various techniques for learners to manage stress (e.g., relaxation, meditation, mindfulness) K. Act as a role model for self-reflection, self-care, and coping skills L. Empower learners to be successful in meeting professional and educational goals M. Engage learners in applying best practices and quality improvement processes	

6. Implement Effective Clinical Assessment and Evaluation Strategies	17%
A. Use a variety of strategies to determine achievement of learning outcomes B. Implement both formative and summative evaluation that is appropriate to the learner and learning outcomes C. Engage in timely communication with course faculty regarding learner clinical performance D. Maintain integrity in the assessment and evaluation of learners E. Provide timely, objective, constructive, and fair feedback to learners F. Use learner data to enhance the teaching-learning process in the clinical learning environment G. Demonstrate skill in the use of best practices in the assessment and evaluation of clinical performance H. Assess and evaluate learner achievement of clinical performance expectations I. Use performance standards to determine learner strengths and weaknesses in the clinical learning environment J. Document learner clinical performance, feedback, and progression K. Evaluate the quality of the clinical learning experiences and environment	

The CNE®cl Test Blueprint is subject to periodic revisions. The most current version of the CNE®cl Test Blueprint will always be published within the NLN CNE®cl Handbook, available on the NLN website.